1 MONTH OF
FREE
READING

at

www.ForgottenBooks.com

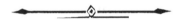

By purchasing this book you are eligible for one month membership to ForgottenBooks.com, giving you unlimited access to our entire collection of over 1,000,000 titles via our web site and mobile apps.

To claim your free month visit:

www.forgottenbooks.com/free874682

ISBN 978-0-265-60612-4
PIBN 10874682

This book is a reproduction of an important historical work. Forgotten Books uses
state-of-the-art technology to digitally reconstruct the work, preserving the original format
whilst repairing imperfections present in the aged copy. In rare cases, an imperfection in
the original, such as a blemish or missing page, may be replicated in our edition. We do,
however, repair the vast majority of imperfections successfully; any imperfections that
remain are intentionally left to preserve the state of such historical works.

PULMONARY CONSUMPTION:

ITS

NATURE, VARIETIES, AND TREATMENT.

WITH AN ANALYSIS OF ONE THOUSAND CASES

TO EXEMPLIFY ITS DURATION.

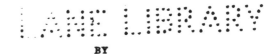

BY

C. J. B. WILLIAMS, M.D. F.R.S.

*Fellow of the Royal College of Physicians; Senior Consulting Physician to the Hospital
for Consumption, Brompton; formerly Professor of Medicine and
Physician to the Hospital, University College, London:*

AND

CHARLES THEODORE WILLIAMS, M.A. M.D. OXON.

*Fellow of the Royal College of Physicians,
Physician to the Hospital for Consumption, Brompton.*

PHILADELPHIA:

LINDSAY AND BLAKISTON.

1871.

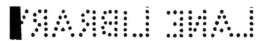

PREFACE.

As some years have elapsed since this book was announced for publication, some apology might be expected for the delay in its appearance. But although I could plead personal excuses for this delay, I hope that our readers will find the most satisfactory apology in the clearer light which we have been enabled to throw on our subjects, derived from some of the most recent discoveries in histology. I have long been led to the general inference, that Consumptive Diseases arise from a defect in the living plasma, or formative material, from which textures are produced and nourished; but it is only within the last few years that the nature and properties of this plasma or germinal matter have been made known through the researches of Lionel Beale, Recklinghausen, Stricker, Cohnheim, Max Schultze, and others; and it is not until now that we have been able to carry our inferences, connecting this matter with consumptive disease, into any precision of detail. The whole subject still teems with matters for further research; and many of the conclusions, to which we have been led by analogy and reason, will have to be brought to the additional test of direct observation and experiment.

A very cursory glance through the pages of this work will suffice to show that its great object is practical: to

it and explain what nature and art have done, and
o, in the treatment of a disease, which has been
only considered one of the *opprobria medici* : and
troduction of theoretical views as to its intimate
: is so far from being unpractical or unprofitable,
hese views are really the results of extensive obser-
and experience ; and without some generalisation
s kind, the multitudinous facts and opinions with
l to Pulmonary Consumption are at the present day
state of incomprehensible and unmanageable con-
. Any reasonable attempt to bring this chaos into
can hardly be objected to ; but the competency of
ndividual who makes the attempt may be fairly
nged.

assuming (or rather resuming) the position of an
tor of the nature of Pulmonary Consumption, I
I may be excused the egotism of alluding to the
—that during a period of nearly fifty years it has
one of the objects of my most constant study :—that

ciples of Medicine,' were analysed and applied the leading facts and opinions in General Pathology and Therapeutics:—and, lastly, that my experience in diseases of the
chest in private practice during the last forty years has
probably not been exceeded by that of any other physician:—all these proofs of qualification being taken into
account, I trust that the present attempt to place in a
clearer light the nature and varieties of Pulmonary
Consumption will not be deemed presumptuous or pre-
mature, and will be not the less favourably received in
conjunction with an account of modes and results of
treatment, which give evidence of considerable improvement on any former experience on record, and afford
encouragement to hope for still further success in the
future.

It is not possible to convey in a few words the views
on the nature of Phthisis, to which I have been led by
observation and reflection on the facts and opinions of
others as well as my own: but the popular terms *decline*
and *consumption* are the most significant which I can
employ to represent them. I believe Pulmonary Consumption to arise from a decline or deficiency of vitality
in the natural *bioplasm* or *germinal matter*; and this
deficiency manifests its effects not only in a general wasting or atrophy of the whole body, but also in a peculiar
degradation, chiefly in the lungs and lymphatic system,
portions of this bioplasm into a sluggish low-lived, yet
irritating, matter, which, instead of maintaining the
action and integrity of the tissues (which is the natural
office of the bioplasm), clogs them and irritates them
or a substance which is more or less prone to decay,

and eventually involves them also in its own disintegration and destruction. This degraded bioplasm, which I will call *phthinoplasm* (wasting or decaying forming-material), may be thrown out locally, as a result of inflammation; or it may arise more spontaneously in divers points of the bioplasm in its ordinary receptacles, the lymphatic glandular system; and then it commonly appears in the form of miliary tubercles, scattered through the adenoid tissue of the lungs.

I would characterise all consumptive diseases heretofore classed under the terms Tuberculous and Scrofulous, together with the products of low and chronic inflammations, as instances of a *lowered vitality of the bioplasm*; and I would strongly insist on their being totally distinct, on the one hand, from cancer and other malignant diseases, the characteristic of which is a new *kind* of vitality, a new growth, perhaps parasitic, with new organic elements, foreign to those of the tissues which they invade and destroy:—and, on the other hand, distinct also from *total loss of vitality*, death of the bioplasm, which would speedily result in decomposition, gangrene, and putrefaction: to such a result phthinoplasms do occasionally lead, but it is not a part of their common history. That this latter distinction is not sufficiently observed by some German writers is evident from their applying the term *necrobiosis* to caseation, which, although a process of decay from *lowered* vitality, does not indicate the absolute death of every living part, as in a slough or gangrene. It will be seen in the chapter on Fatty Degeneration (which thirty years ago was a special object of my study), that I have traced a resemblance to vegetable life in its

process and products; and, although ultimately destructive, it is the most gentle step towards the death of the
tissues. Nay, various proofs will be adduced that fatty
transformation is often a salutary process, assisting materially in the removal of phthinoplasms and other super-
fluous products of inflammation.

The preceding imperfect sketch will, I trust, make it
apparent that the views now offered are not barren specu-
ations; but, if they prove to be well founded, they are
largely suggestive of practical measures. The great
indication to sustain the vitality and sufficiency of the
bioplasm, by all available means, medicinal, regiminal,
and climatic, will be the first suggestion for the preven-
ion and treatment of consumptive disease. A second,
equally obvious, will be the avoidance of all influences
which may injure the bioplasm; generally, by deleterious
action on the whole body; or locally, by exciting low
inflammations in the lungs or other organs. A third
indication, more difficult than the others in its fulfilment,
is to counteract the injurious effects of phthinoplasms
already formed, and to promote their quiescence or removal.

It has been our endeavour in the chapters on the
treatment, and in those containing the illustrative Cases,
to show how these indications are carried out; and,
although in the worst and most rapid forms of disease,
we have still to confess that medicine is almost powerless,
yet in those less overwhelming, and in those more
gentle, which happily constitute the far greater number
of cases, we have been able to adduce many proofs (and
they might be largely multiplied) that much may be

done to mitigate, to prevent, to retard—aye, and even to arrest and cure, this most destructive of human maladies.

And here occurs an opportunity, which must not be lost, of saying a strong word on what renders the practice of our art much less successful than it might be if it had a fair chance:—I mean the fickleness or indocility of the patients or of their friends. Our recorded cases are dry enough to read, being neither smooth in diction nor sensational in narrative: but they teach this lesson, that those patients benefited most surely and most permanently, who early, and at reasonable intervals, sought for advice, and who implicitly and faithfully followed it to the best of their ability, during the several months or years required by the nature of their cases. On the other hand, only irregular and uncertain improvement ensued where the advice was imperfectly carried out; and relapses, serious and even fatal, resulted often from its neglect. This is an old grievance, and we must not cease to raise a warning voice against it. The cause lies very much in the ignorance and conceit of even the educated classes in medical matters, especially of the aristocracy, many of whom consider themselves better judges than medical men; and, if they seek advice, neglect to follow it, or capriciously decide to discontinue the treatment— to change the doctor—or, it may be, to try homœopathy, or some equally absurd form of quackery—at the very time when the patient's life and recovery depend on the steady continuance of a plan of rational treatment. It is awful to reflect on the numbers of valuable lives that are sacrificed to such ignorance and caprice! and until the public intelligence becomes sufficiently enlightened to discern the wickedness and folly of this reckless tampering with health and life, our own profession at least should not cease to protest against it. We have difficulties enough to contend against in our endeavours to correct and control the decaying tendencies of the frail body, without having them fatally aggravated by the officious interference of ignorance and prejudice. The treatment of Pulmonary Consumption involves a long watchful struggle with a strong, subtle, and insidious enemy; and to secure any amount of success, the will, the faith, and the hopes of the patient must be persistently and patiently on our side.

It was mainly the unsatisfactory and inconclusive character of histories of short duration that induced me to select for statistical analysis those cases only, which had been under observation for a period of one year and upwards. A large proportion of the patients who seek the advice of a consulting physician come once, and may never be seen or heard of after. In those who repeat their visits within a few weeks or months, changes for the better cannot be relied on without the test of longer time to prove their permanency; and the cases of death occurring within these short periods belong to those acute and overwhelming forms of the disease which art is never able to control: happily these early deaths are so rare that they only slightly affect the average duration of life in our cases.

The statistical parts of this work have been entirely worked by my son, Dr. C. Theodore Williams, who has bestowed much labour upon them. His assistance in this

department has been the more satisfactory to me, because I
have neither taste nor talent for that kind of work, which
is nevertheless indispensable where precision and accuracy
are required.   It is necessary to explain that his calculations contained in Chapters XV., XVI., and XXIV. are based
on the 1,000 cases selected (as stated) from my note-books
during a period of twenty-two years ; and those only who
are familiar with the numerical method of tabulating and
calculating facts and results can form an idea of the
amount of work required in this investigation.   The results appear to be highly interesting, and, although much
in accordance with the general impressions which I had
previously derived from my experience, it is much more
satisfactory to have determinate figures to rely on, than
the hazy tokens of vague memory.

The abstracts of cases, occupying six chapters, are not
limited to the 1,000 cases above mentioned, but are
taken from my whole experience, private and hospital ;
and are selected chiefly to exemplify the matter in the
text bearing on the nature, varieties, signs, symptoms,
causes, duration, and treatment of Pulmonary Consumption.   In the preparation of these cases for the press, and
in their arrangement into groups, my son joined his
labours to mine, and thus the work has been more rapidly
accomplished.   The task of selection has been difficult:
it would have been easier to have increased them two or
three-fold, as there was abundance of material ; but it was
judged better to give only representative cases, and not
to swell the volume, and try the patience of the reader
by numbers which would probably prove too monotonous
and tedious to be read.   The short fatal cases narrated

are selected chiefly on account of the *post-mortem* appearances; and the chronic cases, many of which are still living, give a longer insight into the nature and course of Pulmonary Consumption than any that have yet been given to the Profession.

The short chapter on the Physical Signs of Consumption is introduced to explain the signs and interpret the terms given in the histories of the cases. It is more than thirty years since the appearance of my last work on the physical signs of diseases of the chest, and it has been for more than twenty years out of print; but I have found no need to change the language which I then used, except in the way of simplification and abbreviation, and to adapt it to describe the varieties in the history of phthinoplasms. I flatter myself that the views given of the pathology and tendencies of these will render their physical diagnosis more intelligible and easy than it has been generally considered hitherto.

The chapters on Family Predisposition and other causes of Pulmonary Consumption and on Hæmoptysis are contributed by my son, the statistics bearing on them being derived chiefly from the 1,000 cases which he had tabulated from my notes. Some important deductions respecting the origin of Consumption and the pathology of Hæmoptysis will be found in these chapters.

The Summary View of the treatment of Pulmonary Consumption is only slightly modified from that which appeared in the *Lancet* three years ago. In the subsequent chapters which consider the treatment in relation to forms or varieties of the disease, I have found it convenient to divide it into the three heads, antiphlo-

, antiphthisical, and palliative. Having sketched
ind of antiphlogistic treatment required in the
amatory forms or complications of the disease, I
taken into consideration the remedies which can be
antiphthisical, including cod-liver oil, tonics, and
ptics. The chapter on Palliative Treatment, and
on diet, regimen, and climate in Pulmonary Con-
tion, I have left to my son, whose experience at
rompton Hospital, as well as taking charge of my
ts in my absence, and whose familiarity with
est climates for invalids, well qualify him for the

remains for me only to bespeak the indulgence of
aders on account of many shortcomings and defects
execution of this work. It does not profess to be
plete treatise on its subject, nor to record all the
rs and opinions of others. Its chief purpose is

CONTENTS.

CHAPTER V.

PATHOLOGY OF CONSUMPTION.

CHAPTER VI.

PATHOLOGY OF CONSUMPTION.

CHAPTER VII.

PATHOLOGY OF CONSUMPTION.

a 2

CHAPTER XV.

FAMILY PREDISPOSITION AND CERTAIN OTHER CAUSES OF CONSUMPTION.

By Dr. C. Theodore Williams.

CHAPTER XVI.

HÆMOPTYSIS AND THE HÆMORRHAGIC VARIETY OF CONSUMPTION.

BY DR. C. THEODORE WILLIAMS.

CHAPTER XVII.

OUTLINE OF PHYSICAL SIGNS OF VARIETIES AND STAGES OF PULMONARY CONSUMPTION.

BY DR. WILLIAMS.

CHAPTER XVIII.

ABSTRACTS OF CASES ILLUSTRATING THE NATURE, VARIETIES AND TREATMENT OF PULMONARY CONSUMPTION.

CHAPTER XIX.

ABSTRACTS OF CASES, &c.—continued.

CHAPTER XX.

ABSTRACTS OF CASES, &c.—continued.

CHAPTER XXI.

ABSTRACTS OF CASES, &c.—continued.

CHAPTER XXV.

TREATMENT OF PULMONARY CONSUMPTION.—SUMMARY VIEW.
BY DR. WILLIAMS.

CHAPTER XXVI.

TREATMENT OF PULMONARY CONSUMPTION.

PULMONARY CONSUMPTION.

—•••—

CHAPTER I.

Definitions—Illustrations of degree—Galloping Consumption—Acute Tuber-
culosis—Scrofulous Pneumonia—More chronic and limited forms—Pro-
gress of the disease—Power of Medicine—Unity but not uniformity of
Phthisis.

THE DISEASE, too well known to the public, as well as to
the medical profession, as PULMONARY CONSUMPTION, is
characterised by the symptoms, persistent cough, expectoration of opaque matter, sometimes of blood; a progressive loss of flesh, breath, and strength; often hectic
fever, night sweats, and diarrhœa; and the common
tendency of the disease is to a wasting of the body and a
decline of its powers, down to its termination in death.

Pathologically considered, pulmonary consumption is
characterised by certain changes in the textures of the
lungs, consisting chiefly of consolidations, granular or
diffused, which irritate their functions and clog their
structures, and which proceed to further changes, of degeneration, disintegration, and excavation of some parts,
and of induration and contraction of others—all tending
to a disorganisation of the lungs, and a wasting away of
the flesh and blood of the body.

It is this tendency to degeneration and destruction,
which stamps the *consuming* character of the disease;
the more strongly this tendency is manifested, the

B

more irresistible and rapid will it be in its fatal course.
In certain cases the disease is so acute and extensive as to
carry off the patient in a few weeks or months. In others
it is more limited and slow, and may not destroy life for
five, ten, twenty, or more years. In the former cases
medicine has little or no control over the disease; decay
and death invade the frame so overwhelmingly, that there
is neither sufficient power in nature to resist them, nor
time for art to aid that power. One of the most vital
organs of the body becomes suddenly invaded by a disease,
changing its structure, obstructing its functions, and
spreading through it the seeds of further decay, which
not only in the organ itself, but by the blood and lymphatics, diffuse its destructive influence through the whole
system.

Let us briefly sketch the two most terrible forms of the
disease.

A man of middle age is attacked with fever, with
pungent heat of the body, cough, viscid expectoration,
extreme oppression, and overwhelming weakness, resembling that of continued fever; and the likeness sometimes
appears also in the coated or dry brown tongue, sordes on
the teeth, and occasional delirium. The vesicular breath-
sound is superseded everywhere by bronchial rhonchi and
mixed crepitation. On percussion, the chest is dull nowhere, but less clear in the posterior than in the front
parts. This case might be supposed to be one of universal
capillary bronchitis, with general pulmonary congestion.
So it is; but this is not all. In spite of blisters and
other remedies, the breathing remains short and difficult;
the pulse becomes more rapid and feeble; the lips, cheeks,
and nails become livid; clammy sweats break out, and the
patient dies in the third or fourth week from his first
attack. The lungs are found congested, and the bronchi
loaded with viscid mucus; but more than this, innu-

merable miliary tubercles are scattered throughout the pulmonary tissue, and these are the obvious cause of the intractability of the case. They break out simultaneously, like the eruption of an exanthem, and by their numbers and bulk induce such an amount of obstruction and congestion in the lungs, as to destroy life before there is time for any considerable degeneration or softening to take place. This *acute tuberculosis* is the worst and most surely and rapidly fatal form of consumption.

The second form of acute consumption begins with pneumonia in one or both lungs. The patient, generally a young subject, is of consumptive family, and may have previously had cough and occasional hæmoptysis. The fever attendant on the inflammation may not be very high at first, and the expectoration by no means so viscid and rusty, nor the crepitation so fine and even, as in simple inflammation of the lungs. But the symptoms are more persistent. The pulse and respiration remain frequent. The heat of the body, particularly of the chest, continues remarkably high, almost burning the ear of the auscultator as he examines the back. But this intense heat is alternated with occasional chills and profuse sweats at night. The cough continues distressing, and the expectoration becomes opaque, purulent, and clotty; the flesh wastes, and the strength ebbs away; and if the appetite does not return, the progress of consumption and decay is rapid. Auscultation reveals the steps of the destructive process in the lung. The affected part, or the whole side, or part of both sides, becomes dull on percussion, only varied with the cracked-pot note from the gurgling within; the loud tubular sounds are replaced by coarse crepitation, in parts amounting to gurgling; and the diffused bronchophony is modified into detached islands of voice, loud and pectoriloquous, or into the snuffling or whispering sounds equally characteristic of a cavity. This form of *galloping con-*

sumption may also prove fatal in a few weeks; and the
lungs are found after death in a state of consolidation
little more dense than the hepatization of pneumonia, but
their red is mottled with grey and yellow patches of tuberculous or aplastic matter, and excavated in various parts
into numerous small cavities communicating with the
bronchial tubes, and containing more or less of the same
compound matter which was expectorated during life,
consisting of mucus, pus, degenerating epithelium and
exudation-matter, with disintegrated fragments of lung-
tissue. This form of acute phthisis, although generally
rapidly fatal, is not universally so. When not too extensive, it may sometimes be arrested and brought to a
chronic state; and the chance of this result will very
much depend on the recovery of the appetite, and the
power of the stomach to bear strong nutriment, tonics,
and, above all, cod-liver oil.

And in a large majority of the cases of consumption
the destructive element is still less extensive and less
active, and its progress is much more slow; and we have
both time and means to resist its inroads and to fortify
the system against its operation to a greater or less
extent. In the greater number of instances the disease
begins with the symptoms of common cold, often referred
to the throat as much as to the chest; and there is, in
truth, more or less of bronchial irritation and inflammation attendant on the development of the disease, and
recurring with renewed intensity at the time of its increased activity. Often the disorder is mistaken for a
common cold, until either its remarkable persistence, or
the occurrence of hæmoptysis, of night sweats, of loss of
flesh, or of some other uncommon symptom, gives intima-
tion of its more serious nature. Then it is found that, in
addition to the signs of bronchial catarrh, there are some
of the signs of consolidation of the lungs, generally near

an apex; slight dulness or raised tone of the stroke-sound at or below a clavicle, or at or above a scapula; a tubular character in the breath-sound and voice; an undue intensity or duration of the sounds of expiration, or a weakness or absolute obstruction of the inspiration; and sometimes the various slight degrees of crepitus substituted for the proper breath-sound; and various other signs which it is unnecessary here to detail. These signs, however, are the indications of *incipient pulmonary consumption*—that is, of a disease which tends, sooner or later, to injure and destroy the structure of the lung, and to deteriorate and waste the flesh and blood of the whole body. And the progress of this work of injury and destruction is marked by signs of increased density and diminished motion of parts of the lungs; by more of the moist crepitus, from augmented humidity, in and around the consolidations; and eventually by signs of excavation at one or more points, which announce the removal of the diseased tissue.

The progress of this disease may vary infinitely in time and in extent. The more extensive the mischief, generally the more rapid will be its progress, which goes on in the worst cases, uninterrupted by any check or pause, attended by the distressing train of symptoms—harassing cough, opaque clotty expectoration, increasing shortness of breath, burning fever alternated with profuse sweats and chills, rapid loss of flesh and strength and colour, sometimes diarrhœa, and aphthous mouth; and terminates in death in a few months.

But in other cases, and these are by far the most common, the destructive lesions are less extensive, and their progress is more slow and intermittent, and often seems in great degree to depend on occasional attacks from cold or other external causes, in the absence of which the disease may be quiescent or stationary, and may not destroy life for years.

Powerless as medicine is in the overwhelming and rapid types of the disease, it has yet considerable influence over these milder forms; and the following pages will give some evidence that under careful treatment life may be prolonged for many years in comfort and usefulness, and in not very few cases the disease is so permanently arrested, that it may be called cured.

It may well be questioned whether a disease which presents such striking differences in form, intensity, and result, can be truly one and the same disease; and there seems to be a growing disposition among modern pathologists to supersede the comprehensive terms *consumption* and *tubercle* by others more specifically applicable to definite forms of the disease. But while I fully participate in the objections to include all forms of phthisis under the head of tubercle, and have long insisted on the origin of many cases in inflammation, I still maintain that all the varieties of phthisical lesion are identified by their common *consumptive* nature; and the following pages will supply numerous proofs that all are characterised by a tendency to degeneration and decay. It will be shown that all are due to the presence of various kinds of *phthinoplasm,*[1] a withering or decaying modification of the proper plasma or formative material of the body; and although for clinical purposes it is useful to note their differences, and group them accordingly, yet we hold it to be most important, in relation to pathology and treatment, to consider them as varieties of one common malady—PULMONARY CONSUMPTION.

[1] I have found it necessary to coin this word, *phthinoplasm* (from φθίω, or φθίνω, ' I waste or decay'—whence also ' phthisis '—and πλάσμα), to give expression to one of the leading ideas of this book, and to avoid the common use of the word *tubercle*, which is quite inapplicable to many kinds of degenerative formation which cause pulmonary consumption. I trust that the utility of the term will reconcile the reader to its novelty.

CHAPTER II.

Pathology of Pulmonary Consumption—Views of Laennec criticised, and compared with those of Andral, Cruveilhier, Alison, and Abercrombie—Original Conclusions of the Author—Consumption produced by defective Vitality and Organisation of the Plasma resulting from Inflammation or Malnutrition.

THE term 'pulmonary consumption' was restricted by Laennec to the wasting disease produced by the presence and progress of tubercles in the lungs. These tubercles he described as existing in the form of grey granulations, or miliary tubercles (of Bayle), yellow tubercles, and tuberculous infiltration, which might be either grey or yellow. But he held that the yellow is only a more advanced stage of the grey, and that the yellow tubercle tends to change further from the crude hard state to that of softening and ultimate excavation. He entirely denied the inflammatory origin of tubercles; and in classing them among 'accidental productions' he associated them with cancer and other formations, which have been subsequently denominated *growths*, although he was well aware of the generic difference between them in regard to both structure and history.

These views of Laennec, characterising pulmonary consumption as an essentially tuberculous disease, and repudiating the previously prevalent notion, that it might arise from inflammation, were adopted by Louis, and by most writers in this country, with very little qualification.

But they were by no means so implicitly accepted by the
cotemporary pathologists of France. Broussais, true to
his system, traced phthisis to varieties of inflammation,
and propounded the notion that tubercles are the result
of chronic inflammation of the lymphatics of the lungs.
Being personally acquainted with the strong antagonistic
feeling entertained by Laennec towards Broussais, I have
little doubt that the former was biassed in his views,
and framed them in opposition to those of his rival.
Another eminent pathologist of that school, Andral, not
less remarkable for his powers of observation than for his
sound and impartial judgment, was also led to differ from
the exclusive views of Laennec, and recognised inflammation as a primary agent in much of the pathology of pulmonary consumption ; and he even sought to trace miliary
tubercles to an inflammation of individual vesicles of the
lung. Cruveilhier also maintained the inflammatory origin
of tubercles, and thought that he had produced them artificially in living animals by injecting quicksilver into the
bronchial tubes. But although it may be admitted that
what is called yellow tubercle may be developed in both
the modes thus indicated by Andral and Cruveilhier, yet
the same cannot be said of miliary tubercles, the general
uniformity of which, in size, shape, and substance, gives
them a character quite distinct from that of inflammatory
products.

The diffused consolidations, which Laennec called infiltrated tubercle, were soon proved to be of inflammatory
origin, a result, in fact, of chronic pneumonia ; and as
these often form a large part of the lesions in phthisical
lungs, the exclusive opinions of Laennec have long ago
undergone modification.

One of the earliest critics of the peculiar views of
Laennec on the origin of tubercles, was my revered
teacher, the late Professor Alison, of Edinburgh, one of

the most careful observers and soundest reasoners of
his day. In a series of papers read before the Medico-
Chirurgical Society of Edinburgh during the years 1822,
1823, and 1824, he brought forward a number of cases and
statistical facts to prove that tubercles and other lesions
met with in the lungs of consumptive patients may originate in inflammation. I quote one sentence: 'I have
also been led to believe that it is not merely, as Laennec
states, a possibility, but a real and frequent occurrence,
that inflammation, acute or chronic (to which I would add,
and febrile action), however produced, becomes in certain
constitutions the occasion of the development of tubercles;
and the facts, which seem to me decisive on this point, I
propose to lay before the Society.' (' Trans. of Med.-Chir.
Society of Edinburgh,' 1824, p. 408.) In the same volume,
p. 682, is a remarkable communication from another eminent physician of that time, Dr. Abercrombie, ' On the
Nature and Origin of Tubercular Diseases.' The views
expressed in this short paper are so important, and have
so apt a bearing on recent researches on tubercle, that I
am induced to give their substance in a note.[1]

[1] After alluding to the complex character of the tubercular masses met
with in the lungs, and the consequent difficulty of tracing their nature and
figures, he mentions the tuberculous disease in the mesenteric and lymphatic glands as strictly analogous in its nature, and as exhibiting more simply and distinctly its states and stages. He traces the change from simple
enlargement (hyperplasia) to increased firmness, and paleness, until it assumes
a kind of semitransparency, and a texture approaching to that of soft cartilage. Then appear opaque white spots (caseation), which seems to be the
latest in these changes, and strictly analogous to the white tubercle of
lungs. In the most advanced stage, the opaque white matter is most
firm, and this afterwards softens and degenerates into the soft cheesy
mass of ill-conditioned suppuration. From the effect of boiling water on
newly enlarged glands, he concludes that the enlargement is due to
effusion of albuminous matter, first soft, but subsequently becoming
hard, and the mass becomes less vascular and less organised; and this
increases in proportion to the advance of the disease from simple
enlargement to grey consolidation and opaque transmutation. Mesenteric
glands, in their natural state, contain hardly any albumen,

These papers of Drs. Alison and Abercrombie appeared
during the period of my study in Edinburgh; and I was
the more interested in them as some of the cases described
by Dr. Alison were under my care in the New Town Dispensary during the years 1823 and 1824. It was not to be won-
dered at, therefore, when I became a pupil of Laennec
in 1825, that, much as I admired and profited by the
clinical sagacity and skill of the discoverer of auscultation,
I did not accept much of his pathology; and from that
time to the present, in all my writings and lectures, I
have consistently repudiated his opinions on pulmonary
consumption and tubercle as unsatisfactory and unsound.

and are almost entirely dissolved in boiling water. When simply
enlarged, about five-sixths are dissolved, the remaining sixth presenting
the properties of coagulate albumen. Glands in the advanced state
of semitransparent consolidation lose one-fourth by boiling, three-fourths
remaining in the state of firm albuminous coagulum; and the white
opaque tubercular matter loses still less by boiling, and, when small portions are detached from other structures, they seem to consist almost entirely
of coagulated albumen. 'There seems, then, to be some ground for the
conjecture that this deposition of albumen is the origin of tubercular
disease. It is in the mesenteric and lymphatic glands that we have the best
opportunity of marking its progress; but betwixt the various stages of disease in them and the various forms of tubercular disease in the lungs, there
is the most close and remarkable analogy. In the bronchial glands we
observe the same forms of disease, and according to Portal and other writers
of the first authority, glands similar to these exist in very great numbers
throughout the whole structure of the lungs, being found at every division
of the bronchiæ, however minute. If this be the case, they must pervade
every part of the pulmonary substance in such numbers as would readily
account for the usual appearance of tubercular lungs, on the supposition
that this disease is seated in this glandular structure. For even the larger
glands which we find at the bifurcation of the trachea are very small bodies
in their natural healthy state; while in the state of tubercular disease, they
may acquire the magnitude of eggs, or even a still larger size. I do not,
however, contend that tubercular disease is necessarily confined to a glandular structure. On the contrary, there seems every reason to believe that
the peculiar deposition which constitutes it may take place from every tissue
of the body; in some cases slowly and gradually, in others as the result of
a low inflammatory action of a peculiarly unhealthy character.'

¹ 'Much as Laennec has done in elucidating the history of phthisis pulmonalis, his opinions on tubercles and other diseased products have always

Adopting, with some modifications, the general opinions
[of] Alison and Andral, I was led by observation and reflec-
[ti]on to conclude that the lesions constituting pulmonary
[con]sumption originate in either some form of inflamma-
[tio]n, or a perverted nutrition, of the textures of the lungs,
[and] tending to further degradation or degeneration, and
[con]sequent decay and destruction, of the affected parts.

[ap]peared to me artificial and unsatisfactory. Tubercles, according to this
[view] an accidental tissue, are produced—or, according to some of his ex-
[pres]sions, spring up—in a healthy tissue without any aid of the vessels of
[the] part, are changed from a greyish semitransparent to an opaque yellow-
[ish] white colour, and pass from a state of cartilaginous hardness, through
[inter]mediate gradations, into that of imperfect liquidity: and all this by a
[mecha]nism perfectly unknown, and in a manner entirely unexplained. It
[is, in] my opinion, without sufficient reason that he identifies the granu-
[la]tions of Bayle with the yellow tubercle—bodies quite different in their
[physi]cal character—only because the one is generally in time converted into
[the other]. As well might cartilage be called bone, or inflamed cellular
[tissue a] stage of pus.'—*Rational Exposition of the Physical Signs of the
[Diseases of the] Lungs and Pleura*, p. 154. By Charles J. B. Williams, M.D.
[&c.]

[I adduce] this quotation to disprove assertions recently made by several
[... German] and English, that the views of Laennec on tubercle have
[... gene]rally adopted, and only called in question by Dr. T. Addison in
[this coun]try, and more fully by German pathologists during the last ten
[years. My views on] this subject were not unknown in Germany, for the
[work above] quoted was translated into German more than thirty years
[... passed through] several editions, having been used, as I have been
[... text-book] at some of the medical schools in that country.

[The only] writer in this country, Dr. W. Stokes, also long ago anti-
[cipated the Germans] in their opposition to the opinions of Laennec, and
[... views] on the inflammatory origin of phthisis, in many points
[... those held] in this volume. The titles by which Dr. Stokes desig-
[nates varieties of] phthisis will sufficiently show this:—
[... Inflammatory] tuberculisation of the lung without suppuration.
[2. ... ve] tuberculisation. 3. Chronic progressive tubercle, with
[... and general] irritation; pulmonary ulceration. 4. Chronic
[... tuberculisation] succeeding to an unresolved pneumonia. 5. Tuber-
[culisation succeeding] to chronic bronchitis. 6. Tubercle consequent
[... on an] empyema.'—*On the Diagnosis and Treatment of
[... the Chest*, 1837, p. 414. Allowing for difference in nomenclature,
[necessary] by advances in pathological science, several of these
[... correspond with] those described in this work.

In scrofulous constitutions, whether hereditary or acq
these results might follow any form of inflammation,
or chronic, membranous or parenchymatous, the pr
of the inflammation being yellow tuberculous (cas
tending to softening and irregular suppuration or u
tion, and infecting the system through the blood, b
ing out in the form of miliary tubercles in other
with or without inflammation.   But consumption
arise also in those previously healthy, from various ot
inflammations of the lungs, either following acute at
imperfectly cured, or arising from the long operati
exciting causes, such as the habitual inhalation of i
ting dust of stone, metal, &c., or prolonged expos
cold and damp.

The prevalent idea to which my study of consum
diseases led me, as expressed in my first little work in
and in several subsequent editions, was that the co
dations of the lung characteristic of phthisis, inst
being, as Laennec maintained, ' accidental producti
' heterologous growths' (like cancer), are really n
degraded modifications of the common nutrition o
tissues of the lung, often, but not always, produc
inflammation; and that their disposition to further d
and decay is owing to their defective vitality and org
tion.   The cause of this degradation is to be refer
the low or chronic type of the inflammation prod
them, or to a depraved state of the blood from
they are formed.

Thus, in a previously healthy subject, consum
disease can arise only from inflammation of a low
or rendered chronic by inefficient treatment, or b
prolonged or repeated operation of its exciting
The result is cacoplastic consolidation, of low organi
red or grey, which tends to undergo the further de
tion into opaque and still more disorganised matter (c
or yellow tuberculous).

But in a scrofulous subject, the cacoplastic or degenerating tendency may have been already manifest in enlargement and caseation of the lymphatic glands, or in the
cutaneous formation of indolent abscesses or ulcers; and
in such a subject, any inflammation of the lung, however
slite, may end in consumptive destruction, through the
imperfectly organised (aplastic), and therefore decaying nature of its products, which go under the designation of caseous or yellow tubercle. In a person of this
constitution also, the grey consolidation, diffused and
granular,[1] may arise in the lungs without further cause
than casual congestions or catarrhs, and sometimes without
even these.

It would take up too much of our space to trace this
subject through all the handlings which it has received
from various observers and commentators during the forty
years which have elapsed since the above stated views
were published; but so much light has been obtained
in certain lines of research, that it will be necessary to
give a brief account of the best ascertained facts concerning, which may be ranged under these three heads:—
The *Nature* and *changes* of tubercle and kindred
, which will lead to the subject of *Caseation, or
Degeneration of tissues*, and, in conclusion, to *the
actual production of tubercle by inoculation, &c.*

CHAPTER III.

ON THE NATURE OF TUBERCLE AND OTHER PHTHINOPLASMS.

Micrology—Gulliver, Addison, Rokitansky, Lebert, Gruby—Histology of Tubercle—Cellular Pathology—Virchow's Views objected to—Tubercle and Cancer contrasted—Burdon Sanderson's conclusions—Portal's anticipation of the lymphatic nature of Tubercle.

THE microscopical observations of Mr. Gulliver on tubercle,[1] published in 1842, '3, and '4, are more original and accurate than those of many others who have succeeded him, and have been confirmed by the most careful recent observers.   He described young or grey tubercles as chiefly composed of cells ; but crude or yellow tubercle of shrinking, blighted, shapeless, degenerating cells, with preponderance of granular matter and oily particles.   The site of pulmonary tubercles (grey and yellow ?) Mr. Gulliver described to be both inside and outside of the air cells ; and their endowments to be very low in the scale of organisation, so that, devoid of inherent power of growth possessed by the cells from which they originated or increased, they only retrograde or degenerate into amorphous lifeless corpuscles, and into granular and molecular fatty matter, all incapable of organisation.

About the same date appeared the independent observations of Dr. W. Addison, which, so far as related to the structure of tubercle, were very similar to those of Mr. Gulliver.[2]

[1] *Appendix to Gerber's Anatomy*, 1842, Plates 29 and 31 ; *Notes to Boyd's Vital Statistics ; Edin. Med. and Surg. Journal*, July 1843 ; and *Willis's Translation of Wagner's Physiology*, 1844, p. 360.

[2] ....parent forms of tubercle and tubercular infiltration owe .... a great relative amount of granulated vesicles ; whereas

Some years later Rokitansky described tubercles as consisting of a more or less pellucid base with elementary
granules of various magnitudes, nucleus formations in
various phases, and scanty nucleated cells. He considered
tubercle, as I had done long before, as an altered fibrinous
exudation from the vessels; miliary tubercle corresponding
with the *fibrinous* (fibrillated), and yellow tubercle with
the *croupous* (corpuscular) variety of lymph. More recently Mandl[1] pushed this view to an extreme, in de-
scribing tubercle as an amorphous matter consisting of
mere granules or molecules, and as unorganised albumen
subject to fatty transformation.

On the other hand, Lebert, Gluge, Gruby, R. Hall, and
others described a peculiar form of cell or corpuscle as
characterising tubercle; just as particular forms of cell
distinguish cancer. Had these last descriptions been accurate, they would have gone far to establish Laennec's
notion of the specific character of tubercle as a heterologous growth, instead of being, as I supposed, a cacoplastic
secretion or product. But these peculiar tubercle corpuscles have not been recognised by subsequent observers; the
formation present in miliary tubercles not differing
from those in inflammatory exudations, or even those normally existing in the lymphatic glands and vessels. (Burdon
Sanderson.)

But a very important influence on the views concerning
tubercle, and all other tissue changes, was brought to bear
by the hypothesis of the cellular physiology and pathology,
originating in the researches of Schleiden and Schwann,
erected into a system by Virchow and others, represented in the axiom, ' omnis cellula e cellulâ.'

Without attempting to enter on a discussion of cellular
histology in general, we quote Virchow's description of

the white forms of tubercle are attributable to great numbers of
granules.'—*Trans. Prov. Med. and Surg. Assoc.*, 1843, p. 287.
Anat. de Méd., 1855.

grey granular tubercle, this being the typical form of this product :—

I am of opinion that a tubercle is a granule or a knot, and that this knot constitutes a new formation, and indeed one which from the time of its earliest formation is necessarily of a cellular nature, and generally, just like all other new formations, has its origin in the connective tissue, and which, when it has reached a certain degree of development, constitutes a minute knot within this tissue, that, when it is at the surface, projects in the form of a little protuberance, and consists throughout its whole mass of small uni- or multi-nuclear cells. What especially characterises this formation is the circumstance that it is extremely rich in nuclei, so that when it is examined as it lies embedded in the tissue which invests it, at the first glance there seems to be scarcely anything else than nuclei ; but upon isolating the constituents of this mass, either very small cells provided with one nucleus are obtained—and these often so small that the membrane closely invests the nucleus—or larger cells, with a manifest division of the nuclei, so that from twelve to twenty-four or thirty are contained in one cell, in which case, however, the nuclei are always small, and have a homogeneous and somewhat shining appearance. *This structure, which in its development is comparatively most nearly related to pus,* inasmuch as it has the smallest nuclei, and relatively the *smallest cells, is distinguished from all the more highly organised forms of cancer, cancroid, and sarcoma, by the circumstance that these contain large, voluminous, nay, often gigantic corpuscles, with highly developed nuclei and nucleoli. Tubercle, on the contrary, is always a pitiful production, a new formation, from its very outset miserable.* From its very commencement it is, like other new formations, not unfrequently pervaded by vessels ; but when it enlarges, its many little cells throng so closely together that the vessels gradually become completely impervious, and only the larger ones, which traverse the tubercle, remain intact. Generally fatty degeneration sets in very early in the centre of the knot (granule), where the oldest cells lie, but usually does not become complete. Then every trace of fluid disappears, the corpuscles begin to shrivel, the centre becomes yellow and opaque, and a yellowish spot is seen in the middle of the grey translucent granule. This is the commencement of the cheesy metamorphosis which subsequently characterises the tubercle. The change advances from cell to cell, farther and farther outwards, and it not unfrequently happens that the whole granule is gradually involved in it.'

' Virchow's *Cellular Pathology,* translated by Dr. Chance, 1860, p. 475–7.

Now, whilst I admit that these observations prove grey
tubercles to have a more definite organisation than I was
wont to ascribe to them in my earlier writings, I would
call the reader's attention particularly to the passages from
this author which I have put in italics. They amount to
an admission that granular tubercle in its form and history
has more resemblance to pus than to the more organised
structures which are properly denominated growths, such
as cancer, sarcoma, &c.; and I therefore, and for many
other reasons, still maintain that grey tubercles have more
affinity to the class of cacoplastic hypertrophies or cacoplastic deposits than to that of new growths. It is true
that Virchow assigns them to a distinct class, under the
term of *lymphoma*, because they possess the same kind of
structure as that found in natural lymphatic glands; and
I am quite willing to acknowledge a close affinity between
lymphatic glandular swellings and tubercles; for they
affect the same subjects, and run a similar course. But
these glandular swellings also have a close resemblance on
the one hand to swellings from inflammation, and on the
other to the simple enlargement of the spleen and liver
occurring in leucæmia. In both these cases there is doubtless hypertrophy or hyperplasia, but this may be in the
way of exudation or cell proliferation, without the development of complex tissue which constitutes a *growth*. If
the addition of cells, fibres, and other products of inflammation in a tissue, constitutes a growth, then common
cutaneous pimples, tubercles, and boils, are growths, and
swelling from erysipelas or cellulitis must be included
under the same term; but surely this would exceed its
acceptation.

Even if it be admitted that tubercles are in any sense
entitled to the appellation of growths, it is of great importance to distinguish them from cancers and other formations, to which the term growth is more commonly and

fitly applied; and it may be useful to exhibit their chief differences in a tabular form, although in doing so here we have to anticipate some of the descriptions which will follow afterwards.

GREY MILIARY TUBERCLES.

Structure.—An aggregation of small nucleated corpuscles, with or without cells (like those in corpuscular lymph and in lymphatic glands), with interstitial hyaline and a few fibres; only slight vascularity, and the adjoining blood-vessels more or less obstructed.

Progress. — No further growth or development beyond the formation of minute knots, which under pressure may somewhat flatten and spread, but no spreading to adjoining parts, or from tissue to tissue.

Termination. — Generally soon undergo cheesy decay and softening, which involve the cells and containing structure in decay, more or less mixed with inflammation of adjoining textures. More rarely the cells dwindle, and the tubercles shrink into obsolescence.

Origin. — Simultaneously appear in several points in one or in many organs.

CANCER AND SIMILAR GROWTHS.

Structure. — Large and highly organised cells, with well-developed nuclei and nucleoli, contained in a distinct stroma, abundantly supplied with blood-vessels, both around them and among them.

Progress. — Grow in any direction, forming increasing tumours, sometimes of large size. Spread and penetrate through all textures, by continuity and contiguity.

Termination. — Generally live and grow on, with a parasitic life of their own, till they prove fatal to function and structure by their bulk, and spoiling the nutrition of the body by irregular ulceration, hæmorrhage, and cachexia. Rarely degenerate into cheesy matter; and then only from injury to their structure by pressure.

Origin.—Generally appear in one part, not spreading for some time; and then by growth and dissemination.

Causes.—Family predisposition. Also other influences deteriorating the nutritive functions: such as poor living; confinement in impure air; damp and cold; prolonged fevers; repeated or imperfectly subdued inflammations; inoculation with tuberculous matter, or with pus, or with the flesh or blood of a tuberculous or pyæmic subject; or the presence of these matters in the body from disease; irritation of lymphatic vessels or tissues by foreign bodies.

Occurrence. — So common that it is the cause of a large proportion of the deaths in all countries, climates, ages, and ranks.

Causes.—Family predisposition. Other causes unknown. Inoculation doubtful.

Occurrence.—Comparatively rare; chiefly affecting persons of adult or advancing life.

Thus the whole clinical and pathological history of tubercle seems to separate it widely from cancer and other specific growths, and to approach it more to common lesions of nutrition, such as pus, lymph, and other hyperplasms, inflammatory or non-inflammatory.

Virchow distinguished miliary tubercle as heteroplastic lymphoma; that is, a new growth of lymphatic tissue where none exists naturally. On this subject I quote the important remarks of Dr. Burdon Sanderson, in his account of recent Researches on Tuberculosis.'[1]

Virchow distinguishes lymphomas into two great classes, hyperplastic and heteroplastic. The hyperplastic lymphoma *par excellence*, is scrofula, for this consists in the

[1] *Edinburgh Medical Journal*, Nov. 1869.

c 2

growth of nodules of material, which have the same structure in parts of the body where no such structure exists. Leucæmia occupies an intermediate position, because in it we have hyperplasia of the spleen and lymphatic glands, heteroplasia of the liver, kidneys, and mucous membranes. I propose to use the word *adenoid* to characterise the tissue, for the following reasons : There are in various parts of the body organs which, like the morbid growths in question, possess a structure exactly resembling, in fact identical with, that of the follicles of the lymphatic glands. These organs are the Peyer's follicles, the *Trachomdrüsen* of the conjunctiva, and the Malpighian corpuscles of the spleen. In addition to these, there are other parts of the body in which the same tissue is met with. Thus in the neighbourhood of the bronchial tubes in the lungs of the guinea-pig there are collections of adenoid tissue, which lie between the bronchioles and their accompanying blood-vessels. In the pleura, immediately under the epithelium, there are gland-like, or as I call them, adenoid bodies, consisting of collections of the tissue in question, surrounding tufts of capillary vessels, and covered with epithelium. In the peritoneum (omentum) there are similar bodies ; in addition to which the vessels are surrounded by sheaths or cylinders of the same structure. Underneath the parietal peritoneum there are similar sheaths, much less massive but not less distinct in structure.

'The reason why I have drawn attention to all these anatomical facts is this. We have seen that all these structures agree in being formed of adenoid tissue ; that tubercle (in the true sense), the new growth in leucæmia, the new growths in tuberculous disease of cattle, have this in common—that they also consist of adenoid tissue ; and that Virchow distinguishes tubercle from the rest mainly in that it is heteroplastic. I have now to say that the tubercle, produced artificially, is, in a certain sense, *hyperplastic,* that is an overgrowth, not a new growth. Thus the parts most apt to be affected with tubercle are those in which the structure in question exists naturally. The tubercle nodules which are formed in the peritoneum and pleura are overgrowths of nodules which existed before; the masses of new growth in the lung are overgrowths of masses infinitely smaller which existed before, &c. • • • • •

'This process of overgrowth of pre-existing adenoid tissue is not, however, all that we observe in artificial tuberculosis. I have already stated that nodules are found not only in the serous membranes, but in the solid organs. In the latter, the constitution of the nodules is somewhat more complicated. I will take two organs to illustrate this—the liver, and the lungs. In the liver there are two very distinct forms, the leucæmic and the miliary serous. In the first the new growth assumes precisely the character of leucæmic enlargement. The organ is enormously enlarged in consequence of the growth of adenoid tissue around the bile ducts. At the same time the epithelium of the bile ducts grows with great activity; so that you have a combination of two things —overgrowth of adenoid tissue round the ducts, of epithelium within the ducts. In the serous form, miliary nodules of adenoid tissue grow underneath the serous membrane.

'In the lung there are also two forms. In tuberculised lungs the lung becomes disseminated with minute nodules of lobular catarrhal pneumonia. Each nodule is exactly translucent. On making sections it is found that it consists of two materials, entirely different from each other anatomically. On the one hand the alveoli are filled with the ordinary roundish cells, which are always found there.[1] The alveolar walls are thickened by the growth in them of adenoid tissue. As the disease progresses these masses of lobular pneumonia coalesce. Each mass caseates in the centre, i.e. becomes opaque and soft. The disintegration goes on till a vomica is formed.[2]

In this masterly summary and interpretation of the results of the researches of himself and others on the artificial production of tubercle in animals, Dr. Sanderson answers more completely than has ever yet been done, the question proposed by me more than forty years ago—what elementary part of the lung is affected to produce the constant shape and form presented by miliary tubercles? He replies, the *adenoid* tissue, which he has proved to exist naturally in minute patches scattered through the lung, of the same structure as miliary tubercle, and requiring only increase in quantity to become the same in all respects.[2] These conclusions have been confirmed by

---

[1] 'These cell-like bodies which occupy the alveolar cavities are often called epithelial. Their relation to the epithelial lining of the alveolar walls is not known.'

[2] The connection of pulmonary tubercle with the lymphatic system, thus proved by the skilful appliances of modern science, has been glimpsed by several old writers, and by none more completely than the celebrated French Professor, Portal, who has anticipated Dr. Sanderson in the following description of adenoid substance throughout the lung :—' Indépendamment de ces corps bronchiques, dont les poumons sont pourvus, il est dans ce viscère, comme on vient de le dire, des véritables glandes lymphatiques d'une nature très-différente, avec lesquels plusieurs anatomistes les ont confondues ; elles ne sont pas, comme les corps bronchiques, toujours placées autour des bronches; mais elles sont indistinctement répandues dans la substance du poumon, principalement à sa face externe. J'en ai vu quelques-unes qui étaient contenues dans la masse des corps bronchiques même, avec lesquelles on les aurait confondues: de même qu'on trouve des glandes lymphatiques autour des glandes parotides et des glandes maxillaires. Les glandes lymphatiques du poumon sont plus petites que les corps bronchiques ; elles sont plus régulièrement arrondies, plus dures au tact; et on voit par l'appareil des vaisseaux lymphatiques qui y aboutissent, qu'elles sont véritablement de la nature de celles que l'on connaît dans les autres parties du corps sous le nom de glandes lymphatiques ou conglobées.'

the independent observations of Dr. Wilson Fox, whose experiments led to the same results, and will be further noticed hereafter.

The conclusions of Drs. Sanderson and Fox appear to me much more correct than the notion of Virchow, that tubercle, as well as pus and all other new formations, has its origin in the cells of connective tissue only : a notion incompatible with the production of tubercle and pus on serous membranes and within blood-vessels and lymphatics. But although I think that Dr. Sanderson has proved that miliary tubercles are modifications of the adenoid tissue, I do not admit that any and every inflammation or overgrowth of the adenoid tissue will produce miliary tubercle; nor do I admit that adenoid tissue is essential to the production of other phthisical consolidations, especially of what has been called yellow tubercle, either in its crude or in its caseous stage.   But this subject and the general relations of inflammation to consumption demand consideration in another chapter.

‘ Pour revenir maintenant aux tubercules qui constituent la phthisie originaire, je pense, d'après l'examen le plus attentif, qu'ils sont formés et par des engorgemens des glandes lymphatiques, répandues dans presque toutes les parties du poumon, ou loin des bronches, ainsi que par des engorgemens lymphatiques du tissu cellulaire des poumons, lesquelles, après avoir pris une consistance plus ou moins grande, terminent fréquemment par tourner en une mauvaise suppuration.'—*Obs. sur la Nature et le Traitement de la Phthisie pulmonaire.* Par Antoine Portal, Prof. de Méd. au Coll. de France, &c., 1809, tome ii. p. 307.

CHAPTER IV.

RELATIONS OF INFLAMMATION TO TUBERCLE AND OTHER PHTHINOPLASMS.

When and how does inflammation produce Tubercle?—The plastic process of Inflammation—Sarcophytes, or Bioplasts: their formation, migration, and changes—Nature of Bioplasm; Cells not essential—Observations of W. Addison, Max Schultze, Stricker, Lionel Beale, &c.—Explanation of production of membrane, pus, tubercle, &c. by changes in Sarcophytes—Examination of other phthinoplasms in the Lung—Chronic Induration—Fibroid—Pathological and Clinical results—Contraction—Dilated Bronchi—Emphysema—Asthma—Bronchial exudations, fibrinous and albuminous.

THE adenoid tissue of the lymphatic glands may inflame, swell, and the inflammation either subside by resolution, or go on to complete suppuration in healthy abscess; and in neither case does tubercle or any other morbid change remain behind. In acute pneumonia also it can hardly be supposed that the adenoid tissue does not partake of the general inflammation; and yet the inflammation may end in resolution and absorption of its products, and leave not a trace behind. It is the scrofulous inflammation of lymphatic glands that makes them enlarge first, and then harden, and at length degenerate into caseous masses, which soften eventually, and discharge from scrofulous sores. It is a similar type of inflammation which may develope miliary indurations in the adenoid tissue of the lungs, tending in like manner to caseation, softening, and spreading, and to the formation of vomicæ. In both cases the death and destruction of the tissue is preceded by induration, and the microscope reveals the nature of this induration in the abundant production of cells, which change their colour from red to grey, and eventually so press on each other and on their containing fibrous stroma, as to choke their nutrition, and they then become cheesy, that is, undergo fatty degeneration and disintegration. It is therefore not the mere inflammation or simple growth of the adenoid tissue that constitutes the destructive changes of scrofula and tubercle, but the excessive multiplication of perishable cells doomed to speedy decay. These cells have the closest resemblance to *leucocytes*, the ordinary corpuscles found in lymph, and circulating also in considerable numbers in the blood; and there are good grounds for concluding that these all are identical in nature. The strong probability is, therefore, still in favour of the opinion which I have entertained, and in general terms expressed during the last forty years, that variations in the plasma, as represented by these bodies, constitute the essential element in the production of lymph, pus, and tubercle.

The coagulable lymph, composing the plastic exudations from inflamed serous membranes, contains more or less of these corpuscles or leucocytes; their greater abundance causing a more opaque appearance, and a lower capacity for organisation in the inflammatory product, and constituting the kind of lymph termed *corpuscular* by Paget, *croupous* by Rokitansky, and by myself *cacoplastic* and *aplastic*, having the further varieties purulent and tubercular.

Now it is in the subjects in which inflammation of serous membranes produces this kind of lymph, that inflammation of lymphatic glands causes induration followed by caseation, and inflammation of the minute patches of adenoid tissues in the lung, produces miliary tubercle. There is even a preference in the lymphatic system for the manifestation of this tendency; and, therefore, lymphatic swellings often precede its development in other tissues, and occur in slight degrees in consequence of wounds or cutaneous eruptions, without necessarily infecting the system. The artificial production of miliary tubercles in so large a proportion of animals, by inoculation or mechanical injury, is another proof of the peculiar susceptibility of this system, to which we shall have occasion to advert hereafter.

But although showing this preference, this degenerating cell proliferation is surely not confined to the adenoid, to the connective, or to any other tissue. In some form or other it may occur in other textures of the body; and in none more surely, perhaps in none sooner, than in the blood itself. I allude not only to the case of leukæmia—the distinctive feature of which is an excess of the pale corpuscles at the expense of the other animal constituents of the blood—but also to all cases of extensive inflammatory disease, especially those of a chronic character.

It was an observation long ago made by Mr. Gulliver,[1] that blood taken from an inflamed part contained an unusual quantity of pale corpuscles. Mr. W. Addison[2] first noticed an increased appearance of these in the inflamed vessels of the frog's web; and soon after I observed, not only their increased production within the blood-vessels, but that they manifested a remarkable adhesive quality, making them stick to the coats of the vessels and in some cases, together with the entangled blood-discs, to cause their complete obstruction.[3]

It was the sudden appearance of these adhesive corpuscles in the blood-vessels of the frog's web irritated with capsicum, that riveted my attention; and after repeated observations I was led to conclude that herein lay the chief cause of that obstruction of the vessels,

[1] Willis's *Translation of Wagner's Physiology*, 1844.
[2] *Med. Gazette*, January 29, 1841.
[3] *Ibid.* July 23, 1841.

sarcophytes in the exudation from inflamed vessels, I was
in doubt how they could pass through the coats of the
vessels, in which no pores had ever been discovered; but
I suggested that small granules or nuclei might so pass,
and then grow into larger. But Dr. W. Addison had,
in 1843, described the actual fact of emigration, by the
sarcophyte first passing into the substance of the wall of
the blood-vessel, and then being thrown out of it. To
Dr. Addison, therefore, belongs the merit of having first
discovered the emigration process. It was again accurately observed in the tongue of the frog, and described
with perfect clearness by my lamented friend Dr. Augustus
Waller.[1]   Although this demonstration of the exudation
origin of lymph and pus cells did not attract notice at the
time, yet many others besides myself adopted the exudation theory—that is, that of the origin of the chief
products of inflammation, cellular as well as fibrous and
fluid, in exudation from the inflamed vessels. This does

---

[1] *Philosoph. Magazine*, 1846, p. 347. Dr. Norris has endeavoured
to refer the passage of sarcophytes through the walls of vessels to a
general fact, which he has beautifully illustrated by experiments, that
colloid bodies can pass through each other's substance without breach
of continuity. But these experiments were made with soap or glycerine
bubbles, formed by a colloid of very different consistence from that of
the walls of blood-vessels, even granting that these do consist of
colloid protoplasm without endothelium, which is more than is admitted
by the latest authors. (See Eberth, ' On the Minute Anatomy of the Capillaries,' in Stricker's *Histology*, p. 282.) It must be borne in mind that the
walls of the capillaries continually resist the considerable pressure from the
heart and arteries, which a soft colloid could not do. The walls must
either consist of a very tough colloid, or be strengthened with endothelium
scales. Observations render the latter alternative most probable, and it is
conceivable that there may be minute interstices between these scales, containing protoplasm permeable to the active sarcophytes, but not pervious to
the mass of the blood. The sarcophytes, when young, consist simply of soft
colloid, which subdivides and passes through the interstitial protoplasm,
and reunites into their original form outside the vessel, just as, in Dr.
Norris's experiments, the bubble and the film regain their continuity after
passing through each other's substance.

most scrupulous full admission on my part that the cell-life
of the tissue is also brought into fuller activity; and that
some inflammatory products arise from that source, as,
for example, connective tissue cells, epithelium and epi-
dermis cells, and others, which are produced in abundance
in inflammation of particular tissues; but I hold that the
more distinctive products of the inflammatory process,
lymph, pus, and tubercle, and albuminous and fibrinous
matters in other varieties of form, are truly *exudations*
from the inflamed blood-vessels; and I was enabled to
trace most of the products to the chemical and physiological properties known to be in operation. It was in
concordance with this view that I was led to class the
products of inflammation as deposits. Similar views were
subsequently brought forward by Rokitansky and other
authors, and were generally adopted in this country, until
within the last ten or twelve years, when they have been,
in great measure, superseded by the cell-growth theory of
the North-German school.

When Schwann and J. Müller propounded the general
axiom that animal, like vegetable tissues, are formed by
their elementary cells, they did not exclude the blood-
vessels of the animal body from their share in the work
by causing variations in the distribution of the nutritious
fluid; but neither they nor most of their numerous followers, in advocating the cell-formation theory, seem to
have sufficiently considered that the nutritious fluid itself
abounds in the elements of cell-life. Consequently, the
main fountain of cell-life was comparatively neglected,
and all microscopes were turned on the tissues and their
nourishing and formative elements. There, in these
parts, was sought the origin, not only of the tissues
themselves, but of morbid products also; and pus, lymph,
cancer, &c. were all referred by Virchow to
conditions of the proliferating power of the elementary

cells of connective tissue, and grouped together, in spite
of their total dissimilarities in structure and history,
under the general term of ' growths.'

But extended observation has already done much to
rectify such hasty and partial generalisation. The very
axiom ' omnis cellula e cellulâ' was upset by the discovery that there is no absolute need of a cell at all in
a protoplasm or parent organism. Max Schultze[1] says
that the embryonal cells (so called), in which ' the unlimited power of tissue formation is most distinctly
evident, consist only of a little mass of protoplasm and
a nucleus.' A cell without a wall! But further, even
the nucleus is not essential. Max Schultze has discovered
a non-nucleated Amœba (*Amœba porrecta*) in the
Adriatic; Haskel, a larger non-nucleated *Protista*, pro-
pagating by division, in the Mediterranean;[2] and Professor
Stricker mentions other instances, proving that the ideal
type of a cell is a little mass of sarcode or protoplasm,
without either cell wall or nucleus. This being the case,
that the essential element of the protoplasm is independent of both cell and nucleus, it is surely a misnomer to
use the word cell, and it is erroneous to suppose that all
living matter must originate in either cells or nuclei. It
appears, therefore, that Dr. Lionel Beale is more accurate
in giving to all active protoplasm the term *germinal matter*
or *bioplasm*, whilst cells and all other formed rudiments
of tissue are expressed by the antithetical term *formed
matter*; and both his language and his descriptions seem
to answer well in their application to the products of
disease.

In their indefatigable researches in the field of nature,
if the German physiologists have not wholly emancipated
their language from the trammels of the hypothesis of
cytology, or cell-doctrine, they have greatly extended our

[1] Stricker's *Histology*, vol. i. p. 7.   [2] Stricker, *loc. cit.*

knowledge of the properties of elementary living matter; and inasmuch as the pale blood- or lymph-corpuscles are samples of this elementary matter or protoplasm, we are interested in these properties in connection with our present subject.

Although a bioplasm or perfect protoplasm may exist without any structure discernible under the highest microscopic powers hitherto applied, yet its vitality is abundantly manifest by its spontaneous motions, external and internal by its nutrition and growth, and by its power of reproduction. Its motions are displayed in its singular changes of shape; hence the term amœba (ἀμείβω, ' I change '). These changes give the amœbal mass a power of irregular locomotion, if floating in liquid; and some species also throw out processes like arms, with which they embrace other objects, and draw nourishment from them. In doing this the bioplasm seems to exert sometimes a solvent power on the matters seized; at others, one of absorbing them into its substance: in the case of colouring matter, its particles can be seen in the interior of the protoplasm, and by their motions show the intrinsic movements which are taking place.

Without dwelling longer on this curious and interesting topic, we have to recur to the white corpuscles, or sarcophytes, which as before said, are of the nature of protoplasm, and under circumstances of excitement exhibit these motions and properties of amœboid matter. In the fresh-drawn blood of the frog, they have been seen to exhibit lively changes of form and locomotive movements, and to take into their interior milk globules and particles of colouring matter. As exudation globules, they show the wonderful power of emigration before mentioned; and when extravasated, their moving and other powers continue, and may aid in explaining some of the obscure changes in the tissues in inflammation and

suppuration.   For example, the disappearance of
blood corpuscles, and of the structure of tissues under the
rapid increase of pus cells, which used to drive us to the
assumption of a marvellous activity of absorption, now
appears as a proof of the amœboid voracity and digestive
power of this active germinal matter.

And if the bioplasm exhibits this potent activity in the
case of rich blood and acute inflammation, are we not to
expect varied results, and less lively actions, when the
blood is depraved, and the inflammation more chronic?
This is a subject well worthy of direct investigation from
this stand-point.   Max Schultze observed the amœboid
cells of freshly drawn human blood increase in activity
when the temperature was raised to between 95° and 104°
F., but above that heat the *movements cease, and the
cells harden.*[1]

How full of suggestion is this single observation!
These little germinal elements are full of life and activity
within a certain range of temperature ; below it their
activity diminishes ; above it, it ceases, and they *harden.*
This range of temperature, thus quelling amœboid life and
activity, is quite within that which occurs in inflammatory
and febrile diseases ; and how does the observation correspond with our clinical knowledge of the grave import of
continued high temperature in pneumonia, bronchitis, or
even febrile catarrh !   It matters not what may be the
cause of the rise of temperature to 104° and upwards in
these cases.   If the above observation is correct, such a
heat injures the vitality of the plastic materials within
and without the blood-vessels, and instead of their undergoing changes, by which they are either properly organised, or are eliminated from the tissues by transformation
into pus globules, or other liquid discharge, they concrete
into little solids, it may be still with the proliferating

---

[1] Stricker's *Histology*, vol. i. p. 414.

.... matter, but of low and decaying
............., and proving a cause of obstruction and
.... to the tissue, both as first formed, and in their
.... decline into caseation and decay. This is but
.... suggestion, arising out of a solitary observation; and it opens up the obvious inquiry, What other influences, besides heat, may impair the activity and plasticity of the germinal matter, and cause its accumulation
in the caeoplastic, degenerating, and decaying form of
......., and kindred consolidations of tissue?

This, then, is the line of argument by which I would
point out that modern researches appear to support the
view which I have always held, that the tuberculous and
.... lesions, which cause consumption of the lungs,
arise from a degradation of the plasma, or nutritive
material, by which old textures are renewed, and new ones
formed. This material, or protoplasm, is seen in an inflamed
..... of a living animal in the form of *sarcophytes*, or
........, multiplying and clinging to the inside of the
........., penetrating their walls, and emigrating by a
.... of their own into the adjoining tissues. Like
...... forms of animal and vegetable protoplasm, these
.... have vital endowments of motion, growth,
...... absorbing and digesting various matters from
...... and of multiplication by division, and probably
.... and endogenous proliferation. There
...... doubt that all these vital properties are con-
..... the processes of construction and destruction
...... inflammation. The conversion of the sarco-
...... containing liquid and nuclei and
...... amoeboid motions of these, and their further
...... and growth, at the expense of the red
...... containing tissues, have been already observed

...... are wanting on the share which

the vital properties of the bioplasm have in the formation of false membranes and cicatrices, and other higher products of inflammation; but it may be presumed that they are here in full activity. Again, in all probability, the reverse is the case in the hard, opaque, cacoplastic products resulting from low inflammation, of which grey consolidation is the type in the lung tissue. Their very density and opacity are suggestive of a change from the soft and pliant substance and gelatinous translucency of the active sarcophyte; and under the microscope, these indurations present the appearance of crowded leucocytes, become solid from induration of their contents, and having lost all their active movements and plasticity.

If the inflammatory process continues, so likewise does the transudation of sarcophytes, together with liquor sanguinis and its consolidating contents—fibrillating fibrin and hyaline with other granules or molecules—causing an increase of substance in the part; and if the vital activity of the sarcophytes fails to maintain the life and functions of the tissues, or even to effect their removal by conversion into pus, a morbid condensation remains, of lower vitality and imperfect functions, causing disorder by its rigidity and mass, and tending, sooner or later, to decay further by caseation and excavation. These results, however, will present considerable variety, according to the quantity of the inflammatory product, the proportion of its constituents, and the extent to which they have lost vitality, or become degraded from a healthy standard. When the sarcophytes and other corpuscles abound, and yet are so deficient in vital properties that they harden and do not even go on to suppuration, then the consolidation is of the most aplastic kind, opaque, curdy, and soon undergoing the caseous softening and disintegration. This is what takes place in the acute form of phthisis, termed acute scrofulous pneumonia. A large part of the lung is converted into a soft solid, of a pinkish-drab colour, with patches of opaque yellow caseation and partial excavation. These patches often begin in the areoles and bronchial tubes, which are stuffed with epithelium cells; but this epithelium does not constitute the whole or the greater part of the solid mass. All the tissues are crammed with exudation-matters—the pleura and the interlobular septa sometimes showing their share, in other cases escaping.

In more chronic cases, and also in those acute ones in which the scrofulous or tuberculous tendency is less strong —in other words, in which the vital powers of the sarcophytes are less impaired, and the exudation-matter less corpuscular and more fibrinous—the consolidation of the lung is less complete. It is redder and less opaque; and although it may show spots of opacity and softening, the greater part remains tough, and undergoes gradual contraction, from an increased development of connective tissue. And thus arises the so-called *fibroid* variety of phthisis, when the first inflammatory exudation has been mainly fibrinous, and results in increased growth of interstitial connective tissue, rather than in deposit in the alveolar texture of the lung. The cause of this variation of result seems to be sometimes a difference in the constitution or crasis of the individual; but in other instances it may be traced to a local cause. In pleuro-pneumonia attended with considerable effusion into the pleura, the pulmonary texture is so compressed, that little or no exudation or epithelial formation takes place into the air cells; but the plastic matter is confined to the interstitial textures, which are thereby consolidated into the state termed by Laennec carnification. This, if not reabsorbed, forms the basis of a dense contractile consolidation, usually of a fibrous nature, which may persist long without passing into further degeneration, and then constitutes disease long since called by Sir D. Corrigan *cirrhosis*

of the lung.   I had previously (in 1856) described it as a
result of pleuro-pneumonia, and explained how the general
dilatation of the bronchi, which often accompanies it,
arises from the atmospheric pressure in inspiration distending the tubes, as it could no longer penetrate into
the agglutinated air cells.   The inflammatory origin of
the disease is proved by the strong pleural adhesions
which always accompany it, and which would not be so
constant if the consolidation depended on a fibrous growth
in the lung, to which it has been referred.   There is, indeed, a fibrous structure, like a condensed connective
tissue, constituting the bulk of this tough induration of
the lung ; but it may be fairly questioned whether this is
not rather from an exudation of fibrin, at once forming
fibres, as in a blood clot,[1] than a true growth of connective
tissue by cell proliferation.

I consider that the fibroid form of phthisis, so well
described by Dr. Andrew Clark, is of the same nature, and
that he is quite right in recognising it as a variety of
phthisis, for it most commonly presents many of the
symptoms of chronic consumption, and is either already

---

[1] Recent histologists, especially the Germans, seem to have overlooked
this fibrillating property of the fibrin of the blood, as exhibited in the clot
of liquor sanguinis. Gulliver and Addison distinctly proved that fibrin
spontaneously consolidates into a series of extremely fine fibrils, which
interlace and cross each other. It has always appeared to me a most natural
inference that these fibres, thus consolidating from the exuded blood-liquor,
form part of the material of the connective tissue of false membranes and
interstitial deposits resulting from inflammation ; and this view has been
adopted by Rokitansky, Paget, and others.   The exclusive cell theory of
Schwann and Virchow, which assumes that every tissue springs from cells,
threw it into the shade until recently, when the observations of Beale and
others have proved that cells are but the produce of simpler germinal
matter, which may form other elements of tissues besides cells ; and these
primary fibrils may be of this nature. The most recent writers who adhere to the cell theory have great difficulty in explaining the formation of
all the fibres of connective tissue from fusiform cells. (See Rollett on ' Connective Tissues,' Stricker's *Histology*, p. 88.)

combined with partial consolidations and excavations of a
tuberculous nature, or, eventually lapsing into these, it
passes into common phthisis. For this reason I have
always viewed it as only a variety, not a distinct species,
of phthisis. This, which I have termed *cacoplastic* deposit, presents a degree higher in the standard of vitality
and organisation than any of the softer and more opaque
phthinoplasms, which are *aplastic*, and pass soon into
caseation and excavation. The cacoplastic abounds more
in the chronic forms of phthisis, having a certain vitality
and persistence; but the aplastic has no self-preserving
power, and tends to more speedy decay.

If any other proof were wanting to establish the fact
that the fibroid consolidation of the lung is in its nature
allied to miliary tubercle, and this, again, to yellow or
caseous tubercle, we may find it in the fact that, in most
cases of chronic phthisis, all three conditions are met
with in different parts of the same lung.   Thus it sometimes happens that the lower portions of a lung, that have
been long ago consolidated by inflammation, exhibit
patches of a more opaque and grey aspect, with spots of
caseation and even excavation, marking the progressive
steps of decay.   Again, we have something like the converse of this in the patches of dense contractile tissue
often found hedging in and circumscribing old cavities in
the upper parts of the lung; and the process of cicatrisation of such cavities is almost always effected by the production and contraction of a fibrous tissue of similar
character.

Many of the symptoms and physical signs of the more
chronic form of phthisis arise from the condensation and
obstruction of the pulmonary tissue caused by this cacoplastic or fibroid material in different parts of the lung.
When resulting from pneumonic inflammation, it commonly affects more the lower part of one or both lungs, as

lately described; and dulness and hardness on percussion,
and restricted movements with diminished capacity of
the corresponding walls of the chest, are the result;
often, also, with the loud and diffused bronchophony
and tubular breathing, caused by extensive dilatation of
the bronchial tubes.

When, on the other hand, the disease arises out of
severe and prolonged bronchial inflammation, this affects
rather the roots and upper parts of the lungs; the inflammation becoming deeper seated, reaches the submucous
and connective tissue around the large bronchi; and as
the parts become thickened with this peribronchial deposit, there may be little or no dulness in the walls of
the chest, but the constriction of the tubes will cause
wheezing rhonchi and prolonged expiration of the asthmatic kind; in fact, if this state of things continues, the
lungs may become emphysematous, and the disorder
pass from the category of consumption to that of asthma.
But if the tendency to decay be greater, the tight, prolonged wheezing is soon replaced by loose crepitation,
with shorter but easier breath; more or less dulness will
be manifest at or near an apex or root of a lung, with
tubular voice and expiration; whilst the expectoration of
opaque matter, shreddy or purulent, abounding in dead and
decaying corpuscles, disintegrated fibrin, and epithelium
cells, indicates the removal of some of the consolidating
matter.   Such cases may terminate favourably or un-
favourably, according to whether the lung texture to
which the deposit has reached does not or does participate in the decay and disintegration by which the deposits
are removed. If the lung does break down, fragments of its
tissue may be found in the expectoration, when carefully
examined by the microscope;[1] and signs of softening and
excavation will become apparent in the affected part of

[1] See Dr. Fenwick's Paper, *Med.-Chir. Trans.* vol. xlix. p. 209.

the chest. Yet I can recollect several instances of deep-
seated bronchitis in which the signs of lung consolidation
threatened the destruction of its texture, but they have
been completely removed after free expectoration of a
quantity of very ugly-looking opaque matter, differing in
no particular from phthisical sputa, except in the absence
of filaments of lung tissue. Some of these cases, having
thus narrowly escaped from lung disease in one attack,
have been less fortunate in a subsequent one, and have
eventually lapsed into phthisis. All these facts point to
the conclusion that the diseases included under the term
consumption present many degrees, and that however in-
tractable and hopeless those may be, in its worst and most
extensive forms, yet that much may be done to counteract
and arrest the more limited and milder degrees of the
disorder. And as we have found that in many instances
the development of the disease may be traced to inflammation, and that this also often has an aggravating
influence on its course, the prevention and removal of
inflammation will be among the chief indications in the
treatment. And yet we have found that there must be
something more than inflammation to produce consumptive disease; and *that something* we have been led to
trace to a defective vitality, and therefore a decaying
tendency, in the plasma, the nutritive materials of flesh
and blood. The most recent researches seem to point to
the *sarcophytes* (alias *bioplasts*, *leucocytes*, or *pale corpuscles*) as the representatives of this living protoplasm
('bioplasm,' Beale); and any means by which their vital
and euplastic properties can be exalted and preserved may
be deemed of paramount importance, above and beyond
the mere prevention and treatment of inflammation.

CHAPTER V.

CONSUMPTION INDEPENDENT OF INFLAMMATION. SCROFULA; A DISEASE OF THE LYMPHATIC SYSTEM.

Sarcophytes of the Lymphatics ; subject to the same changes, and producing the same results, as those from blood-vessels—Leucocythæmia.

WE are now brought to the consideration of the consumptive or scrofulous diathesis or constitution, in which the
seeds of decay may arise *independently of inflammation.*
And guided by what we found the sarcophytes, as representatives of protoplasm, capable of doing in connection
with inflammation, we have to enquire, Are these or
similar bodies to be met with elsewhere, existing independently of this process?

These sarcophytes, or pale corpuscles, exist in the blood
in health, but in very small numbers. It is in the lymphatic system that they are commonly found in the
greatest abundance; in fact, this is their normal source
and habitation; and they constitute the multitude of organic particles, contained in lymphatic vessels and glands,
in Peyer's patches, in the lacteals and mesenteric glands,
and in the pulp and Malpighian bodies of the spleen.

'The lymph corpuscles are now universally admitted
to be identical in all their characters with the colourless
corpuscles of the blood. They show in particular the
same constantly varying form, and the same phenomena
of contractility as long as they are living; whilst they
assume the spheroidal form, which was formerly considered to be their natural shape, as soon as they die. The

manipulations, that up to a recent period were adopted for microscopical examination, very easily kill them; and thus a fatal effect is produced by evaporation, by the addition of water, or of saline solutions containing more than two per cent. of salt. Even mechanical agencies, as the weight of the covering glass, are sufficient to rapidly extinguish all indications of life.' (Von Recklinghausen. Stricker's ' Histology,' vol. i. p. 34.)

The lymphatic system, then, seems to be the nursery or seed-bed of these flesh-germs, these primary elements of flesh and blood; and, as in that exaggeration of the nutritive process—inflammation—we found these sarcophytes to be the chief agents in the formation of its products—euplastic, cacoplastic, and aplastic—so we may he prepared to expect the same bodies to manifest similar tendencies, in all these varieties, in the lymphatic glands and tissues where they mostly do congregate. And this is what we see completely answered in the diseases of the lymphatic system, which form some of the principal features of what is called scrofula. Take, for instance, enlargement of the glands, which may proceed to such enormous extent by rapid multiplication of these lymph corpuscles as to form large tumours (*lymphomata*), particularly in the neck, armpits, groins, mesentery, and bronchial glands. These swellings are for the most part indolent, until they become hard or inflame; and then they undergo various changes of caseation, irregular suppuration, and ulceration, with the discharge of a variety of bloody, cheesy, and purulent matters, resulting from the fatty degeneration and disintegration of the enlarged and softened gland, together with the inflammatory products of the more vascular connective tissue and skin involving the swelling. In Peyer's patches, and other adenoid tissues of mucous membranes, similar changes occur on a smaller scale, producing tuberculous ulcerations.

In these several lymphatic enlargements, there is considerable difference in the consistence and tendencies of the swelling. It may be simple hypertrophy, consisting of increase of lymph corpuscles and containing tissues in equal proportion; and the result is a soft indolent body, which may attain a large size without causing much discomfort, and may be dispersed without undergoing further change. It is different where the swelling is hard, from the excessive crowding of the lymph cells, and probably also from their harder condition, together with an overgrowth of their fibrous stroma. This crowding must have the effect of lowering their vitality; and if, in addition, they have become hardened, there must be a loss of those remarkable properties of mobility and other vital endowments which distinguish these sarcophytes in their state of healthy activity. Therefore, in preportion as they are crowded and indurated, they will be prone to decay and disintegration, in the way of caseation and softening, a process to be considered hereafter; and their decay may cause the irritation, inflammation, and ulceration of the adjoining tissues.

Thus we find in the morbid changes to which the lymphatic glands are subject another illustration of the rapid production, accumulation, and decay of the protoplastic material, the sarcophytes: in this instance, not necessarily induced by inflammation, but often resulting from hypertrophy or excessive production in the proper receptacles of these corpuscles. But to complete the history, we have to add the notable case of grey or miliary tubercle, which, as we have found, Dr. Burdon Sanderson and Dr. Wilson Fox, in independent investigations on their artificial production, were led to identify with the same lymphatic or adenoid tissue. But they are not merely overgrowths of this tissue. Their hardness and grey colour denote an altered structure, which the micro-

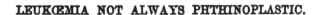

scope discovers in the overcrowding of hardened cells,
which have lost their plastic and self-sustaining power as
sarcophytes, and so become causes of obstruction and
irritation to adjoining tissues, and are themselves prone
to an early decay.

That an excessive abundance of lymph corpuscles alone
does not suffice to produce the decaying tumours, which
characterise scrofula and tuberculosis, is evident in the
disease called *leukœmia,* or *leucocythœmia,* in which they
not only are found in unusual proportion in the blood, but
by their accumulation they cause *lymphomata,* great enlargements of the lymphatic glands, spleen, and liver;
but these are all soft swellings, tending less to the decay
of their substance, than to the exhaustion of the frame by
monopolising the nutritive material of the body in its
protoplastic state, so that the victims of the disease die
of anæmia and asthenia before there is time for the lymphatic swellings to go into decay.   But the vital properties of the sarcophytes in leukœmia require further
investigation before we can be sure of the true nature of
this disease.

In conclusion, we may say that as there seems to be
good reason for regarding the lymphatic and chyliferous
system as the source of the plasma from which both
blood and flesh are formed, nourished, and renovated, it
becomes quite intelligible that any disease in the plasma,
or germinal matter, or in its representatives, the sarcophytes, will manifest its effects commonly, and at an early
period, in some part of this system.

CHAPTER VI.

ON CASEATION AND FATTY DEGENERATION OF TISSUES.

Fatty Degeneration discovered by Gulliver—Proved to be a chemical change —Causes maturation and softening of Tubercle, Fibrin, &c.; and an extensive agent in Pathology—The most gentle step to the death of tissues.

THAT the texture of certain organs are sometimes transmuted into fatty matter was noticed by Laennec and other older authors; but the common tendency of many tissues and morbid products to fatty degeneration was first distinctly pointed out by Mr. Gulliver,[1] who found an abundance of fatty matter in the atheromatous patches in arteries, in diseased testicles and kidneys, and in chronic inflammation and tuberculous disease of the lungs.

Even at that early period he hints that these changes were evidences of decay of animal matter, induced by age or disease; and in the same year (1843) I first suggested the formation of adipocire from flesh kept moist without access of air as an analogous instance of the chemical conversion of flesh into fat.[2] Subsequently Mr. Gulliver

[1] *Med.-Chir. Trans.* vol. xxvi.; and *Edinb. Med. and Surg. Journ.* vol. xl., 1843.

[2] Some years after, Dr. Alison, in his essay on 'Vital Affinities' (*Trans. of Royal Soc. of Edinb.*, 1847), proposed a formula to explain the chemical conversion of albumen and water into fat and carbonate of ammonia. Mr. Gulliver had previously stated that Dr. John Davy had found an increase of oil, with the formation of carbonic acid and ammonia, in the liver of the cod, after it had been kept twenty-five days in a damp place. We may bear in mind that the common representative of living animal *catamorphosis* (downward change of form), urea, has the same elementary composition as carbonate of ammonia, and that the excessive excretion of urea is often observed in the same wasting diseases in which fatty degeneration invades the textures.

duced several instances of the production of fat in albuminous and fibrinous matters after death;[1] and both Dr. Hodgkin and myself noticed in several instances a decided increase of fat globules in morbid specimens after death.

This chemical view of the nature of fatty degeneration was afterwards completely established by the observations of Dr. R. Quain.[2] He produced the fatty conversion in healthy muscle by simply keeping it for a sufficient length of time in water, to which a little spirit or nitric acid had been added to prevent putrefaction. After some days, oil globules appear in the fibres of the muscle, and gradually increase until much of the sarcous element is converted into them, and under the microscope, or by the action of chemical tests, the change is proved to be identical with fatty degeneration as it occurs in the living body.

That which Dr. Quain conclusively established with regard to fatty degeneration of the heart—that it is a chemical conversion of muscle into fat from imperfect supply of blood, or malnutrition—has since been generally adopted and acknowledged to be a process common to most textures and morbid products in the body; and one playing a very important part in pathology. In the first and second editions of my 'Principles of Medicine' (published respectively in 1843 and 1848), I had already advanced a similar view as to the nature of fatty degeneration, and as to the large share which it has in producing the maturation and decay of tubercle and other products of inflammation and malnutrition.[3] This is now the

[1] Vide in Hewson's Works, Sydenham Soc. edit., 1846.
[2] 'Fatty Degeneration of the Heart,' Med.-Chir. Trans., 1850.
[3] After noticing Mr. Gulliver's recent discovery of increasing fat globules in tubercle, the general inference follows:—'The formation of fat, as it appears in atheroma of arteries, and in gangrene of the lungs, seems to be sometimes a débris of animal matter, as in the conversion of glycerine. The detection by Dr. Davy of olein and margarin

generally received opinion, and may be expressed in this
proposition :—That all proteinaceous matters and tissues
in the animal body, whether albuminous or fibrinous,
under various circumstances which impair their vital
nutrition, are prone to a chemical transformation into
fatty matter.

This change of material is, in fact, a partial chemical
decomposition, and incapacitates the parts for the functions of life ; but it is not rapidly or suddenly destructive,
like putrefaction, which not only rots and disintegrates,
but spreads a septic poison into surrounding parts. Fatty
transformation, on the other hand, is a gradual decay ; it
is a step downwards from highly organised to imperfectly
organised matter, more like vegetable than animal in
composition ; and with this change are lost the higher
vital properties of the part—contractility, healthy nutrition, and the power to resist further decay. An organ or
tissue thus degenerating may be said to *vegetate* awhile
before it loses all vitality ; and there may be for a time
even increasing cell-proliferation and growth, but of an
imperfect, perishable material, soon turning to fatty decay
and disintegration.

It would lead too far from our present subject to enter
into the history of fatty degeneration as affecting individual tissues and organs. Our concern is chiefly with that
occurring in inflammatory or other deposits or growths,
and especially in those in the lungs connected with the
progress of pulmonary consumption.

The fibrinous products of acute inflammation will supply
a good example of the manner in which a plastic material,

in opaque exudation corpuscles shows a tendency to the production of fat
in all degenerated plasma.' (*Principles of Medicine*, 1st ed., 1843, p. 321.)
This was, I believe, the first announcement of the general fact of fatty de-
generations. It was further developed and illustrated in succeeding editions,
and in the meantime the same views were entertained and extended by
Rokitansky, Virchow, Quain, Paget, and others.

which under favourable circumstances is capable of organisation, degenerates and decays by this chemical change,
when it is either wanting in vitality or when it is cut off
from the nutrient influence of the circulating blood and
of living tissues. The coagulable lymph, exuded in
moderate quantities by an inflamed pleura in a healthy
subject, is either reabsorbed or is organised into loose
adhesions of connective tissue, which may not interfere
with the motions of the part. But if the lymph effused
be excessive in quantity, or bad in quality, as manifested
by its opacity and a large predominance of the corpuscular
elements, it may either form only a dense tough solid, of
low organisation, binding down and impairing the movements, or it may not become organised at all, but degenerate and disintegrate into a cheesy or curdy mass,[1]
tending to further decomposition and mischievous results,

[1] Case I.—The following case exemplifies this kind of inflammatory product:—Master ——, æt. 4½ years. Feb. 9, 1847. Father (middle-aged)
lived long in India. Mother subject to liver disorders. The child has
always been precocious and delicate. Last summer had a feverish attack,
and has ever since been failing in appetite and flesh. For the last eight
months has had slight cough, and feverishness at night, sometimes ending
in perspiration. Bowels formerly costive; now irritable, and fæces pale and
clay. Right side tender, both at and below ribs. Pulse 120, weak.
Urine turbid and very acid.
   *Dulness; no motion or breath in lower half of right chest, which is larger
than the left; bronchophony in middle region, egophonic in parts; breath
and above; obscure crepitus on deep breath. Liver dulness two or three inches
below ribs; abdomen distended, with superficial fluctuation and dulness on
percussion.*
   A small dose of hydrarg. c. cretâ, digitalis, and Dover's powder twice a
day; chlorate of potass three times; iodine ointment to abdomen, with a constant wearing of piline.
   After a week of this treatment, the urine became more abundant, bile appeared at times in the fæces, and the abdominal tenderness, distension, and
dulness subsided, with improvement of appetite and cessation of cough;
the pulse continued frequent, with feverish accessions at night, and
chest signs remained the same. In March and April there was a
improvement in flesh and strength, especially after leaving off milk,
which was found always to stop the flow of bile. In June appetite again

or terminating in calcification, which is mineral degeneration.

Perhaps the simplest example of caseation or fatty
disintegration of fibrin is that occurring in the contre of
clots of fibrin within vessels, the true nature of which was
first pointed out by Mr. Gulliver.[1] The appearance of

failed, and intestinal irritation and hectic fever increased. Cod-liver oil was
then tried, and agreed, but with no good results; and after repeatedly
passing by the bowels sudden discharges of fœtid matter, with blood and
mucus, the patient died (July 12), in extreme emaciation.

On examination thirty-six hours after death, the abdomen was found distended, chiefly by gas in intestines. Very little fluid in peritoneum, and so
lymph or tubercle. Right lung closely adherent to anterior and upper wall of
the chest, its tissue compressed and congested, with patches of yellow tubercle; and the whole lower lobe, and a large part of the upper, converted into a
caseous mass, with layers of the same opaque curdy matter on the pleura
covering the caseated portions. Few traces of the lung tissue could be distinguished in the most opaque cheesy parts; but bronchi were found ab-
ruptly terminating in it in irregular excavations, comparatively dry, and
without any membrane or vessel, and only here and there could a tinge of
blood be seen. Deposit, tissue, and all, seemed degenerated into a mass of
opaque, yellow, friable, tuberculous matter. Similar caseous matter was
found in the bronchial glands, and spread under the costal pleura, and even
under the peritoneum lining the lower ribs. Left lung generally crepitant,
and free from adhesions, except near the root, where were several small
yellow and friable tubercles, and a small patch of opaque yellow lymph on
the pleura over one of these tubercles. Heart small and flabby. Bronchi
pale and dry. Liver lay low in abdomen, being somewhat enlarged, and also
depressed by the caseous deposit in right lung and pleura; it was closely
adherent to diaphragm. Tissue rather tough; red, not mottled. Nothing
remarkable in other organs.

This case presents a clear example of what has lately been regarded as
scrofulous pneumonia. At the time I considered it a striking instance of
caseous degeneration of the products of inflammation both in the lung and
on the pleura. The fatty transformation and disintegration of both products and containing tissue here superseded all vascular action or irritation; so that consumption did its destructive work almost without pain,
cough, or expectoration.

[1] Med.-Chir. Trans. vol. xxii., 1839. I promptly availed myself of this
discovery in showing that 'this softened fibrin in aspect and microscopic
composition differs in no essential particulars from those of softened tubercle.' (Princ. of Med., 1843, p. 324.) The subsequent observations of
Virchow on the same subject have not given due credit to Mr. Gulliver's
discovery.

..... of opaque softening in the emboli of veins had ... previously mistaken for pus; but Mr. Gulliver ... under the microscope that they contained no pus ..., but merely broken-down fragments of fibrin, with an abundance of oil globules, the formation of which ..... the disintegration.

Instances of a similar change may be seen in fibrinous vegetations on the valves of the heart, and in the shreddy lymph covering the pericardium and pleura, when prolonged inflammation of these membranes reduces their products from plastic to aplastic. In fact, in some cases, called empyema, the fluid effusion is not truly purulent, but consists of serum, holding in suspension numerous minute flakes of opaque degenerated fibrin, whilst large shreds of the same material still adhere to the pleura or pericardium. In true empyema there is little or no coagulable lymph, or curdy matter. All the plasma is converted into pus globules and liquor puris; and this transformation of the sarcophytes, the suppurative, demands a .... notice in this place, as contrasting with their more .... condition in tubercle. This we will consider .... next chapter.[1]

.... decided tendency thus shown in tubercle to spontaneous change .... the results of ultimate analysis of its composition uncertain. I am .... with any accurate analysis having been made since that of ..... which is as follows:—

.... pulmonary tubercle yielded little fat or extractive matter. An .... analysis, after the most careful removal of foreign constituents,

....	.	.	53·888	} which corresponds with the formula
....	.	.	7·112	
....	.	.	17·237	$C_{42} H_{33} F_6 O_{13}$.
....	.	.	21·767	

.... may be regarded as protein ($C_{48} H_{36} N_6 O_{14}$), from .... of carbon, one of hydrogen, and one of oxygen have been ....'s *Animal Chemistry*, by Dr. Day, vol. ii., p. 479.

CHAPTER VII.

ON THE NATURE OF PUS AND SUPPURATION.

Pus cells modified Sarcophytes; partly liquefied by oxidation—Circumstances favouring it—Result aplastic and destructive, but with salutary intent—Favourable issues—Termination of abscess in Caseation and Petrifaction—Gradations of lymph, pus, and tubercle.

ACCORDING to several observers (Beale, Von Recklinghausen, and others), pus globules exhibit the living properties of germinal matter, or active bioplasm, in their spontaneous motions, in their rapid proliferation, and in their power of absorbing and assimilating other matters. But we cannot understand fully the process of suppuration without due consideration of the chemistry of the process, which has a chief share in determining the liquid condition and disintegrating properties of pus. ' The chemical change which accompanies and probably causes this disintegration and liquefaction in the formation of pus seems, according to the researches of Mulder, to be an increased oxidation of the protein, whereby it passes from the state of a solid deutoxide into that of a tritoxide, which is readily soluble in water or serum.[1] But this further oxidation and solution implies also ' a frustration of the vitality of the exuded corpuscles, which, although still moving and multiplying, ' lose their organising power, and degenerate into a diffluent aplastic material. Probably, in some instances, the corpuscles' (sarcophytes) 'are originally defective in organising power, and are, therefore,

[1] Simon's Animal Chemistry, by Day, vol. i., p. 12.

prone to degenerate; whilst in others they become so from depraved nutrition or other circumstance spoiling their plastic power.

'The circumstances which determine suppuration as a result of inflammation are chiefly three :—(1) A certain intensity and duration of the inflammation ; (2) the access of air to the part ; (3) a peculiar condition of the blood. 1. Intensity and continuance of inflammation comprise the persistence of the two chief elements in the process, determination of blood and obstruction ; and as we have seen that the physico-chemical effect of these is first to direct the force, and to exaggerate the influence of the red corpuscles (which convey oxygen) on the liquor sanguinis, so that more of its protein passes into the state of solid deutoxide '—the material of sarcophytes—' fitted for organisation and reparation, so we may infer that the excessive degree or continuance of the same action may overdo the change, give chemical properties an ascendency over the vital powers, and, by turning the most recently formed solid into a fluid tritoxide, it may effect a werk of segregation and destruction, involving the blood in the obstructed vessels, and extending to the albuminous matter of the containing texture. Such a result is most likely to ensue in complex and highly vascular structures, in which the effused matter is retained in intimate contact with the blood-vessels ; hence intensity and continuance of inflammation in the true skin, connective tissues, glands, and most parenchymatous organs, pretty surely lead to suppuration. In serous and fibrous membranes, on the other hand, suppuration is a rarer result, because the vessels are few, and the effused corpuscles (sarcophytes) placed less within their influence.'—' Principles of Medicine,' 3rd ed., p. 364.

Referring to the above work for the further explanation and substantiation of this view, I would now add that

mature reflection and modern research have not shaken my
belief in its correctness. Recent observations have given a
clearer insight into the vital properties of the plasma and
its representative sarcophytes, and have supplied more definite facts in the process of histogenesis; but the chemistry
of the inflammatory process has not made similar ad-
vances, and has been too little considered by the most
modern writers. It is a subject that requires further experimental investigation; but in the meantime I propose
this view as consistent with our present knowledge concerning the chief varieties of abnormal nutrition.

The rapid increase of the germinal matter or sarcophytes in inflammation is the result of that combination
of increased flow of blood to the part, with obstruction to
its passage through it, which characterises inflammation.
The sarcophytes, thus supplied with abundance of pabulum, increase and multiply rapidly; and under the exciting influence of the oxygenating arterial currents, and
of the heat evolved by it, this multiplying germinal matter displays all its lively properties of motion and migration, through the coats of the obstructed vessels, into the
surrounding textures, where it exerts its digestive and
assimilative powers, which are communicated also to the
germinal matter already existing in the cells of the connective and other tissues; and if the inflammatory orgasm
(determination of blood, with obstruction) continues, the
multiplying, digesting, and oxidating process goes on until
the whole mass is converted into pus, in which the sarcophytes have become loose cells, with liquid tritoxide of
protein within and without. Such is the result in complete suppuration, or abscess; in which the somatic life and
integrity of the part is sacrificed to the molecular life
and chemical action, ending in destruction of the tissues.

This process of suppuration, although thus destructive
to the part, and often producing other mischievous results,

is nevertheless one salutary for the body; being Nature's
mode of removing a part so much injured by disease as to
be incapable of living, and therefore liable to a much
worse kind of decay, by putrefaction. In their active
proliferation and power of assimilation, pus globules
evince the vital attributes of germinal matter, which resist
the common chemical tendencies to putrefactive decomposition. But if by its own solvent and penetrative action
pus does not make its way to the surface, to be discharged
outwardly, it after a time becomes inert: the cells collapse and form a curdy or cheesy purilage, closely resembling, in aspect and chemical composition, the softened
cheesy matter of lymphatic glands and yellow tubercle.
As in these instances, this change is accompanied by a
considerable increase of fatty matter; and it has long
been noticed that the matter of old abscesses abounds
in fatty globules. So the latter end of chronic abscesses
is a closer approximation to the end of tubercle and such
aplastic matters, involving the parts affected in a destruction more gradual than that caused by suppuration and
gangrene.

But there are many situations in which the formation of
pus does not involve the destruction of tissue. Inflammation of mucous membranes causes an abundant formation and shedding of epithelium and mucus cells, which
after a time present all the characters of pus globules; and
the free discharge of these may terminate the inflammation.
This is the common course of catarrhal inflammations.
And further, where the inflammation is deeper, involving
the submucous tissues, and even the connective tissue and
parenchyma, so long as the sarcophytes, proceeding from
the blood-vessels and proliferating in the tissues, retain
their vital properties of motion and migration, they may
series escape to the surface, and be thrown off; and
that the products of bronchitis and pneumonia may be

cleared away by free mucous and purulent expectoration.
But if the sarcophytes are deficient in these subtle properties of migration, and prematurely form granular cells
('formed matter,' Beale), which cannot escape, but choke
up the tissues, then is produced the red and grey hepatisation, which, if the inflammation continue, may pass
on to the state of purulent infiltration, or may otherwise remain solid, as in caseous pneumonia, and other
cacoplastic consolidations of the lungs, subject to the usual
processes of fatty softening and decay. One or other of
these evil results is to be feared, when, after the active
stage of pulmonary inflammation, the pulse continues frequent, the heat keeps high, and the physical signs of
obstruction and consolidation of the lung persist, with
perhaps increasing liquidity and coarseness of the crepitation in parts.[1] On the other hand, a favourable issue may

[1] Such cases as the following are uncommon, but they teach us not to
condemn all such as hopeless :—

CASE 2.—A married lady, aged 44, of consumptive family, was attacked,
in Dec. 1869, with double pleuro-pneumonia. I had attended her in a
slighter attack on the right side two years previously. Two-thirds of the
left lung, and the lower third of the right were now involved; and in spite
of blistering and other treatment, the disease went on to hepatisation, with
dulness and large tubular sounds on both sides, but on the left extending
through nearly the whole lung. The strong vocal vibration showed that there
was no liquid in the pleura. The orthopnœa was distressing, and aggravated by a very sick stomach, which rendered the exhibition of food and
medicine very difficult. In the third week from the beginning of the attack,
there was no amendment. Pulse 120. Heat, above 100°. Sweats and
purulent expectoration followed, with great loss of flesh; and the increased
liquidity of the crepitus in parts of the left lung seemed to threaten softening and excavation. Just then a boil in the left axilla, which followed the
blistering, began to assume large dimensions, and in a few days a large
abscess formed, and being opened by Mr. Squire, of Orchard Street, discharged a large quantity of healthy pus. From this time the stomach
recovered its tone: food and stimulants, and cod-liver oil and tonics, were
well borne; the pulse and temperature fell, and the chest symptoms subsided. But the most remarkable change was in the rapid restoration of
the lung to a nearly healthy state, the chest sounding much clearer, the
vesicular respiration returning, and the only sign of disease remaining was

... for the present at least, when there is a re-
... of the frequency of the pulse and heat of the

... dulness and a little crepitus at the left base. The abscess continued
to discharge for six weeks, but the general health has since continued good,
without cough, with increased flesh, and with only some remaining shortness of breath. This lady is now (June 1871) stout and well, except
some shortness of breath. The sudden subsidence of the lung disease on
the occurrence of the large abscess externally is strongly suggestive of a
translation of the sarcophytes—by some way or other—perhaps by some
migratory process more direct than through the blood-vessels.

Case 3.—Mr. ———, æt. 45. March 3, 1866 (seen with Dr. Humby).—
Strong and active, and in constant habit of lecturing to large assemblies.
A fortnight ago, after a chill, had a rigor, followed by pain in chest, cough,
and rusty expectoration, with signs of consolidation of left lung (lower two-
thirds). To-day there is *less dulness, but large liquid crepitus, impaired
breath, and bronchial rhonchi in lower half of left lung.* Cough violent; sputa
mucopurulent. Profuse sweats. Is taking Dover's powder, and has been
blistered. Nitric acid, calumbo, and glycerine three times daily. Morphia
lotion at night.

10th.—Was better till two days ago; after talking on business, the cough
has become more violent, with much purulent expectoration; the pulse weaker
and more frequent; and there is great failure of strength and appetite. Has
wasted much. Clammy sweats.

*Dulness, with large tubular sounds and gurgling at and below left scapula;
coarse crepitation, and tubular sounds are heard now above right scapula also.*
To take cod-liver oil, with nitric acid, strychnia, and calumbo; back to be
painted with iodine. Wine and nutriment increased.

March 22.—After a few more doubtful days, began to amend: taking
more food, and cough and expectoration moderating, especially in the last
week. Pulse reduced to 80. Perspirations have ceased.

*Less dulness, and more vesicular sound in left lung; loud bronchophony at
and within left scapula; right lung clear.*

April 5.—Convalescent; rapidly regaining flesh and strength; cough
slight; expectoration mucous.

*Dulness and tubular sounds much diminished, and a rough vesicular
sound in left lung.*

———.—In two months resumed his lectures, and has been strong and
well ever since.

For about a week both general symptoms and physical signs seemed to announce breaking up of the lung; but this happily was averted.

Case 4.—Mrs. ———, æt. 30. April 29, 1868 (under Mr. Theoph.
———. Without any previous ill-health except menstrual irregularity,
... ten days ago, was attacked by vomiting and sharp pain of right
... the pain was supposed to be from gall-stones, as there was

body; when the cough either subsides, or becomes looser
and accompanied by easier and sometimes more copious
expectoration of opaque matter, abounding in corpuscles,
more or less of the pus-cell character, but presenting
considerable variety in size and form. The occurrence of
this expectoration is by no means constant, for in many
cases, especially in the young, pneumonia subsides without
cough or expectoration, the inflammatory products being
dispersed by absorption. When it does occur, it gives us
some insight into the changes of these products which
accompany their dispersion; and in the bland inadhesive

absence of bile in the fæces, but cough followed, with catch in breath, rusty
expectoration, scanty dark urine (slightly albuminous), and hot skin.

Dulness in whole right chest; most in lower half (which is tender on percussion), *with crepitation in several parts; fine in axilla, near sternum, and
above scapula; tubular sounds at and above scapula.* The case (obviously
pneumonia), was treated with effervescing saline with nitre, calomel and
morphia at night, and repeated blisters. It went on to *complete hepatisation
of the lung, which at the end of the second week showed no signs of resolution,
the dulness being still extensive, with large tubular sounds, and no crepitus or
breath in the whole side.* In a few days the expectoration became purulent,
and *coarse gurgling crepitus was heard in the large tubes.* The pulse was
still 120, and the weakness and perspirations increasing, although wine and
liquid nutriment had been freely supplied. The patient had a strong prejudice against cod-liver oil, and it was only after much persuasion that she
was induced to take it, which she did without difficulty in a mixture of
nitric acid and orange infusion. The improvement in the general symptoms
was striking, the pulse coming down in frequency, the sweats ceasing, the
cough and expectoration moderating, and the appetite increased. *The chief
change in the physical signs was in the diminution of the liquidity of the
large crepitation; but the large snuffling bronchophony, simulating pectoriloquy, at and above the scapula, and the persisting intense dulness over a great
part of the right lung,* made it for a long time doubtful whether it would
recover its normal state. The flesh, and in some degree the strength, were
restored several months before the breath and the healthy sounds of the
lung.

In the spring of 1869, a year after the attack, an examination was made,
and there was *only slight dulness and deficiency of motion of the right
chest, and a general vesicular breathing less soft and uniform than on the
left side.* There has been no recurrence of pulmonary symptoms since:
(1871).

······· with a diminution of the viscid and
······· and an increase of the granules and
···· we can trace a resemblance to the process of fatty
········· and disintegration of larger deposits; only
in the latter case the lung tissue is involved in the decay,
whereas in the case under consideration the matter expectorated contains the exudates only, and shows no fragment
of the lung tissue under the microscope.

The resolution and dispersion of the inflammatory consolidation may be complete, leaving no trace behind; or
it may be partial, sufficient to remove present danger of
destructive suppuration, or of caseation, but leaving
patches of consolidation; and these, if not gradually dispersed by the improved circulation and respiration of
restored health, may prove sources of future irritation and
obstruction, and become the nuclei of recurrent disease.
The signs of these remnants of consolidation are commonly
patches of dulness, with weaker or partially obstructed
breath-sound, sometimes with roughness or slight remaining
crepitus in the affected part. But a very common sign of ·
remaining disease is a tubular sound, often loud, above
one or both scapulæ, most frequently the right; and this
comes on sooner or later, even when the lower lobes of
the lungs alone have been previously the seat of disease.
I believe this sign to arise from enlargement of the bronchial glands, which, pressing on the lung, conduct the sound
of the tracheal breath and voice through it. I have had few
opportunities of verifying this by examination after death,
as patients rarely die at this stage; but it is almost proved
by the seat and nature of the bronchial sound, and the
fact that it seldom supersedes the vesicular sound of the
lung; and if it affects the stroke-sound, it is by adding
somewhat of a tubular note, rather than deadening it. I
note these observations here because, if my inference is
right, it throws light on the pathology, in showing the

share which the lymphatic system has in the subsidence,
as well as in the development, of this class of diseases ; the
corresponding lymphatic glands swelling as the reabsorbed
matter passes through them.   It is rare to find the bronchial glands free from disease in chronic tubercle of the
lung ; and I have long been in the habit of pointing to
this in the dead-house, as one of the proofs of absorption
of tubercle.   In these chronic cases, the matter found in
the glands is commonly old, being cheesy or calcareous ;
but the examples I have cited above are recent, and show
how these glands may be first affected.

After the preceding analysis of consumptive diseases of
the lungs, we shall be able to construct a table, with com-
ments, presenting a synthetic view of the inflammatory and
tuberculous lesions of the lungs which are met with in
the consumptive.   This may serve as a key to explain the
varieties, contrasts, and complications in the morbid appearances, and the very great diversity in the symptoms,
signs, course, and duration of the malady in different
cases.   As strictly bearing on this subject, I quote the
following propositions, to which I was led more than thirty
years ago, and which I venture to believe are now receiving their detailed demonstration :—

' Lymph, pus, and tubercle are the same albuminous
matter, and differ from each other in mechanical condition and susceptibility of organisation, rather than in
their chemical nature. . . . . .   We can readily perceive
that these different properties, although possessed by matter chemically the same, and from the same source, must
lead to all that variety of results which we know to follow,
respectively, organisable, purulent, and (yellow) tuberculous deposits.   But the characters of these matters are
not always distinct: lymph is not always equally organisable, nor perfectly free from the greenish colour and
disintegrating globularity of pus, nor even from the

the curdy particles of (yellow) tubercles; and tuberculous matter often contains flakes or fibres of imperfect lymph. The diffused tuberculation or infiltration of the lung from inflammation generally presents a matter in this transition state. It is neither good organisable lymph, nor is it wholly unorganised tubercle; and the albuminous (curdy) effusions on serous and mucous surfaces not unfrequently present such an intermediate state that it is difficult to determine to which class they most belong. *Lymph, pus, and tubercle pass by imperceptible gradations into each other.* The history of the intermediate products has yet to be more fully studied; and it is a subject of immense importance, for they probably constitute those forms of phthisical lesions which it is most within the power of medicine to control.'[1]

In accordance with the view here given, it may be stated that, although the protoplasm, from changes in which all these morbid products proceed, does take the distinct forms defined in the following table, and in different examples, one or other of these forms may so predominate as to distinguish the disease into characteristic groups, yet most cases present less marked distinctions, and comprise a mixed history of various proportions of lymph, pus, and grey and yellow consolidations, in the varying course of the consumptive malady.

[1] *Pathology and Diagnosis of Diseases of the Chest*, 4th ed., 1840, p. 166.

Tabular view of Elements of Consumptive Diseases, and their results.

Elements	Condition	Products	Ulterior results
I. Hyperplasms from blood-vessels inflamed or congested.			
(Liquid Fibrin. Sarcophytes.)	Healthy, or euplastic. Healthy and active.	Fibrils in connective tissues. Tissue cells and nuclei.	Well organised; or reabsorbed. Well organised; or reabsorbed.)
1. Liquid Fibrin.	Unhealthy, or cacoplastic.	Fibroid or scar-tissue.	a. Dense, tough, and contracting. b. Degeneration and caseation.
2. Sarcophytes, or germinal matter.	Unhealthy. A. Active, with over-oxidation by arterial blood.	Pus-cells, with liquid trit-oxide of protein; proliferating and assimilating other tissues into pus.	a. Discharging from free membrane. b. Suppurating into abscess, and discharging. c. Imperfectly suppurating and caseating.
Ditto.	B. Proliferating, but concrete and inactive.	Red, pale or grey indurations of lung and other tissues.	a. Withering and corrugation. b. Decay by caseation and softening.
Ditto.	C. Inactive and splastic.	Caseous hepatisation.	a. Early softening and cavernation. b. Obsolescence and calcification.
3. Albumen; mucus; epithelium and other cells and granules; red blood corpuscles, &c.	Combined with the above, and partaking of their changes and results.		
II. Hyperplasms in lymphatic system.			
1. Sarcophytes and trabecula in glands.	Multiplied and increased.	Enlarged and indurated glands.	Suppuration, caseation, calcification.
2. Sarcophytes in minute adenoid tissue of lungs, &c.	Multiplied and concrete.	Miliary tubercles.	Caseation and softening, calcification, obsolescence.
3. Sarcophytes in lymph tissue.	Multiplied, with deficiency of red corpuscles in the blood.	Soft, swellings of lymph tissues in glands, spleen, &c.	Occasional suppuration or caseation. Atrophy of other tissues.

CHAPTER VIII.

CLINICAL AND PATHOLOGICAL VARIETIES OF CONSUMPTIVE DISEASES, EUPLASTIC AND CACOPLASTIC.

Phthinoplasms, or elements of Consumptive disease—Their origin and results —Divided into those of the blood-vessels and those of the lymphatic system— Clinical and pathological varieties of Consumptive diseases, euplastic and cacoplastic—Of inflammatory Phthinoplasms ; the fibroid is the highest, tending to contract, and endure long without decay—But it dwindles, and is attended with evidences of wasting—Effects of fibroid in the lung ; scars ; dilated bronchi ; emphysema.

The preceding table will supply a key to explain the leading varieties of consumptive disease with which clinical experience makes us familiar, by referring them to the predominance of one or other of the elements here specified.

The first two on the list, representing the most healthy hyperplasms produced by inflammation, do not in themselves tend to induce consumptive disease. They are supposed to occur in otherwise healthy subjects ; and, although they are morbid in their superfluity, yet they have in themselves either sufficient vitality to assimilate them to the natural tissue, or sufficient vitality and divisibility to be removed by reabsorption. But what begins as healthy formation may become deteriorated through mistreatment, neglect, or other unfavourable circumstances, or by repeated application of the exciting cause ; and then one of the more unhealthy results follow ; and so the healthy hyperplasms may be combined with, or turned

into, cacoplastic or aplastic products. The converse takes
place more rarely. A person previously unhealthy recovers health ; and then an accidental inflammation may
produce euplastic results, to be well organised or dispersed without any evil consequences.

Unhealthy inflammations evolve two classes of hyperplasms, with less or more of a degenerative or consumptive
tendency : (1) the fibroid and (2) the corpuscular, each
of which has several remarkable varieties.

1. Fibroid hyperplasms are probably in part formed
from the fibrillæ of the fibrin exuded from inflamed vessels ; possibly also by hypertrophy of pre-existing connective tissue. A great part of the tough consolidations
produced in the lung by prolonged subacute or chronic
inflammation consists of a fibrous material, which assumes
the form of irregular connective tissue. They may owe
their origin to the variety of pulmonary inflammation
which I long ago [1] distinguished as the interstitial kind,
and leading to a non-granular form of hepatisation. To
this variety, without recognising its cause, Laennec gave
the term of carnification. It occurs in pleuro-pneumonia
when the pressure of the pleural fluid on the lung restricts
the plastic effusion to the interstitial texture, without any
granular formations in the air cells. This is the most
common origin of extensive fibroid disease of the lungs ;
and its nature is evident in the accompanying proofs of
previous inflammation,—the general adhesions (often of
the same tough character) of the pulmonary and costal
pleura of the affected lung. But there is also, probably,
a peculiarly fibrinous state of the blood, which Rokitansky
calls a *fibrinous crasis*, in certain cases, rendering the
products of inflammation more fibrinous than usual, and
with smaller proportion of the corpuscular elements ;
and tending, therefore, to produce more fibroid or con-

[1] *Cyclopædia of Medicine*, Article ' Pneumonia,' 1833.

corpuscles, and less of the purulent and opaque curdy deposits which originate in the corpuscles or sarco-phytes.

In whatever way fibroid disease of the lung may have originated, its ultimate tendency is either to contract and condense the textures in which it is formed, or to degenerate and disintegrate into cheesy matter.   The remarkably different effect of this condensation and contraction, according to its seat, has already been pointed out. When affecting the upper parts and root of the lungs, it contracts and constricts the large bronchi, causing an asthmatic difficulty of inspiration and expiration, and an emphysematous distention of the lower and peripheral vesicular texture.   When, on the other hand, the condensation and contraction affects the lower lobes and obliterates the peripheral air cells, the bronchi become generally dilated by the pressure of the inspired air within their walls, as it cannot penetrate to the cells beyond.   This is the explanation which I originally gave of the dilatation of the bronchi which follows contractile pleuro-pneumonia, and which was subsequently ascribed by Corrigan and his followers to a new tissue called *cirrhosis*, to which was imputed the paradoxical power of *dilating the bronchi by contracting around them*!   But it is obvious that the dilating power is the pressure of the air in inspiration, which, failing to penetrate beyond the tubes, is exerted in distending them.

The contractile property of the fibroid tissue is manifested in the shrinking of the lung, and in the drawing towards it of the walls of the chest, the heart, and the opposite lung, to occupy its place.   Thus, when the left lung is affected, in addition to the collapse of the ribs, the heart is drawn upwards, and may be felt with its apex beating at or above the fourth rib, and its body in contact with the ribs to the third costal cartilage ; and the right lung may reach to the left of the sternum above. When the right lung is contracted, besides the flattening of the walls of the chest, the heart is drawn over to the right of the sternum, with its apex beating between the fourth and fifth costal cartilages, with the left lung sounding clear above it. So, likewise, other adjacent organs, the stomach and the liver, may be drawn up into the chest by the contractions of the lungs above them; and the upper and posterior walls of the chest may show depressions or flattenings from the same cause.

This contractile disease of the lung, consequent on inflammation, although an evidence of cacoplasis and degeneration, does not in all cases end in decay or consumption. In some instances, especially in young subjects, it may give way to a gradual re-expansion of the affected lung, and a restoration to the normal state. [Cases will be given afterwards.] Yet fibroid disease may properly be grouped among the varieties of phthisis; both because in most instances it is attended with symptoms of decline, and shows a tendency to degenerate further by its own caseation, and by the production of miliary tubercles in other parts of the lung; and also because in other varieties of phthisis, already tuberculous or caseous, inflammation of the lungs commonly produces more or less of this fibroid tissue in the more healthy parts of the decaying lung. It is, in fact, a modification of this which constitutes the scar-*tissue* around and between tubercles and their vomicæ, and which tends, by its condensation and contraction, to pucker up and cobble together the wounds and breaches of the more destructive decay. In almost all of the more chronic kinds of phthisis there are proofs of the presence and operation of this contractile tissue during life, in flattening or hollowing of corresponding parts of the chest-walls, or in the signs of partial emphysema in the adjoining portions of lung; and after death, in puckered scars on the surface and in the substance of the lung, around cavities or remains of caseous or tuberculous matters. In the more rapid forms of consumption there is neither time nor material for the formation of this fibroid scar-tissue. The exudations and deposits are corpuscular, more destitute of vitality, and therefore aplastic ; passing speedily into disintegration and decay. But in chronic cases there is an attempt to limit and hedge in the work of destruction ; and although this is done by a cacoplastic material, and in a clumsy and irregular manner, it may be looked on as a proof that nature is capable of exerting some resistance to the consuming malady.

In such cases the clinical history of the malady will show the symptoms and signs of partial emphysema and bronchitis in addition to those of phthisis. Occurring, as tuberculous lesions commonly do, mostly near the apex and root of the lungs, the puckering and contraction of the scar-tissue around them may shorten and narrow some of the chief bronchial tubes, with the effect of causing more rhonchi and wheezy prolonged breathing instead of tubular, and more emphysematous stroke-sound in patches, instead of the general dulness of consolidation. We were before led to this same conclusion, that chronic cases of consumption frequently assume more or less of an asthmatic character, which has some tendency to divert the disorder from the substance of the lungs to the bronchial surface.

But to complete the history of these fibroid productions, and to prove their connection with phthisis, we have to point to the other ulterior results mentioned in our table : they are themselves liable to degeneration and reaction. In most cases of confirmed phthisis, even of the chronic kind, sooner or later there comes a break up— a failure of the vital powers and a sudden increase and violence of the work of decay. It may be occasioned by weakening or greatly disordering influence—an

r

exhausting hæmorrhage or diarrhœa; a harassing inflammation; any cause of severe mental depression or bodily
weakness; or the decay may be gradual and progressive.   But the change is manifest in the increasing weakness, pallor, emaciation, and colliquative sweats; in the
occasional hard cough and wheezy breathing giving way
to constant loose expectoration and panting breathlessness,
the sputa being copious, opaque, and heavy; in the substitution of more moist and cavernous sounds in the breathing
for the bronchial or wheezing rhonchi which existed before.
Then come increasing weakness of circulation, œdema and
lividity, and the end is not far off.   In the lungs of these
genuine victims of chronic consumption are found the
evidences of decay, not only in the old cavities spreading,
and tubercles softening and forming new, but also in the
opaque spots of caseation mottling the fibroid masses, and
proving their degeneration; and in the numerous plump
and soft (therefore newly-formed) miliary tubercles scattered through the less diseased parts of the lung.   These
are the signs and seeds of decay spreading and invading
both the healthy tissues, and the frail barriers which nature
had raised against it.

CHAPTER IX.

CLINICAL AND PATHOLOGICAL VARIETIES OF CONSUMPTIVE
DISEASE—*continued.*

Inflammatory Phthinoplasms—Corpuscular, from change in the Sarcophytes—Suppuration, if healthy, not Phthisical, but unhealthy often so; and also often part of the Consumptive process—Purulent Phthisis—Causes.

But although we thus find the fibrous element of hyperplasms amenable to the law of degeneration and decay, it is in the corpuscular element, the sarcophytes or bioplasts, that we can more commonly and constantly trace its workings. These, which in their healthy and vigorous state, are so lively in their moving, self-nutrient, assimilating, organising, and proliferating powers—in their unhealthy and enfeebled condition fail in these manifestations of vitality, and form a material more or less perishable and prone to decay, spreading degeneration and dilapidation in the adjoining tissues.

It will be an interesting subject for further investigation to trace the operation of this bioplasm in the more normal variations from healthy nutrition in mere determination of blood to a part, and in simple membranous inflammation, soon terminating in increased secretion, resolution, and the dispersion of its products; and still further to observe it working in adhesive inflammation, and in the healing of the simplest wounds by ' first intention.' In all these operations the bioplasm exercises its vital properties, and the result is a living struc-

ture abiding and conforming to the nature and habits of
the tissue of the part.   This is all *euplasia* (healthy healing) hardly differing from normal nutrition, and tending
to no decay.

But when inflammation becomes intense, or endures
long, the hyperplasia exceeds the bounds of euplasia, and
the bioplasm suffers in its vital properties, and tends
to form products more or less prone to disorder and decay ;
in other words (as I expressed them forty years ago), the
results of the inflammation are less vital and less susceptible of lasting organisation, and constitute a material
producing further disorder, and sooner or later falling
into decay.   We are now able to define more precisely
the kind and form of these degraded products of the
plastic process, and some at least of the particulars in
which they differ from each other, and from the healthy
sarcophyte or bioplast, which is the representation of
healthy nutrition.   For in declaring the corpuscles of
the fibrinous exudations of inflammation, pus-cells, and
grey and yellow tubercles to be only modifications of the
same sarcophytes, which are known as the pale corpuscle
of the blood and the lymph globule of the lymphatic
system, I only express what all the most recent and most
careful observations have concurred to establish.[1]   In the
remarks preceding the table, and in the table itself (p. 60),
an attempt has been made to explain the nature of these
variations from the healthy sarcophyte ; the truth of this
explanation has to be tested by further investigation.   In
the meantime, a brief further consideration of these elementary variations will supply an intelligible clue to the
diverse forms and phases which we meet with in consump-

---

[1] In Dr. Burdon Sanderson's interesting lectures on Experimental
Pathology, in the *Medical Times and Gazette* of the present year, and in
his able essay on the *Process of Inflammation* in *Holmes's System of Surgery*,
the reader will find an admirable summary of the most recent researches
which have been made on this and kindred subjects.

tive diseases, and may help us better to understand their nature.

The first morbid variety of the sarcophyte presented in the table is the pus-cell, which, although still lively and proliferating, is distinguished by its solvent and disintegrating power. This is undoubtedly a frequent element of consumptive disease; for there is more or less of suppuration or ulceration, mixed up with the advancing work of phthisical destruction in the lungs and other parts of the body. But the formation of healthy pus in suppuration and abscess, although consuming and destroying tissues, does not carry with it the progressive habit of destruction, such as we find in true consumptive disease. On the contrary, suppuration tends to rid the body of the destroyed matter; and under the protective and repairing power of the healthy and active sarcophytes and tissue cells of the empty abscess-walls, the breach is repaired and the part is healed. Healthy suppuration, therefore, has no tendency to produce consumption; and I can cite numerous cases of abscess of the lung ending in complete and comparatively speedy recovery.

It is far different in scrofulous abscess, or in any kind of suppuration in unhealthy subjects. Not only is the pus in these instances imperfectly formed, and mixed with flakes and curdy matter, which render the suppuration incomplete and the abscess cold and chronic, and as likely to caseate as to discharge, but the surrounding consolidation is formed of cacoplastic material, tending either to contract or to caseate, according to its degree of degeneracy, and perhaps, too, according to the predominance of the fibroid or of the corpuscular constituents. These results must be referred to defective vitality of the sarcophytes, which, instead of actively completing the process of clearing, resolution, or suppuration, choke up the tissues with an obstructing and decaying matter, which leaves them in continued disorder and consumption.

Undoubtedly, also, suppuration and ulceration are largely concerned as *secondary* results of the softening and breaking up of tubercles and other cacoplastic consolidations of the lung. Where there is intervening healthy tissue with sufficient circulation, inflammation may be excited, and go on to the more complete formation of pus and partial abscess; and often in phthisical lungs little abscesses containing chiefly pus may be found between the tuberculous cavities. The common, and sometimes abundant, presence of pus in the expectoration of the consumptive might be supposed to be another proof in point, but it must be admitted with some reserve, as much of this often proceeds from the bronchial membrane. Still, this is part of the general process of consumption; and where the larynx is also affected with ulceration, we have exemplified another form of the disease—*laryngeal phthisis*.

There is another relation, which the formation of pus bears to consumptive diseases, which must not be overlooked. . The outbreak of pulmonary consumption, even in its most destructive forms — acute tuberculosis and scrofulous pneumonia—has, in some instances, been preceded by the existence of an abscess or purulent wound in some other part of the body. The most common case is that of *fistula in ano*, but I have known the sequence after abscess in the jaw, in the cervical glands, in the inguinal glands, and lumbar abscess, and not always in cases distinctly scrofulous.[1] The sudden healing of old ulcers, and of the suppurating wounds of setons and issues, is often quoted by authors as a cause of pulmonary consumption; but it is not clear that the cessation of the discharge may not be due to the morbid change in the lungs having already begun. Compared with the artificial production of tubercle in animals, which we shall hereafter notice, it appears as likely that the presence of

[1] Examples will be given in the abstracts of cases.

part, whether by production or inoculation, have a deteriorating influence on the sarcophytes of the blood and lymphatics, as that the cessation of suppuration should have a similar effect. But it is quite rational—and, perhaps, the safest view—to admit both influences in different cases. A comparatively healthy subject may, under some unknown conditions, get his blood contaminated by the occurrence of suppuration in any part of the body. A scrofulous subject, whose blood already abounds in sarcophytes of low vitality, which have been habitually drained off by a suppurating wound, is likely to suffer from their accumulation and mischievous effects in other parts, if this wound be suddenly healed. In the latter case, the decaying material, which was escaping from the body, is retained. In the former case, a deteriorating or decaying influence set up in a part is communicated to the contents of the lymphatics or blood-vessels, and results in a degeneration of sarcophytes into pus-cells or concrete adenoid corpuscles; and thus, under certain unknown conditions, a suppurating wound may produce pyæmia or tuberculosis—I say *unknown* conditions, for the sequence is rare compared with the very common process of local suppuration; but as the occurrence of pyæmia seems to be promoted by close habitations, foul air, and concentration of animal effluvia, so it may probably be found that similar influences, associated with damp soil and malnutrition, favour the production of tuberculosis as a result of the deteriorating influence of a local suppuration on the living sarcophytes. The zymotic character of these developments of pyæmia and tuberculosis may be further argued from the increasing evidence which we have of the preventive and salutary influence of antiseptics, and, above all, of the pure dry air of a healthy locality; or, better still, of a high mountain. This subject will claim our attention again under the head of Treatment.

CHAPTER X.

VARIETIES OF CONSUMPTIVE DISEASE: INFLAMMATORY
PHTHINOPLASMS—*continued*.

Red and grey Indurations of the lung; consist of multiplied concrete Sar-
cophytes, with more fibroid, tending to contract and wither; with less
fibroid, tending more to caseate and excavate—Varieties and Results—Obso-
lescence and Calcification.

LEAVING the suppurative element of consumption, we now
come to that which consists in the sarcophytes becoming
concrete and comparatively *inactive*, although they retain at first their proliferating powers, so that they multiply into numerous cells, which stuff and condense the
containing tissue. This, in the pulmonary texture, forms
a consolidation, at first red and of moderate firmness and
consistency; but as the multiplying cells supersede the
blood-vessels and their contents, the solid becomes harder
and of a light buff colour, which may be rendered more
or less grey by the black pulmonary matter which is not
removed. This consolidation may occur in small spots, or
in lobules, or may extend to one or more lobes. The
latter more diffused variety commonly arises from pneumonia or pleuro-pneumonia of a subacute or chronic
type, and occurs chiefly in the lower and middle lobes;
whilst the lobular or more limited variety may originate
in phlegmonous bronchitis, and affect the upper lobes in
preference. It is this last kind of consolidation which is
induced in persons habitually exposed to cold and damp,
or to the inhalation of an atmosphere containing dust of

an irritating nature, as in the occupation of stone-masons, coal-miners, dry-grinders, feather-cleaners, and millers. The cold in the one case, and the dust in the others, excites bronchial inflammation, which, on continued operation of its cause, gets deeper and deeper, affecting first the bronchial membrane, then the connective tissues underneath, and eventually the pulmonary texture of individual bronchial bunches. As the inflammation penetrates deeper, the hyperplasm which it produces is less readily thrown off. The sarcophytes thrown out by inflamed mucous membrane pass off in form of mucous and pus-cells and epithelium; but those in the deeper tissues are retained in a concrete form, and by accumulation constitute the consolidations of the pulmonary texture. This latter result is favoured by any constitutional cause lowering the vitality of the sarcophytes, such as scrofula, syphilis, irregular living, and other influences which degrade the standard of nutrition.

The different forms and varieties of red and light or grey induration of the lung—texture thus induced, correspond with the carnification and grey tubercular infiltration, chronic hepatisation, red and grey, of Laennec and Andral, and with the albuminous pneumonic solidification of Dr. T. Addison; the iron-grey induration of the last author being a more chronic form of the same lesion. In those varieties resulting from the inhalation of dust, the presence of particles of the dust may add another anatomical character; and in the case of coaldust, the very striking one of completely blackening the consolidations. Without dwelling further on their details we go on to notice the ulterior results to which they tend, mentioned in the table (p. 60)—a withering and cornefaction, and decay by caseation and softening.

It has been before mentioned that red consolidation in lung becomes pale from the multiplication of its con-

stituent cells superseding the blood-vessels and their
coloured contents; and subsequently grey by accumulation of black pulmonary matter; and if the consolidation
endures in its low vitality, without going into caseation
and decay, it undergoes more or less of a withering or
dwindling process, somewhat like the contraction and
hardening of the fibroid or scar-tissue; but being much
more corpuscular than fibrous there is less shrinking and
more drying up of the material, so that it becomes more
leathery or horny in substance, and of darker hue, from
the increase and approximation of the black pigmental
matter of the lungs. The grey consolidation thus withers
and darkens with age, and passes into a state of obsolescence not liable to further change. This result, to a large
extent, is not very common, and occurs chiefly in old
subjects, and renders them less liable to more destructive
and consuming changes; the disease is therefore at this
age more generally chronic. But limited specimens of
this grey withering of old consolidations, without any
scar or remnant of yellow tubercle, are not uncommonly
found at or near the summits of the lungs in persons who
die of other diseases, and may be considered evidence of
phthinoplastic deposits arrested in their earlier stage.

But the more common tendency of the chronic consolidations of the lung tissues is to caseation and softening;
which we now identify with fatty degeneration and disintegration, and which was mysteriously characterised by
Laennec as a new stage or change from the infiltrated
grey tubercle to the yellow crude and softened tubercle.
That the diffused grey induration of the lung is of inflammatory origin was generally concluded, in opposition to
Laennec's views, by many of his contemporaries, and this
view was adopted and extended by Dr. T. Addison, who very
ably traced the inflammatory origin of several varieties of
solidification of the lung, distinct from tubercle, and yet

[...] same consumptive decay.[1] He described these
[...], produced by inflammation, as persisting for
[...], and then either becoming more indurated, or being
[...] into cavities resembling those of tuberculous
phthisis, yet sometimes quite distinct from them; in
[...] cases combined with them and affecting their
course. He specifies the three kinds of inflammatory
consolidation: the uniform albuminous, the granular,
and the iron-grey induration. The albuminous and
the iron-grey correspond with the pale and grey indurations which I have been in the habit of designating
sacoplastic, and form the varieties of chronic induration
which have just been described. The granular induration is that state of lung tissue corresponding with
granular hepatisation, more aplastic, and tending to
break down soon, and to form cavities. It appears to
me that the albuminous and grey indurations are only
different phases of the same change at different periods
and in different subjects; the albuminous pale consolidation affecting younger subjects and at an earlier stage;
[...] the grey being the result of longer duration and at
[...] older age.

But all these consolidations are produced by sarco-
[...] multiplying and becoming concrete in the lung
[...] with more or less tendency to disintegration and
[...] in the way of fatty degeneration and softening.
[...] tendency to this change is in the more uniform
[...] and fibroid indurations, which have been recently
[...] in their converse disposition to chronic contrac-
[...] withering. The greatest disposition to the
[...] change is manifested in opaque consolidations,
[...] more or less granular on section; and under
[...] showing a great crowd of corpuscles or

[...] of the *Writings of Dr. T. Addison*, New Sydenham Soc.,

granular cells, in which fat globules already show themselves in considerable numbers, portending the organic
instability of the material and its proclivity to break up
and decay. If with this we contrast the character of
euplastic matter, as manifest in the sarcophytes or
bioplasts of a healing process or of a healthy inflammation—all transparent, gelatinous, teeming with vital properties of motion and formative and nutrient power,—we
can form some conception of the different tendencies of
the two products—the one bringing new life and living
material to a work of reparation, the other clogging the
tissues with opaque, sluggish, inorganisable corpuscles,
either lifeless or of the weakest vitality, and doomed to
speedy dissolution and decay. Let us bear in mind also
how these cacoplastic products of inflammation injure
the nutrient power of the textures in which they are
crowded. Compressing the blood-vessels, they deprive
the nuclei or bioplasts of the tissue cells of their pabulum
from the blood, these consequently starve and waste, and
soon partake of the decay of the encroaching material,
and all break down together into a caseous mass, which
softens and makes its way into the bronchi for expulsion.

CHAPTER XI.

VARIETIES OF CONSUMPTIVE DISEASE. INFLAMMATORY
PHTHINOPLASMS—continued.

Caseous Exudation—Sarcophytes lifeless—Scrofulous Pneumonia—Soon softening and ulcerated, or drying and calcifying — Infecting, or en- . . .

THE advanced or caseous stage of the pulmonary induration, noticed in the last chapter, is in some cases presented
from the first in what may be called the *aplastic* or *caseous*
consolidation of the lung, the direct result of acute scrofulous pneumonia. The effused matter is at first in a
dully opaque condition, without signs of plastic activity
apparently in its constituent elements, which are numerous
minute, irregular cells, and their fragments, so loosely
cohering together that they form only a soft cheesy mass,
breaking up the proper tissues, and speedily running into
fatty decay and partial suppuration. This caseous consolidation, being not circumscribed by induration, may
extend to a large part of a lobe, a whole lobe, or more;
but sometimes it is confined to lobules, not extending
through the interlobular divisions. A variety of it seems
to have its seat in the bronchial tubes and alveolar texture; and it has been stated that the effused matter consists chiefly of epithelium; but this is of rare occurrence,
and does not warrant the assertion which has been made,
that all cheesy deposits are to be referred to 'catarrhal
phthisis.' In all probability, any acute form of pneumonia or broncho-pneumonia in a scrofulous subject may

end in caseous consolidation, and thus produce an acute phthisis or 'galloping consumption;' and we here have occasion to refer its rapidly destructive tendency to the lifeless and aplastic nature of its products, and their consequent proneness to early decay.

But caseous consolidation may be so limited that although it destroys the part, yet it may not extend to other parts of the lung or infect the system at large. Clinical instances of this may have occurred in those cases in which after an attack of inflammation signs of excavation become evident in conjunction with the expectoration of opaque matter; after which the cavity contracts, the wound heals, and the patient recovers. More common is the necroscopic evidence met with in the bodies of those, who, after having recovered from an attack of inflammation, have died of some other disease; and there is found a cavity, lined with adventitious membrane, either empty or containing cheesy matter. If old, this exhibits more or less of the calcareous transformation, or calcification, a change to which all effete animal matter retained in the body is subject in time.[1] This calcareous matter is chiefly phosphate of lime, and may be either the mineral ash or residue of the deposit after the animal matter has been dissolved or absorbed away; or it may be the result of a chemical concretion from the pervading fluids, like urinary calculi. In all these cases of partial caseation of the lung from inflammation the aplastic matter is hedged in by a plastic process in the surrounding texture, which forms a membrane or cyst, and the softened caseous matter may either be discharged through an opening into the bronchi, or being retained, it becomes obsolete and may petrify. Small

[1] CASE 5.—Miss F. M., æt. 28; brother and sister died of phthisis. In 1839 was attended by Dr. W. for cough, with opaque expectoration, which lasted several months, with considerable loss of flesh. Slight partial

... but not always
... found in the lungs of adult

... breathing were found at the summits of both
... there had been occasional pain. Under the
... and sarsaparilla, with external counter-irritation,
... flesh and strength were pretty well restored.

... abdominal disease came on, attended with pain and in-
... extent of the small intestines and colon, ending
... of the ileum, and death. This was diagnosed
... disease; and so it proved on examination after death,
... had spread between the coats of the intestines to a
... both stricture and ulceration in several parts. It is
... this part of the case, which is cited in reference to
... the lungs.

... partially adherent, especially at the summits of the
... of the left lung was a thick fibro-cartilaginous patch,
... the lung-tissue around its edge; and underneath was a
... partly calcified tubercle, not completely filling
... by a dense membrane forming a cyst around the
... right apex there was also some puckering of the
... patches, and slight condensation of tissue under-
... these were dark grey in colour, with several minute
... seeds. There were no other tubercles in the lungs,
... nodules near the roots.

... the residue of tubercle, perhaps superseded and
... by the revulsive influence of the more malignant disease

... dark, age 25. First seen September 18, 1847. A
... had syphilis, and was treated by mercury for three
... ago an eruption appeared on the skin, followed by
... afterwards becoming violent, with purulent ex-
... accompanied by sweats, and loss of flesh, strength,
... below left clavicle, extending to mammary
... around. Loud tubular sounds within and
... oil; and counter-irritation with iodine

... oil regularly all the winter, and has quite
... Cough slight, with scanty opaque morning
... in upper left chest, with dry cavernous sounds
... or crepitation; bronchial sound faintly heard
... sounds in right lung.
... well, and taking active exercise. Dulness much
... sounds in upper left chest, front and back. No
... heard.

and old persons who die of other diseases, that they may be taken as proof that there is nothing specific or peculiar in their nature, but that they are among the common lesions of nutrition, which are injurious by their extent rather than by their kind. A reference to the table will show that caseation and calcification is a result in which most of the phthinoplasms may end and become obsolete. The frequent occurrence of caseation to a limited extent, without any evil effects, sufficiently sets aside the notion, recently propounded in Germany by Buhl and others, that acute tuberculosis is always produced by infection from caseous matter.

Dec. 26, 1856.—Heard from Dr. Carlill that this patient had just died suddenly of peritonitis from intestinal perforation. He had been apparently well, and actively engaged in business, till ten days before his death; subject only to occasional attacks of headache and costiveness. After walking a mile he was seized with sudden and severe pain in the abdomen, with collapse and other symptoms of perforation, and died in two days. A post-mortem examination was made by Dr. (now Sir W.) Jenner. The abdominal walls were found to be covered with fat an inch thick. The ileum just above the cœcum was perforated by ulcers of tuberculous character, of which there were several.

Both lungs were strongly adherent at their apices, especially the left; and in both cretaceous matter was found; in the right in tubercles, varying in size from a pin's head to a pea; but in the left lung there was a large mass of the same material, which quite filled an ancient cavity at the summit of the lung.

This patient had been free from chest symptoms for eight years.

This case is less remarkable for the duration of life after recovery from the third stage of consumption, than for the completeness of the cure of the chest symptoms, and for the demonstration it afforded after death (from another cause) of the arrest of the tuberculous disease which had made rapid strides eight years before.

The phthinoplasm at the left apex must have been long in a caseous state, before it petrified, without giving rise to fresh tubercles; and those which formed at last in the intestines, and were the cause of death, are rather to be ascribed to constitutional causes than to the influence of the obsolete phthinoplasm.

CHAPTER XII.

VARIETIES OF CONSUMPTION FROM INFLAMMATORY EXUDATION—*continued*.

Varieties distinguished by expectoration — Catarrhal, albuminous, and haemorrhagic — Catarrh may precede or follow Phthisis — Peribronchial and fibroid variety—Albuminous, mucopurulent, and pellicular—Haemorrhagic.

ALTHOUGH in all inflammatory consolidations of the lung leading to consumption, the sarcophytes and fibrin constitute the basis or essential element, there are other contingent matters belonging to the hyperplasms which give a variety to the course of the disease and to the character of the consolidation. These are noticed in the second column of the table (p. 60), as a third class of morbid elements, including albumen, mucus, epithelium, and other cells and granules, red corpuscles, &c. These are thrown out in various proportions during the inflammation of the lungs and bronchial tubes, and may be studied in the expectoration, where they are often blended with the consolidating materials, and partake of their changes and results. It is chiefly, however, in the expectorated matter that these contingent products are seen; and an examination of this, in different cases, suggests three chief varieties which may be connected with phthisis, under the terms catarrhal, *albuminous*, and *hæmorrhagic*.

By the *catarrhal* variety I would designate those forms of inflammatory phthisis preceded or attended by mucous secretion from the bronchial membrane, with an unusual amount of cough and expectoration. There is more or

G

less of bronchitis in all cases of phthisis; but in some, the early history is completely that of bronchial catarrh; and the affection of the lung becomes apparent only through the persistence of the disease, and the additional physical signs and constitutional symptoms.　In some cases the bronchial inflammation precedes the lung affection, and eventually induces it by penetrating deeper, in the manner already described.　In others, the consolidation of the lung is evident from the beginning, but is attended with bronchial inflammation or bronchial flux to an unusual extent.　This occurs especially in connection with the fibroid or cacoplastic consolidation of the lung.

The expectoration is often abundant, with various degrees of frothiness and viscidity, and contains chiefly water, with saline matter and more or less hyaline mucus, and nume- rous epithelial cells, ciliated and pavement, from the bronchial membrane.　To these at times may be added pus-cells in various proportions, giving the expectoration the mucopurulent character, which increases with the occurrence of any suppurating or softening process in the lung.　Sometimes this opaque appearance of the expecto- ration is attended with a diminution of the bronchial irritation.　In other instances, it brings no mitigation, and only adds to the weakness and emaciation.　In fact, these catarrhal varieties of phthisis are often more dis- tressing than those of more rapid and unresisted decay. The harassing cough, exhausting expectoration, and oppressive dyspnœa, are most painful, and are sometimes very little controlled by treatment.

Under the head of *albuminous* expectoration of in- flammatory phthisis, I would include that containing *albumen*, either uncoagulated or coagulated.　The expec- toration in the first stage of pneumonia, and in bronchitis attended with much pulmonary congestion, contains a considerable amount of liquid albumen, which may be coagulated by heat and acids.　This was noticed long

since by Drs. Brett and Bird, and may be considered the
result of the exudation of serum from the over-distended .
blood-vessels. In the advanced stages of inflammation,
the sputa become opaque, either from pus cells multiplying, or from the albumen coagulating into a curdy matter.
In some cases the albumen coagulates as secreted, forming opaque films or flakes; and where these occur to a
large amount, they unite to form the pellicular or croupous
matter, which may take the forms of the bronchial tubes,
ramiform, or arborescent. When thus tough and consistent, they probably contain also fibrin and sarcophytes,
being like the false membranes thrown out on serous
surfaces; but in the looser and more curdy varieties, these
exudations have a nearer resemblance to the albumen or
casein coagulated from eggs or milk. In the expectoration of certain phthisical patients, this curdy or shreddy
matter predominates so much as to constitute a variety;
and it probably proceeds from a croupous or albuminous exudation from the parts of the bronchial membrane contigu-
ous to cavities, rather than from the cavities themselves.

The *hæmorrhagic* variety of phthisis is that in which,
more or less constantly, blood appears in the expectoration.
As this subject will be noticed in a special chapter, we need
not dwell on it here further than to point out its connection with the first stage of pneumonia, in which the sputa
are tinged with hæmoglobin, often altered; and the common persistence of red corpuscles in their entire state
in certain other varieties of phthisical sputa in connection
with scurvy and purpura. In all these different cases, the
hæmoglobin, like the other matters, may be superseded by
the pus formation or caseation. The abundance of this
hæmatin is the cause of the dark brown or green colour
of phthisical sputa sometimes brought up before death.
The colouring matter exuded by the moribund congestion
perishes then undergoing conversion.

CHAPTER XIII.

VARIETIES OF CONSUMPTION—*continued*.

*Phthinoplasms in the lymphatic system—Production of Tubercle by inocula-
tion—Observation of Laennec—Experiments of Villemin, Andrew Clark,
Sanderson, and Fox—Analysis of results—Causes of success and failure
considered—The most infecting matters either phthinoplastic or septic—
Local effects of inoculation—Lymphatic or adenoid system first infected—
then organs—Observations of Drs. Sanderson and W. Fox—Infection
aided by septic influences in the body or in the air.*

WE have now gone through the consumptive elements
which originate from the sanguiferous system — the
phthinoplasms from inflamed or congested blood-vessels.
We have next to notice those which have their origin and
chief seat in the lymphatic system—that remarkable supplementary apparatus which is at once the feeder and the
scavenger of the flesh and blood of the body. We have
already, at some length, endeavoured to trace the origin
of disease in the lymphatic glands and other portions of
the so-called adenoid tissue to a change in their most
vital and characteristic element—the germinal matter, or
sarcophytes. And to enable us to understand how this
change may be brought about independently of inflammation, we now have to bring to our aid the subject of infection, and the modern discoveries on the artificial production
of tubercle.

The idea of the possibility of producing tubercle by
inoculation originated with Laennec. I have several
times heard him relate what happened to himself twenty
years before : how that, in opening some vertebræ affected

with tubercle, the fore-finger of his left hand was slightly
scratched by the saw.   The next day a little redness
appeared, and there formed gradually after, a little swelling under the skin, of the size of a large cherry-stone.
In eight days the skin opened at the scratch, and there
appeared a yellowish compact body, exactly like crude
yellow tubercle.   After cauterising it with butter of
antimony, which gave hardly any pain, he gently squeezed
out the contents, which, being softened by the liquid
caustic, exactly resembled softened tubercle.   After re-
peating the cauterisation to the remaining little cyst, the
wound healed, without further inconvenience.   I may remark that Laennec died of phthisis; and during the year
before his death, when I attended his clinique, although
full of vivacity and intelligence, he had the wasted aspect
of one in advanced disease.

The subject seems to have received no further attention
till about seven years ago, when M. Villemin, led by various considerations to suspect the infectious nature of
tubercle, performed experiments on animals to determine
whether it could be produced by inoculation.   The matter
of tubercle, grey and yellow, was inserted under the skin
of rabbits and guinea-pigs; and in the course of from two
to six months the animals were killed, when tubercles,
both grey and yellow, were found in the lungs, liver,
spleen, lymphatic glands, peritoneum, and other parts,
the yellow being most manifest in the animals that lived
longest.   These experiments have been repeated and
varied by many competent observers in France, England,
and Germany, and with a concordance of results so general,
that no doubt can be entertained of the fact that grey
tubercles, in all respects resembling those spontaneously
occurring in the human subject, affecting the same structures, and liable to the same changes, may be artificially
produced in certain animals by the insertion of tubercu-

lous matter in any form under the skin. This result seemed at first to countenance M. Villemin's idea that tubercle depended on a specific poison, the infection of which was communicated from one animal to another. But as experiments were multiplied and varied, it was found that the subcutaneous introduction of not tubercle only, but of other matters, as pus, putrid muscle, and diseased liver, from non-tuberculous subjects, was equally followed by the production of tubercles in several organs. This was first announced by Dr. Andrew Clark,[1] and confirmed, subsequently, by Drs. Burdon Sanderson[2] and Wilson Fox.[3] Further, it was proved by both the last experimenters that, without any inoculating matter at all, the introduction of a mesh of clean cotton thread, as a seton, into the skin of a guinea-pig, was followed by the production of tubercles in the lungs and other organs. Dr. Fox has given a tabular view of the results of his experiments, and from this we will give extracts, from which some estimate may be formed of what agents prove most efficient in producing artificial tubercle.

Of 8 inoculations with tubercle, 6 succeeded, 2 failed.

Of 11 inoculations with various pneumonic products (red pneumonia in tuberculous patient, grey infiltration, 'scrofulous,' yellow, cheesy, and chronic), all succeeded.

Two inoculations with sthenic pneumonia failed.

Four inoculations with sputa of chronic bronchitis and acute pneumonia failed.

Of 2 inoculations with phthisical sputa, 1 succeeded, 1 failed.

Of 17 inoculations with pus from various sources, 7 succeeded: comprising, 1 each from injury to knee, sup-

[1] *Med. Times and Gazette*, 1867.
[2] *Tenth Report of the Medical Officers of the Privy Council*, p. 150 (1868).
[3] *The Artificial Production of Tubercle in the Lower Animals* (1868).

purating bone, and lumbar abscess; 3 out of 5, of foul pus; 1 out of 2, from scrofulous bone.

Of 11 inoculations from acute inflammations, 4 were successful, 2 being from pyæmic abscess of spleen; 1 out of 2 from unaffected part of same spleen; and 1 out of 2 from sloughy wound.

Of 9 inoculations from matters from 'chronic inflammations, &c.,' 6 succeeded: 2 of gelatinous inflammation of knee; 3 of lardaceous liver; and 1 of cirrhosis of kidney.

Of 12 cases of reinoculation from tuberculated animals, all were successful.

Four cases inoculated with vaccine matter succeeded.

Of 5, with putrid muscle, 4 succeeded.

Of 4, tried with seton, 1 succeeded.

Of 3, with cotton thread, 1 was successful.

Of 10 trials with matter from syphilis, typhoid intestine, and cancer, all failed.

In these trials, we find that the materials most efficient in producing artificial tubercle were those from low pneumonia, pyæmic abscess, gelatinous inflammation of knee, lardaceous liver, reinoculation from artificially tuberculated animals, and vaccine matter. Less constantly successful were human tubercle, phthisical sputa, foul pus, putrid muscle, and cotton thread and seton; whilst no results were obtained from material from acute sthenic pneumonia, pneumonic and bronchitic sputa, healthy abscess, diphtheria, various inflammations in rabbit, syphilis, typhoid intestine, and cancer.

Whatever be the influence which determines the production of tubercle, that it is nothing specific in the materials which succeed in producing it is obvious from their varied nature—tuberculous and non-tuberculous, animal products and mechanical injuries. But it is impossible to avoid seeing the close analogy which this pro-

cess bears to suppuration. When Mr. Simon's experiments
on the production of tubercle in the rabbit were discussed
at the Pathological Society in the spring of 1867, my
opinion was asked whether the experiments did not prove
the specific nature of tubercle. My reply was in the negative ; and that I believed it would be found that tuberculisation bore more analogy to suppuration; and that acute
tuberculosis had its parallel in pyæmia. But it is not
healthy pus, or other sthenic inflammatory products,
which surely produce tuberculosis, but the pus of pyæmia, foul pus, putrid muscle, and such septic matters as
must be injurious to the vitality of the bioplasm; these
have the same effect as tubercle itself, and the kindred
forms of deteriorated bioplasm found in chronic condensa-
tions and caseations of the lung, lardaceous liver, &c.

The occasional production of tubercles from more
healthy materials, and from the wound of a seton, must
be referred to some additional septic influence acciden-
tally acquired, and giving a foulness to the material or to
the wound; and here we can perceive how atmospheric
hygienic agencies may operate, as in acute suppuration
infecting the blood by pyæmia, so in chronic injuries infecting the lymph and blood with tubercle. On this
point the following observations of Dr. Burdon Sanderson
are very important, and call for further investigation.

' With reference to the traumatic origin of tuberculosis
in the guinea-pig, another possibility claims consideration, namely, that of the influence of the air and of the
organisms which it contains. It has not yet been proved
that injuries which are of such a nature that air is completely excluded from contact with the injured part are
capable of originating a tuberculous process. The following experimental results seem, indeed, to suggest that
they may not be so. Setons, steeped in carbolic acid,
were inserted in ten guinea-pigs, on September 24, 1868,

animal receiving two. At the same time, extensive fractures of both scapulæ were produced in five others, care being taken not to injure the integument. No tuberculosis or other disease of internal organs has resulted in either case.'[1]

Before noticing some of the details of the process of artificial tuberculisation, I must again advert to the subject of the very different degree of susceptibility shown by different animals. Rabbits and guinea-pigs have been generally selected as affording the most frequent results, and therefore must be considered to be somehow predisposed to artificial tuberculisation, although Dr. Sanderson declares that they are not liable to the natural disease. Attempts made to produce tubercle in other animals—dogs, cats, goats, sheep, and birds—have rarely succeeded. Again, Dr. Fox has remarked that tuberculisation succeeds better with guinea-pigs than with rabbits; and ascribes M. Villemin's repeated failures with other materials than tubercle to his using the latter animals. In several of these experiments the rabbits died of pyæmia, before there was time to produce the more chronic result, tuberculisation; and in others, a local suppuration occurred, without being followed by any appearance of tubercle in the organs. In others, there was a slight appearance of pus, often offensive and becoming cheesy, and this was more generally followed by tuberculisation.

Drs. Sanderson and Fox have given the most complete and minute descriptions of the process of artificial tuberculisation in the guinea-pig, and these should be carefully studied. We can here give only a brief abstract of the principal points, chiefly relating to the primary local effects, and to those in the lymphatic glands and the lungs.

The most common result of the introduction of the

'Further Report on the Inoculability and Development of Tubercle,' . . . Report of the Medical Officer of the Privy Council, 1869, p. 92.

matter under the skin is the formation of masses of cheesy matter, which are dry and friable ('débris of fattily degenerated material') and often encapsuled. But in addition to these are small granulations, varying in size from that of a poppy seed to that of a hemp seed, irregularly scattered in the subcutaneous tissue. These masses, sometimes transparent throughout, sometimes opaque in the centre, present to the naked eye and under the microscope a striking resemblance to the changed lymphatic glands. In their denser and more central parts they consist of nuclei imbedded in a homogenous tissue; in their less dense parts a fibrillated tissue which forms bands or trabeculæ, between,which the cells lie, the whole forming a structure which has the strongest resemblance to the elementary composition of a lymphatic gland. Throughout the granulations many of the cells and also of the nuclei are seen in various stages of fatty degeneration.[1]

Dr. Sanderson also describes the local effect of the inoculation in the guinea-pig to consist in the production of small subcutaneous knots, which at first appear to be composed of round cells, like lymph corpuscles (sarcophytes). At a later period these cells are enclosed in a meshwork of fibres, thicker and coarser than the reticulum of a healthy lymphatic gland, but so exactly 'resembling that of a gland enlarged and hardened by disease, that the two are indistinguishable under the microscope.'

According to Dr. Sanderson, 'the first step in the dissemination of tubercle consists in its being absorbed primarily by the lymphatics (which convey it to the lymphatic glands of which they are tributaries), and secondarily by the veins. Having thus entered the systemic circulation, it is distributed universally by the arteries. The serous membranes seem, however, by preference to

---

[1] Dr. Wilson Fox, *op. cit.*, p. 8.

~~appropriate it,~~ and from them it extends by contiguity to the superficial parts of the organs which they cover.'[1]

Of lymphatic glands, those supplied from the inoculated part may soon become enlarged and congested, with such an enormous multiplication of corpuscles as to impair the consistence of the gland, and sometimes to run into suppuration. When more slowly affected, they enlarge, harden, and caseate. The enlargement is chiefly from multiplication of cells, the induration partly from the same cause (why not from their hardening also ?), and partly from the rapid growth of their fibrous reticulum, or trabecular stroma. The caseation is from fatty decay and disintegration of the indurated mass.

The internal lymphatic glands are affected in consequence of secondary production of disease in the organs from which they receive their afferent lymphatics. Their change is also chronic, and tends never to suppuration, but to enlargement, induration and caseation, referable to the same increased cell formation with fibrous degeneration, and eventual fatty or calcareous necrobiosis. Very similar changes affect the spleen, the structure of which bears a close analogy to that of lymphatic glands.

In Dr. Fox's observations, the lungs were affected with tubercle in fifty-nine cases out of sixty-four—the same proportion as in those invading the spleen. The following is an abridgment of his description :—' The chief state I have to describe consists in the lungs being permeated more or less thickly by scattered granulations, varying in size from a millet seed to a hemp seed.' Some are hardly visible specks, and all gradations can be found between the smaller and the larger. Generally they are scattered, sometimes confluent in groups ; even in the larger groups there is evidence that they have been originally composed of distinct granulations. The granulations do

[1] *Loc. cit.* p. 117.

not project much from the cut surface, and they blend
more or less intimately with the surrounding pulmonary
tissue, from which they tear with difficulty. They are
firm, and all marked by a peculiar semi-transparent, hyaline, cartilaginous looking margin, and a cheesy centre,
which is sometimes soft in the larger ones, and when
evacuated leaves a cavity.   Some of the smallest are
semi-transparent throughout.   They are more common
on the pleural surface than deep in the lung, but are
distributed pretty equally through the lobes.   Sometimes
when there is a group of these granulations clustered together, an appearance is presented, which is also occasionally seen in the human lung, of a fibrous network running
between the granules, as if the intervening tissue was
becoming fibrous.   In addition to this there is a general
induration of the lung tissue, affecting in a variable degree the whole organ.   Signs of pneumonia and of general
infiltration, independent of the granulations, is exceed-
ingly rare.

The microscopic examination of these growths in the
lungs presents the following features:—There are three
main points in which they appear to originate—around
the bronchi, around the blood-vessels, and in the lung
tissue unconnected with either.   Around the bronchi they
seem to extend from little masses of a lymphatic character (adenoid tissue), which normally exist in the bronchial sheath, and are also stated by Kölliker to ' exist in
the human lung.   These granulations around the bronchi
consist of masses of cells 1–2500 to 1–3000th of an inch
in diameter, mostly round ; but sometimes, when densely
packed, showing nothing but nuclei.' ' In the perivascular
sheath of the pulmonary arteries, the growth is nothing
more than an accumulation of the cells lining the perivascular canal.   The growth may extend for a considerable distance in length along both peribronchial and

perivascular sheaths, and from both these sources of origin a rapid extension ensues into the surrounding walls of the alveoli and smaller bronchi. A thickening of these is thus produced apparently by a double mode of growth—by a rapid development of fusiform cells at the margins, clusters of which are seen passing among the capillaries, and by an increase of rounder cells which are seen nearer the centre of the new formation ; coincidently with this growth a change of great importance occurs in the neighbouring capillaries of the lungs : their nuclei enlarge, and the vessels otherwise apparently unchanged, contain no blood—that is to say, no injection will pass into them ; and yet their outline is still marked by lines of nuclei. This obstruction of the capillaries takes place through very much wider areas than the space apparently occupied by the tubercle. So also with the thickening of the walls of the alveoli. Around the grey granulations, and for a space of three or four times their area, there is a circumference of thickening affecting the walls of both the alveoli and the smaller bronchi. This appearance is more distinct in the guinea-pig than in many specimens of tubercle in the human lung ; but it can sometimes be distinctly seen in the latter, and is a fact of great pathological importance, explaining the increase of density and loss of elasticity in the lung, which occurs in the early stage of tuberculosis, and which cannot be satisfactorily accounted for by the mere presence of the grey granulations."[1]

In his second paper, Dr. Sanderson confirms his conclusion that the tubercles and consolidations artificially produced in the various organs of animals consist essentially in overgrowth and induration of the adenoid tissue naturally existing in various parts of the textures ; but as regards the semi-transparent and iron grey nodules in the

---

[1] Dr. Wilson Fox, *op. cit.*, p. 10–12.

, that they comprise also an accumulation of the
commonly found in the alveoli, and which have
generally but erroneously considered epithelial.
alveolar cells are nucleated bodies consisting of a
envelope of transparent substance collected round a
refractive central part, and contain pigment and
granules. The true alveolar epithelium cells are
smaller, and are very difficult to demonstrate; but
in the terminal bronchii can be made evident by
of silver, and appear as oval plates, with spherical
about half their width. 'In animals killed at an
stage of tuberculosis, that is to say about four weeks
inoculation, no change is observed except that the
bronchial adenoid pulp is increased, or in other words
true miliary granulations are formed in the neigh-
of the terminal bronchioles.' Subsequently the
lar cells become multiplied, and, filling the aveoli,
lete the mass of iron grey nodules. 'Whether the
ing up of the air-cells is merely a mechanical result

branes or textures, appear first as a rapid multiplication of lymph cells or corpuscles, with a fibrous network, all of which increase and harden, and eventually caseate and break up by fatty degeneration and disintegration, with variations in course and concomitants, according to the structure and functions of the parts.

The perfect resemblance of tubercle thus artificially produced to human miliary tubercle, in seat, general distribution, intrinsic structure, and in course and effects, removes all doubt as to their identity. But as regards their modes of origin, and comparative power of affecting different animals or species, there may be yet a great difference; and we must be cautious, therefore, before we apply all the facts of an artificial tuberculosis to the spontaneous occurrence of tubercle in man. The closest analogy lies with those cases of tubercle which are of constitutional nature, not arising from a visceral inflammation or any local cause, nor affecting one organ in particular, but scattered through several in the form of miliary granulations, and having their origin in the circulating lymph or blood. We comprehend them, therefore, under the second division of the Table of Elements of Consumptive Disease (p. 60).

CHAPTER XIV.

GENERAL CONCLUSIONS ON ARTIFICIAL TUBERCULISATION OF ANIMALS, AND ON THE CAUSATION OF PHTHISIS IN MAN.

Nature and Conditions of Infection—Causation of Phthisis—Specific or Common Septic?—Parallel between Experimental and Clinical Origin of Tubercles—Predisposition necessary—Defective Vitality of Sarcophytes, and corrupting Influences in the Air—Analogy between Pyæmia and Acute Tuberculosis—The latter developed by Heat and Damp—Inflammatory and Chronic Phthisis produced more by Cold—The former more diffusive, the latter more circumscribed—Influence of Climate and Altitude on different forms of Consumptive Diseases.

WE may sum up the chief facts of the process of the production of tubercle by inoculation in the following conclusions :—

1. With regard to the material necessary for inoculation, it is no specific form of tubercle, nor even tubercle at all ; for some non-tuberculous matters are equally successful, and, in a minor degree, matters formed in an open wound in the same animal. But those materials are most sure to produce tubercle which either resemble it in its tendency to decay, or show a septic character, as foul pus, putrid muscle, carious bone, and the like. On the other hand, healthy pus or other product of acute inflammation, has no effect ; and although a seton or other open wound sometimes produces tubercles, yet setons dressed with an antiseptic, and wounds secluded from the septic influence of the air, have no such result.

2. The local effect of successful inoculation is not active inflammation, suppuration, or sloughing, for these always

prevent the tuberculisation; but either low inflammation, slowly producing a slight abscess, often offensive or cheesy; or the direct formation of little nodules at the point of inoculation, consisting of adenoid indurations, and which may be considered a primary tuberculisation. And what are these but sarcophytes or bioplasts, proliferating and hardening in their fibrous network, and tending to early death and decay by caseation?

3. The next effect is found in · the lymphatic glands supplied by the absorbents proceeding from the seat of inoculation.   These are enlarged, indurated, and soon become cheesy in points, but never suppurate (in the guinea-pig), even where there may have been partial suppuration in the primary wound.   Most natural is it that the lymphatics should convey injured sarcophytes (lymph corpuscles) to their usual receptacles, and with them that deteriorating influence on the myriads of sarcophytes contained therein, which take on the same degenerative course of rapid proliferation and induration, ending in early decay.

4. After the lymphatic glands, various organs and membranes of the body become invaded by the indurations, chiefly in the granular form of grey tubercles, but some, as the liver, in larger masses.   But in all forms and sites the careful examinations of Drs. Sanderson and Fox have detected the same structure, that of the adenoid or lymphatic glandular tissue, hypertrophied and indurated by multiplication of corpuscles and fibrous reticulum; tending to obstruct and irritate the natural structures, and to infect them with their own degeneration and decay.   The channel of dispersion may be both the lymphatics and blood-vessels, communicating, as they do, not only through the thoracic duct, but more directly in the spleen, and possibly also in the lymphatic glands, in which the blood and lymph corpuscles are either intermingled or

H

brought into close proximity. And thus the infection of the system becomes complete.

It remains yet a question open for further inquiry, what is the influence in the inoculating matter or open wound which appears thus to affect the vitality of the sarcophytes in the part, and make them proliferate in a concrete perishable form, and communicate a like tendency to other sarcophytes in the adenoid tissue of the body through which they circulate? From its infective power it would appear to be of a zymotic nature (whatever that may be, whether a chemical catalytic force or an organic spore or germ). And the notion has been propounded even recently by Dr. Madden, of Torquay, and Dr. W. Budd, of Bristol, that tubercles are the result of a specific poison, like scarlatina, typhoid fever, and other zymotic diseases. We are, perhaps, as yet hardly in a position to accept or to reject this notion, for there are many facts for and against it, which we cannot afford space to consider at length ; but at present it seems to me more probable that the influence which causes tubercle is something more *common* than a specific poison—something more analogous to putrefactive matter, which may proceed from various materials, and even from the decomposition of a part of the body itself. It may, indeed, be said that putrefaction and other kinds of decomposition are promoted, if not produced, by the presence of vibriones, bacteria, and other septic organisms ; but if so, it is in the way of common corruption, and not through any specific agency engendering or engendered by disease. If I am correct in my inference that tubercles arise from a degraded vitality and concrete state of the sarcophytes, whereby they lose their mobility and plasticity, although they retain their proliferating power, it can be easily conceived that, without assuming the existence of any specific poison, various noxious agencies may be capable of so injuring them. The observation of Max Schultze has been already noticed, that heat above 104° Fahr. is sufficient to stop the movements of the sarcophytes and make them harden. It may be a question how far this power of heat is concerned in developing tubercles in exanthematous fevers, especially measles and scarlatina, which are not unfrequently followed by tuberculosis. This power of heat to injure the sarcophytes may also have some share in the difficult healing of wounds from burns and scalds, and in the very cacoplastic character of the scars which they leave behind them. But both eruptive fevers and burns have other effects besides this direct operation of temperature; and it is easy to perceive that foulness or tendency to corruption of any kind may similarly injure the vital properties of the bioplasm, and degrade its constituent corpuscles to the condition of tubercle.

And if we revert to the miscellaneous matters found capable of producing tubercle by inoculation (for example, in Dr. Fox's experiments, tubercle; red, grey, and cheesy pneumonic matter; foul pus; pyœmic pus; lardaceous liver; putrid muscle; vaccine matter; and, less successfully, seton wounds, &c.), we find further proof that the cause seems to be some common corrupting influence, rather than any specific poison.

Again, we must not lose sight of the different susceptibility to the morbific operation of this cause in different individuals, and still more in different species of animals. In most carnivorous and herbivorous animals, inoculation commonly produces mere inflammation and suppuration, and very rarely tubercles. In rabbits, inflammation and suppuration are as commonly excited as tubercle, and often prevent the production of tubercle. In guinea-pigs, on the other hand, suppuration is rare, and tuberculisation is the common result. In their indisposition to suppuration they resemble birds and reptiles, in which Mr.

Gulliver doubted that true pus is ever produced. This must depend on a natural difference in the sarcophytes of these respective classes of animals, and suggests the probability of similar variations between different individuals of those animals capable of both suppuration and tuberculisation.

We are now in a position to consider the spontaneous occurrence of miliary tubercles in the human subject, and the light which it may derive from the above experiments. The grey miliary tubercle of Laennec, of size varying from a millet seed to a hemp seed, remarkable for almost cartilaginous hardness and some degree of translucency, occurring scattered through the pulmonary tissue or gathered into groups, which in relation to the bronchioles resemble little bunches of berries, is the production which most distinctly characterises the tuberculous form of pulmonary consumption. Laennec noticed that these little bodies tend to become opaque and to soften, just as diffused consolidation do, and, therefore, he concluded all, granular and diffused, under the common term tubercle, which presents the different conditions of grey, crude yellow, mature and softened, as successive stages of the same accidental production. Whilst, with Laennec, we acknowledge the identity of the granular and diffused consolidations in their composition and changes to the opaque and softened states, we reject his notion that they are accidental or heterologous growths like those of Cancer, following special laws of their own; and we adopt the much simpler and more obvious view that they are only results of the degradation of the ordinary material and process of histogenesis or textural nutrition, and that their changes are no other than the successive steps of decay, the natural consequence of gradual declension of life and organisation.

With regard to the diffused consolidations of the lung

In particular, we found reasons for regarding them as the results of inflammation, and have endeavoured to trace them from the observed operation of that process in its different varieties. Miliary tubercles may probably also sometimes originate in inflammatory irritation; for example, when they break out during the febrile stage of an exanthem, measles or scarlatina, from the febrile poison acting as an irritant, in points of the pulmonary tissue, as it does outwardly in the eruption in the skin. Probably we may also refer a certain number of cases of miliary tubercle to prolonged or repeated bronchial inflammation, under circumstances, which deteriorate the blood plasma, such as poor living, damp air, and close habitations.

But in the greater number of instances miliary tubercles seem to arise independently of inflammation, by a spontaneous dissemination through the lungs and other textures, as if scattered by means of the blood-vessels or lymphatics. These are the cases that are so precisely imitated by the experiments of artificial tuberculisation that we can hardly avoid the conclusion that the process is similar in the two cases. Let us trace the analogous cases of tubercle spontaneously arising from infecting causes in the body.

1. We are abundantly taught by clinical experience that miliary tubercles form in the lung after various kinds of *unhealthy local suppurations:* for example, after scrofulous suppuration of the cervical and other lymphatic glands; after abscesses and unhealthy wounds connected with diseased bones; after fistula in ano; after ulceration of the intestines from typhoid fever; and after empyema and pyoperitonitis. 2. Miliary tubercles form in the lungs and other organs also after *caseation* taking place in the lungs; in the bronchial, cervical or other lymphatic glands; in the liver, kidneys,

spleen, or serous cavities. (Buhl and other German writers have taken too partial a view in limiting the paternity of miliary tubercles to this cause.) 3. Miliary tubercles form also in consequence of the presence of various consolidations in the lung or other organs *when these consolidations have a decaying tendency.* Thus various chronic indurations of the lung (among which may be included pre-existing miliary tubercles), larda-ceous liver, granular kidneys, and disintegrating fibrinous emboli in blood-vessels, may become causes of new miliary tubercles. 4. And lastly, we learn from Drs. Sanderson's and Fox's experiments that *common wounds in the integuments,* such as that of a seton or issue, may, in rare cases, determine the production of miliary tuber-cles in the internal organs.

But as in the experiments, so in the natural develop-ment of disease, it is not in every case that tubercles are produced from their supposed causes. If all kinds of animals are included, inoculation with the most potent materials, such as tubercle itself, or the matter of pyœmia, had no effect in many instances, and in others caused suppuration and not tubercle. Even in guinea-pigs, which these experiments prove to be naturally disposed to tubercle, the effect was not certain when matters less allied to tubercle, or less foul, were used; and no result was obtained from healthy pus or other products of healthy inflammation. So in clinical experience we find many instances of the presence of even scrofulous sup-puration, of caseation, of chronic indurations of organs, including tubercle, without any further speading or in-fecting the body; and quite exceptional are the cases of a common wound or healthy suppuration being followed by internal tuberculisation.

There must, therefore, be some co-operating cause which renders inoculation in the one case, and the products of in the other, effective in producing tubercles. In the absence of any direct evidence on this point, we may be guided by certain facts and analogies to the inference that this co-operative cause may exist in the body of the subject, or in the atmosphere, or in both. Where the sarcophytes in the blood and lymph are deficient in vitality, although abundant in quantity, they are more easily injured in their plastic powers by any noxious influence which may affect them; and, proliferating in concrete masses in their adenoid receptacles, form the little tumors, prone to decay, which are called tubercles. On the contrary, where the bioplasm is vigorous and not redundant, it may resist the operation of these noxious influences, and maintain the blood and the lymph in their proper condition for nourishing and invigorating the tissues of the body. The air, too, may convey subtle influences or organisms with septic properties, injurious to life and tending to promote decay; and these may co-operate with the disordering action of any morbid matter previously existing in the body, or introduced into it by inoculation. Take the parallel case of pyœmia, or hospital fever. Wounds and suppurating sores of all kinds have little tendency to infect the system, so long as cleanliness and free ventilation carry off decomposing matters, and supply abundance of pure air for the active performance of the processes of respiration and sanguification; but in close habitations, with an atmosphere tainted with foul effluvia, every sore becomes both an inlet and a source of poison, which is spread by proliferating and septic pus-cells throughout the body. This is a rapid and more acute form of cachœmia. That inducing tuberculosis is more chronic; probably arising from a less potent septic power in connection with humidity of air, and operating on a less active bioplasm, it palsies and coagulates the lymphatic sarcophytes, which, aggregating in little nodules, form spots of degenerating and decaying matter in scattered points of the adenoid tissue of the lungs and other organs.

And here we are led to a position from which we may perceive that the local cause of tubercle by inoculation, or by previous existence of either tubercle or some other degenerating matter in the body, is not indispensable. The septic or deteriorating influence of impure air and bad blood may itself be enough to degrade the bioplasm, and engender tubercle, without any additional exciting cause; and thus may arise the constitutional form of pulmonary consumption. Nor are impure and damp air and septichœmia the only causes of constitutional phthisis. Insufficient or improper food, bad digestion, malassimilation, venereal excesses, exhausting discharges, and perhaps the secondary effects of febrile poisons, diabetes, and urœmia, have been noticed as antecedents of phthisis—often enough to entitle them to be considered as causes; and it is quite intelligible that they may so injuriously affect the bioplasm as to give parts of it a spontaneous tendency to degeneration and decay. To these must be added family proclivity or hereditary disposition to tubercle. This is regarded more commonly as a predisposing cause, requiring some additional influence, as an exciting cause, to bring it into operation. But some families seem doomed to be cut off by tuberculous disease, which sometimes arises without any obvious exciting cause; and thus tuberculous meningitis in infancy, mesenteric disease in childhood, and pulmonary tubercles in adolescence, attack the members of these families at certain ages, who so fall victims to an inbred decay. Happily, such cases are much more rare than they are reported to have been formerly; and it may be hoped that timely preventive measures, hygienic and medicinal, may still further succeed in averting these untimely tragedies.

spontaneous or sporadic cases of acute tuber-
which sometimes present characters almost malig-
as if from the presence of poison in the system.
prostration of bodily and mental powers; very
pulse; constant pungent heat of the body,
rising five or six degrees above the natural stan-
; depraved secretions; furred tongue, and sometimes
on teeth and lips; occasional low delirium; and
wasting of the body,—mark the acute tuberculous
in addition to the cough, dyspnœa, and other pul-
symptoms, and the signs of suffocative bronchitis
parts of the lung, often masking those of the nume-
tubercles scattered through them. Such cases may
fatal in from two to six weeks, by suffocation or ex-
before there is time for the tubercles to go
softening and excavation.

miliary tubercles found in these acute cases are
for their general dispersion over all parts of
a lung, not as in the chronic disease, chiefly confined to
per lobes or parts; and also for their plumpness and
parative softness; so that, although they feel as solid
nodules in the lung texture, they can be crushed by firm
pressure, and have not the cartilaginous hardness of older
tubercles. They consist almost entirely of aggregations
sarcophytes multiplied in points of the adenoid tissue,
with little of the fibrous stroma which time would form
round them, and which gives the greater hardness to
older tubercles. It may be the soft looseness of these
sarcophytes which favours their dispersion and
multiplication in these acute cases, even to infecting the
blood with matter prone to decay. In chronic
on the contrary, the decaying material is hedged
by tough connective tissue, which limits its disper-
and in a measure protects the system. We can
fail to see here an analogy with the erysipelatous

and phlegmonous modes of pus formation, another phase
of sarcophytic history.

If we turn to the external circumstances in which this
constitutional form of tubercle occurs, we shall find that,
besides damp and foul air, a high temperature seems to
favour its production, and in this respect it contrasts with
the inflammatory forms of consumptive disease. The latter prevail especially in cold seasons and climates; but
consumption is frequent also in hot climates, and often
assumes the acute or febrile form, with less marked cough
and other pulmonary symptoms. M. Guilbert goes so far
as to assert that phthisis increases in frequency from the
poles to the equator, and from the highest mountains to
the sea-shore. This assertion seems to have been founded
chiefly on observations on the South American continent,
where the prevalence of the disease in the low, hot plains
of Peru and Brazil contrasts strongly with its almost absence in the high table land of Peru and Bolivia, which
rises ten thousand feet and upwards above the level of the
sea. The climate at this height within the tropics, is
much as that of the temperate countries of Europe; and,
considering the general prevalence of phthisis in the
latter, we must refer the exemption of the mountainous
regions rather to their elevation than to their low temperature.

Since the late Dr. Archibald Smith first called attention to the preventive and curative influence of high altitudes
on phthisis, his statements have been corroborated
by several observers. In Lima, and other of the lower
towns of Peru, pulmonary consumption is very prevalent,
and it has long been the practice to send invalids up the
Andes, to altitudes of from 8,000 to 10,000 feet, and with
most beneficial results. Dr. Guilbert gives similar accounts of the efficacy of the high places of Bolivia, and Dr.
Jourdanet of the high plateau of Mexico, in preventing

curing phthisis. In Europe also the greater immunity of high Alpine inhabitants from phthisis has been
observed by Lombard, Brehmer, Küchenmeister, and
others; and in this country, Dr. Hermann Weber has
directed the attention of the profession to the subject in
reference to the causation and treatment of phthisis.

The general result of recent statistical observations is
that pulmonary consumption is most common in damp,
low situations, and those liable to great transitions of
temperature, in all climates; that it is of less frequent
occurrence in dry places, even although very cold; and
that it is still more rare at great altitudes, varying from
10,000 feet in the torrid zone down to 2,000 feet in the
cooler temperate regions.

These facts render it most probable that the causation
of consumption is two-fold: one class comprising the influences which excite and keep up inflammatory affections
of the chest, which end in cacoplastic products, such as
transitions of temperature, and prolonged operation of
cold and damp; the other class includes septic agencies,
which tend to blight or corrupt portions of the bioplasm
of the blood or of the lymphatics, and thereby to sow the
seeds of decay: these comprise combined warmth and
humidity, foul air, bad nourishment, depraving habits or
diseases, and the like. And when these two classes of
causes co-operate, the effect is more certain; for example,
when a person, with bioplasm deteriorated by a foul atmosphere, or by enervating heat, is exposed to a chill, or
when the subject of an inflammatory attack is confined
in a room tainted with impurities, or deprived of the invigorating influences of pure air, light, and proper

It thus becomes manifest that whether we are considering the intimate nature and causation of consumptive diseases, or are seeking for means to prevent or cure

gard to its prevention a

CHAPTER XV.

FAMILY PREDISPOSITION AND CERTAIN OTHER CAUSES OF CONSUMPTION.

By Dr. C. Theodore Williams.

Causes, general and local—Family Predisposition—Consumption proved to be hereditary—Opinions of Niemeyer, Virchow, and Waldenburg—Family Predisposition explained—Hereditary Tuberculosis in Sheep, Cattle, and Guinea-pigs—Offspring of Gouty, Syphilitic, Aged, and Asthmatic Parents often Consumptive—Prevalence of Family Predisposition—Evidence of Louis, Copland, Cotton, Fuller, Pollock, Briquet, and the Author—Its more frequent occurrence among Females than Males—Paternal and Maternal Transmission—Influence on age of Attack—Private and Hospital Practice —Influence on Symptoms—Cases—Influence on Duration—Relations of the—Age at Death—Conclusions—Other Causes of Consumption— Impure Air and Improper Food—Continued Fevers—Scarlatina and Measles—Cessation of Discharges—Unfavorable Confinements and over-lactation—Mental Depression—Damp—Buchanan and Bowditch's Researches—Dusty Occupations—Consumption not infectious.

Some of the causes of consumption have been glanced at in the preceding chapters in their pathological relations: in this we propose to discuss some of the more important ones which have not yet been considered. Looking at the subject broadly, the causes may be classed as follows, as :—

1. *General causes*, which, by their weakening influence on the constitution *generally*, predispose to consumption: such are family predisposition, want of pure air and good food, continued fevers, scarlatina, measles, cessation of discharges, miscarriages, bad confinements, and over-lactation, mental depression, dampness of habitation.

2. *Local causes*, the effects of which are limited at first to the lungs, but may at a later date extend to the

character of phthisis is the presence of tubercles, often demonstrated in the lungs of a fœtus or of a young infant[1] of consumptive parents; another, though less striking one, is to be found in instances where a consumptive and healthy person marry, and the children become consumptive; but, on the death of the affected parent, the sound one marries again and the offspring of the second marriage is healthy.

Niemeyer admits that the tendency to consumption is inherited only if the parents were consumptive at the time of begetting the offspring. ‘But it is not,’ he says, ‘the malady which causes inheritance, but the weakness and vulnerability of constitution, which had already laid the foundation of the consumption in the parents, or which had arisen in them in consequence of that disease.’[2] Waldenburg[3] denies the direct hereditariness of consumption by means of a specific contagion, and only allows, in any case, the transmission of the phthisical *habitus* and innate disposition of the parents to phthisis. Both these authors, regarding tuberculosis as a secondary product, and never a primary one, hold that tubercular consumption can never be directly inherited, but that the caseous deposits from which it arises may be produced hy the scrofulous or phthisical *habitus*.

[1] Waldenburg and Virchow deny this as regards miliary tubercle. We would draw their attention and that of our readers to the following passage in Sir Charles Scudamore's work on *Pulmonary Consumption*, p. 55:— ‘I examined the body of an infant which died of extreme emaciation at the age of four months, the mother having been in the last stage of tubercular phthisis when she gave birth to it. I never witnessed so remarkable and extensive a display of tubercles, both miliary and of a larger size, the former semitransparent, the latter *grey* in colour. The lungs on each side, both upper and lower lobes, the liver and spleen, the mesentery and peritoneum, were universally studded with tubercles.’ The italics are our own, but the description needs no comment.

[2] *Text-Book of Practical Medicine*, vol. i. p. 213.

[3] *Die Tuberculose die Lungenschwindsucht und Scrofulose*,' p. 524.

Waldenburg cites an instance of six brothers and sisters, who, when they

...... to family predisposition, as the origin is probably endemic; but we must bear in mind, that this objection applies, to some extent, in nearly all cases of family pre-disposition, as when the son of a consumptive father is attacked with the disease, it is often difficult to say for a certainty that the son's disease is hereditary and has not been acquired, especially if, as may be the case, his brothers are quite exempt.

We must therefore take into consideration all degrees of family predisposition, and try to estimate each at its proper worth.

It may be remarked in passing, that man is not the only animal cursed with hereditary consumptive disease. Delafond states that a phthisical ram in a flock of merinoes transmitted his disease to sixteen or twenty of his pro-geny. Dr. Sanderson told me that at the great cattle breeding establishment at Lyons, the offspring of a Scotch bull whose lungs were found to be stuffed with tubercle, after his death, were also infected with the disease, and several of the guinea-pigs who were tuberculized in the late experiments have produced tuberculous offspring.

We must not overlook the fact, that it is not necessary for parents to have consumptive disease in order to produce phthisical offspring. The children of very aged parents, of syphilitic, gouty, or asthmatic[1] parents, or of those whose constitutions have been greatly weakened by drink, sexual indulgence, or other debilitating causes, are prone to phthisis. We cannot agree with Niemeyer, that

[1] The tendency of asthmatic parents to produce phthisical children is ...... sufficiently recognised. Among my out-patients at Brompton I found ...... instances, and our tables include several cases.

...... reason of this probably is, that many cases of asthma were at their ...... cases of limited phthisis, which have been arrested. In the ...... induration at the root of the lung has taken place, ... contraction of the bronchi, and giving rise to asthmatic symptoms. ...... The children of these patients, if phthisical at all, are gene-...... decidedly so than the parents.

I

the preceding generation: e.g., 'mother and brother' affected is entered under 'mother,' 'father and sister' under 'father,' and so on. The greater number of duplicates occurred in those of the same generation as, brothers, sisters, and cousins.

Our percentage of *family* predisposition was 48·4, but, as will be seen by the above table, the number of purely hereditary cases, that is, with parents alone affected, was only 12 per cent., thus differing greatly from the percentages of [1] Drs. Cotton and [2] Fuller, and of the first Brompton Hospital Report, which was about 25. The only explanation we can offer of the discrepancy, is a difference in the *class* of the patients, from which our statistics are taken, and of those on which the above authorities found their estimate. Their calculations were based on hospital practice, (except Dr. Fuller's, which included some private patients): ours are based entirely on private practice.

Great pains were taken by Dr. Williams to arrive at an accurate result. The patients were all closely questioned as to their dead and living relations. In many instances, the existence of consumption in the family was at first denied; but after cross-questioning, not only was its existence admitted, but undoubted cases of death from that disease were traced among their relatives.

On the whole, we think that an average of 12 per cent. for direct hereditary predisposition, and of 48 per cent. for family predisposition, are not unfair estimates for the upper classes, and that the average of the above authorities is probably correct for the lower classes; and we think it also likely that our smaller percentage in a class, which from its wealth is able to banish many of the most fertile causes of phthisis, gives a more just estimate of the influence that hereditary predisposition, unaided by poverty and exposure to divers pernicious influences, exercises on

[1] 24·1.　　　　　　　　[2] 25·7.

the first Brompton Hospi[
in this particular, the re[
were as two to one. Our [
tion show similar, though, [
wider list of relations inc[
Fifty-seven per cent. of the[
per cent. of the males, we[
common occurrence of this[
among males is to be accou[
the sedentary and less invi[
offers less opposition to the [
the malady ; whereas the m[
of a man tends to fortify [
and render the predispositic[
sons of phthisical fathers lea[
very common it is for them t[
tion at an early age, and oft[
This observation thus confir[
with regard to the hereditary

(2). The transmission of
through the mother than
Ancell[1] states that, as far [
evidence on this point is stro[
to confirm this state[

the blood, this result might have been predicated, since there is only one period at which the father's influence could be exercised, viz., that of conception ; whereas the influence of the mother is exercised at that period, and also through uterine gestation.'

(3). Fathers transmit more frequently to sons, and mothers to daughters, than the converse. This important fact was first established by the first Brompton Hospital Reports, and having been amply confirmed by numerous competent observers, may now be said to be matter of every-day experience.

How does family predisposition influence *age* in consumption? This is a very important question, bearing intimately on the prognosis of the disease, and deserves a fuller discussion than we have time or space for. Our researches [1] have, we trust, cleared up some of the mystery in which the connection of age and family predisposition was enveloped. We have demonstrated clearly that the chief influence which family predisposition exercises is on the age at which the patient is likely to be attacked.

It hurries the onset of the disease. This conclusion was arrived at by careful investigation of the age at which the 1,000 private cases were attacked. This having been ascertained, we pursued a similar enquiry with regard to those affected with family predisposition; and lastly, with reference to those who were free from it, as far as could be ascertained at the time of their being under observation, that is to say, who up to the last date had had no relatives affected with phthisis. The result is shown on the next page :—

[1] 'On the Duration of Phthisis, and certain Conditions which Influence it,' *Medico-Chir. Trans.*, vol. liv.

Average age of attack in mal	
Family Predisposition .	
Average age of attack in femal	
Family Predisposition . .	

This table shows that th
number affected with famil
was earlier than the avera
number by $2\frac{1}{2}$ years in the
females.   There is also show
of those free from family pre
the males, and by $6\frac{1}{2}$ among
This is very striking; bu
statistics were of the upper
apply to certain circumstanc
determined to pursue the sar
classes, and for this purpose I
ton note-books.   Among 400
as follows :—

Average age of attack in males free f	
Predisposition	
Average age of attack in females free	
Predisposition	
Average age of attack	

position, but the relative influence on the two sexes differs greatly from what we found among the richer classes. In the out-patients' class the age of attack was about the same for males and females, the males being attacked earlier than among the rich, the females later. The age of attack in those free from family predisposition was for both sexes considerably later, and the influence in the male sex greater than in the female—a result exactly opposite to that obtained among the upper classes. This remarkable influence of family predisposition in hurrying the onset of the disease, does not seem to have attracted much attention; and the only authority I can find who seems to have noticed it is M. Briquet,[1] who, in the smaller number of 95 cases of consumption, arrived at the conclusion, that 'hereditary tuberculosis developes itself in the form of phthisis at an earlier period of life than the disease does when acquired. In 89 of the cases with the history of hereditary transmission, 26 became phthisical before 30 years of age; while of 56 cases born of perfectly healthy parents, 31 did not become phthisical until after 30.'

M. Briquet's cases were rather too few to afford strong evidence, and he makes no attempt to separate the sexes, and trace the influence in each sex; but we have little doubt that his observations, as far as they went, were correct, and that the fact 'that family predisposition hurries the onset of phthisis,' as ascertained by his and our own researches, is one not to be disputed.

Let us now consider whether the presence of family predisposition exercises any decided influence over the type of phthisis. Have cases with family predisposition any distinguishing features?

We must confess that it is hard to trace any feature

[1] 'Recherches Statistiques sur l'Histoire de la Phthisie.' (*Revue Médicale*, 1862.)

which cannot also be found in other cases of consumption.
In many instances, great transparency of skin, with veins
clearly visible, and a delicacy of outline, is noticeable;
in others, marked want of development, or else distortion
of the thorax; in many, glandular enlargements come on
at an early age.   These and other features are to be
found, often strongly marked, in hereditary cases; but
they are not invariably present, and, on the other hand,
they are to be seen occasionally in non-hereditary cases.
We are afraid we cannot point to one distinguishing point
of hereditary phthisis.   Dr. Pollock remarks that in
acute cases of phthisis the influence of hereditary predisposition is undoubted, and he says that of 179 cases, only
34 could positively state that there was no family taint
either parental or remote.

We subjoin a few well-marked instances of hereditary
origin, some of which were attacked early and some later
in life.   We think they will be found instructive, as
showing that the strongest hereditary taint does not hin-
der the beneficial effect of remedies, if persevered with.

Case 7.—A lady, aged 34, first consulted Dr. Williams, June 20, 1859.
Had lost her father and mother, and ten brothers and sisters, from consumption, and had herself been always liable to cough, and had one constantly
since December.   Three years previously she had hæmoptysis, amounting to
a tablespoonful.   At the time of her visit the expectoration was streaked
with blood.   She had lost much flesh and strength, and complained of pain in
her chest: catamenia irregular and deficient. *Dulness and tubular sounds in
the upper part of both sides of chest, most marked on the right, where there
was crepitation.*—Ordered cod-liver oil in a mixture of hydrocyanic and
phosphoric acids, with infusion of calumbo and orange; counter-irritation
with acetum cantharidis; and a linctus containing morphia.

May 21, 1860.—Greatly improved under the above treatment, and has
grown stout. Has hardly any cough or expectoration, but lately suffers from
oppression of breathing and frequent boils.—Ordered oil in a mixture of
chlorate of potash, nitric acid, and glycerine.

July 30, 1861.—Continued to improve till the winter, when had inflammation of the lung; and since the attack the expectoration has been sometimes gritty and sometimes fœtid.   Is still stout and strong, but breath

died. Has taken oil regularly, combined with strychnia. Dulness, tubular sounds in upper left back and right front.

April 19, 1866.—Has always wintered in Cornwall, and out a great deal in the open air; but lately stomach weak, and has not been taking much oil. Has lost much flesh; but cough and expectoration are less than during last winter, when they increased, and there was some hæmoptysis. Suffers from piles. *Dulness, large tubular sounds in upper right chest.*—To take oil, with phosphoric acid and hypophosphite of soda. An electuary of sulphate and bitartrate of potash.

October 1, 1870.—Returned to Cornwall, and improved again so much that for the last two years has taken no oil. Last February took cold, and cough again returned, and has been troublesome since, with frequent sickness. In July went to North Wales, there caught fresh cold, and has been very ill ever since, with sickness, pyrosis, disgust at food, and great loss of flesh and strength. Urine pale and copious; sp. gr. 1010; no albumen. A number of red scaly spots on skin. Cough, and opaque expectoration. *Dulness and tubular sounds in both upper regions. Collapse under left clavicle, with defective breath. Crepitus in lower half of right lung.*

Heard of her death in December, about 12½ years after her first marked symptoms.

CASE 8.—A young gentleman, aged 16, whose mother and sister had died of phthisis, saw Dr. Williams, August 28, 1855. He had had repeated hæmoptysis since Christmas, sometimes amounting to an ounce, and also cough, with some loss of flesh, and lately pain in right shoulder. *Dulness and tubular sounds above right scapula.*—Oil ordered, with sulphuric acid, and infusion of roses, &c., and acetum cantharidis liniment.

September 29, 1856.—Wintered at Hastings, and improved in flesh, strength, and health. Oil has been taken steadily, except for about three weeks, when it was omitted, and he lost flesh. Hæmoptysis has occurred several times, generally after some exertion, and once amounted to ℨvi. *Dulness, tubular and obstructive sounds in upper right chest, with subcrepitus.*

October 9, 1857.—Was ailing in May, but now better and free from cough. In last month has suffered from lowness of spirits, sleeplessness, and confused head. *Chest clearer, but still some tubular sounds, with obscure breathing in upper right chest.*

January 11, 1859.—Sleeplessness gradually improved, and spent spring at home; but, after three months in the Regent's Park, cough increased, and hæmoptysis came on to the amount of ℨii. *Some dulness and tubular sounds in upper right chest, crepitation sounds above scapula.*

July 11.—Went soon after to Madeira, and rode out a great deal. Lost cough, and ascended the Peak of Teneriffe. Now strong, ruddy, and able to walk six miles.

October 16, 1861.—Last two years have been spent in London. Has recovered from cough and hæmoptysis, and his condition has been good, but slightly short. Oil has been taken regularly for nearly two years. Still *loud crepitation, left front and right back, with dulness and tubular sounds above right scapula.*

September 7, 1863.—Had been studying at Cambridge for a year, when had hæmoptysis, ʒiii., after bathing; and pain in right chest. After Easter 1863, nursed his father (who died of Bright's disease), and had hæmoptysis to ʒii. daily, for a week in July; has left off oil and is taking cream, and is much reduced in strength, though not in bulk. *Much dulness, and obstructive sounds in upper right back. Tubular sounds both upper sides of chest.*

April 8, 1864.—At St. Leonards; wonderfully improved in flesh, colour, strength, and breath. Walks fourteen miles at a time. Oil in sulphuric acid has been taken all the winter.

October 4, 1864.—Improved at Tunbridge Wells, and was able to walk ten miles briskly: physical signs became drier. Then returned to keep terms at Cambridge. Remained well till on a visit to Liverpool, had hæmoptysis to amount of ʒiv. In February, 1865, was sent to Madeira, and gained strength, 7 lb. in weight, being much out riding; then spent summer in Hants; and returned to Madeira in following winter, there remained till April, when had fever and congestion of the lungs. Since then weaker, with more cough and expectoration, and often chills and heats, and her some expectoration, sometimes opaque, sometimes calcareous. *Tubular and crepitation sounds in both backs, most in the right.*

October 15, 1867.—Remained at St. Leonards till February, then went to Mentone till May, and gained 8 lb.; improving also in strength and apppetite. Had been taking oil, ʒvi. once a day. In warm weather improved in weight, strength, and breath, but worse lately. *More crepitating and obstructive sounds in left front and right back.*

CASE 9.—Miss F., aged 24, consulted Dr. Williams, September 17, 1857. She had lost her mother, two brothers, and one sister from consumption, and had herself suffered from cough for 1½ year, accompanied by expectoration sometimes streaked with blood. Catamenia had been absent for 3 months, and she had lost flesh, strength, and breath. *Extensive dulness, obstruction, and croaky sounds in upper left chest. Pectoriloquy below clavicle. Tubular sounds upper right chest.* Oil ordered in tonic, and use of acetum cantharidis.

October 31st.—Under these means has much improved in flesh, strength, and appetite. *Cavernous croak below left clavicle; more breath below.*

September 20, 1858.—Continued better, taking oil till May, when omitted it for two months, and lost flesh and strength. Then resumed it for two months, and has improved, but has not yet regained the loss. *Cavernous sounds in upper left chest, tubular and crepitating sounds upper right.*

March 29, 1859.—Heard that she had been better till last two months, when she has had more weakness and sickness. No catamenia since May.

CASE 10.—Miss T., aged 21, whose mother had died from consumption, was seen by Dr. Williams, August 26, 1857. From the age of 14 to 16 had been delicate, and taking cod-liver oil. Often subject to cough in the last three winters; now one since March, with yellow expectoration, and lately a little blood. Has been losing flesh and strength. *Collapse, dulness, tubular sounds in left front and back.* Bronchocele 6 months.—Oil ordered, with tonic.

March 29, 1864.—Took oil, and improved very much, having cough only in winter; but now has one lasting since Christmas, with yellow expectoration, breath shorter. Oil has been discontinued on account of sickness, and no tonic taken. *Dulness, tubular sounds and crepitation, in upper left chest, less crepitation upper right.*

Case 11.—Miss V., aged 16, who had lost her mother and sister from consumption, was seen by Dr. Williams, March 22, 1859. Had cough and cold in December, which has continued, though to a slight extent, ever since, with opaque expectoration, and yesterday some blood. Breath short. *Dulness, large tubular sounds, and gurgle in upper right chest, front and back.* Oil ordered in tonic of phosphoric and hydrocyanic acids, with calumba and orange tinctures, the use of acetum cantharidis liniment, and a morphia linctus.

June 10, 1860.—Taken oil, &c., and much better. Last summer had measles; cough was violent for three weeks, but subsided under the use of oil, and has remained moderate since. Wintered at Cannes, and out much. *Still decided dulness, and marked tracheal sounds in upper right chest.* After measles, coarse crepitation there and below.

October 16, 1862.—Well, and free from cough till a month ago, when it was violent for two weeks, and subsided under oil and iodine paint. Now has no cough or expectoration. Hard dulness at and above right scapula, with loud tubular sounds. Back rounded.

1871.—Not seen since; but heard of as tolerably well, having passed a winter at Mentone.

Case 12.—Mr. N., aged 42, consulted Dr. Williams, July 31, 1860. He had lost his father, mother, and a brother from consumption, and had been subject to cough for the last seven years. Two years ago he had hæmoptysis to ʒii. and breath has been shorter ever since. Cough has been constant for the last nine months, and hæmoptysis to amount of ʒss, has occurred once. Has taken oil regularly (ʒss ter die) for nine months. *Dulness and tubular sounds in upper right chest. Tubular sounds above left scapula.*—Oil was ordered with phosphoric acid and tinctures of calumbo and orange; counter-irritation with acetum cantharidis, and a morphia linctus.

April 5, 1867.—Has kept pretty well and stout, but breath has always been short, and he has cough with opaque expectoration, which has been less in last winter, but patient is hoarse. No oil taken last year. *Still dulness upper right, tubular sounds above scapula. Subcrepitus and tubular sounds below.*—Ordered oil, with nux vomica, phosphoric acid and

June 8, 1868.—Tolerably well, but always has slight cough, and some hæmoptysis occurred last spring; oil taken last winter. Spata opaque and tinged with blood. *Some dulness at and above left clavicle with tubular sounds, but breath weaker above right scapula; crepitation down left front.*

Here the strong family predisposition did not tell till comparatively late in life, and did not prevent the remedies used from having a beneficial effect. The patient has been about eight years under observation, and the disease seems to have diminished in right lung, though some increase has taken place in the left.

CASE 13.—Mr. R., aged 17, whose father had died of consumption, saw Dr. Williams, May 7, 1857. For three years he had had swelling and discharge from the cervical glands, and cough off and on for two years; lately has had cough for six weeks, accompanied in last fortnight by pain in the side, and short breath. The scrofulous sores in the neck are still discharging. Oil taken till two months ago. *Dulness, obstructed breath, and much crepitation in front of left chest, mostly in upper portion and above the clavicle. Some dulness above right scapula.*

Oil ordered in nitric acid and tincture of orange: a liniment of strong tincture of iodine.

April 13, 1864.—Took oil, and states that he got quite well in six months, and then omitted oil, except an occasional dose. Throughout last winter has had cough and expectoration, and three times brought up blood to the amount of ℥ii. Has lost much flesh and strength. *Dulness, cavernous sounds in upper half left chest, with obstruction sounds below.*

What effect has family predisposition on the duration of phthisis? Is the duration curtailed by it? Do patients thus affected die earlier than other consumptive patients? These questions are of considerable importance in the prognosis of the disease; and we have attempted to answer them in the following statistical results, extracted from our tables:—

Average Duration from the Commencement of the Disease in 198 Deaths.

	Yrs. Mths.	No. of Cases
Average duration of cases affected with Family Predisposition .	7—5·8	87
Average duration of cases free from Family Predisposition	7—10·9	111
Average duration of total number of deaths .	7—8·7	198

Here it is shown that the average duration among the
87 deaths of those affected with family predisposition
was 7 years 5·8 months, an average not greatly differing
from that of the cases free from this influence, or again
from that of the total deaths. A difference of only a few
months is noticeable, and does not indicate that family
predisposition exercised any decided influence in shortening the duration of the disease.

The evidence of 397 living cases of family predisposition supports the same conclusion; for among these the
average duration already reached was 7 years 11 months;
that of all the cases free from predisposing taint being 8
years 7¼ months, and of the total living 8 years 2 months.

It would seem, therefore, that family predisposition,
without reference to sex, exercises but a slight influence
over the duration of phthisis.

Does it influence the duration of the disease in one
sex more than another?

We have seen that the age of attack is influenced
differently in the sexes, and also that phthisical females
live a shorter time than phthisical males; and the following question should now be solved: Is the duration of
the disease shorter among phthisical females affected
with family predisposition than in others not so affected?
This may be seen by a glance at the table below:—

*Relative Duration of Diseases in the two Sexes in
Family Predisposition.*

	No. of Cases	Dead	No. of Cases	Living
		yrs. mo.		yrs. mo.
Males . .	54	8 — 2	216	8 — 2·7
Females .	33	6 — 7.3	181	7 — 6·7
Total .	87	Total .	397	

The inspection of this table will show that the sexes

are equally influenced as to the duration of the disease, and that family predisposition exercises no particular influence—a conclusion which contrasts with that arrived at with reference to the age of attack; and is entirely at variance with the old views of hereditary phthisis being more rapidly fatal than acquired phthisis.

To this conclusion it might be replied, by those who still believe in the curtailing influence of hereditary taint, Perhaps family predisposition, as a whole, does not influence the duration of phthisis, but do not some of its various degrees do so? We had hoped to answer this point satisfactorily, but, unfortunately, lack of materials prevents our doing it completely. Such information as our cases afford is to be found in the following table:—

	Dead	No.	Living	No.	Total
	Average yrs. mo.		Average yrs. mo.		
Grand-parents affected	*16—7·00	2	*10—6·62	8	10
Father „ .	*7—5·28	7	7—9·25	36	43
Mother „ .	8—3·54	11	7—10·75	56	67
Both parents „ .		1	*6—9·11	9	10
Brothers and sisters .	7—6·02	44	8—2·24	180	224
Uncles and aunts .	*12—6·00	4	7—6·18	44	48

The evidence here furnished is chiefly of a negative kind, and must be viewed as proving that some forms of predisposition do not curtail the duration of the disease, and not as demonstrating what influence other forms may have on it. We see in 11 deaths where the mothers were consumptive the duration was 8¼ years, that 56 living patients similarly situated had lived 7 years 10¾ months. Among these few cases maternal influence had no effect in curtailing the duration, which in the 11 deaths was rather higher than ordinarily.

* Numbers too small to yield fair average.

In the case of brothers and sisters where the numbers, warrant our speaking more decidedly, what do we find?

In 44 deaths, the duration was 7 years 6¼ months, slightly below the whole average of deaths; while of 180 living cases in this category the mean duration was 8 years 2¼ months, about the same as the common average. Here again family predisposition seems to have exercised little or no influence. The other numbers are too small to furnish even negative evidence.

Our last point to consider is the *age* which these patients affected with family predisposition live to. Do they die earlier than other consumptive cases? The grounds for determining this question have been already to some extent settled; the age of attack and the duration in these cases having been ascertained, and therefore the following result was easily arrived at :—

		No. of Deaths
Average age reached by Males free from Family Predisposition	41·51	65
Average age reached by Males affected with Family Predisposition	35·29	54
Average age reached by Females free from Family Predisposition	34·92	46
Average age reached by Females affected with Family Predisposition	30·74	33

Family predisposition, therefore, though it does not materially curtail the duration of the disease, has considerable influence in shortening the duration of life, such limitation amounting in males to more than six years and in females to not quite five years. But we must remember to assign this cutting short of the span of life to its proper cause—not to hereditary phthisis being more virulent and rapid in its progress, for that idea has been disproved—but to the fact that those who come of a consumptive stock are liable to be attacked earlier than others whose families are free from taint.

Our conclusions on the subject may be briefly summed up:—

1. Family predisposition occurs more commonly among, and exercises a more decided influence on, females than males; and the former have a greater power of transmission than the latter.

2. Fathers transmit more frequently to sons, and mothers to daughters, than the converse.

3. Family predisposition does not directly shorten the duration of the disease.

4. It precipitates the onset of the disease, and thus shortens the duration of life.

We have entered thus fully into the relation which family predisposition bears to phthisis, because we believe the subject has hitherto been considered as rather obscure, and not because we think the other causes of the phthisis less important. But the action of these is better recognised, and therefore needs but a passing mention.

Impure air and *improper food* are well-known general causes of consumption. Among the lower classes in crowded cities, evidence of their effects is only too common. Of 3,214 men who became inmates of the Brompton Hospital in ten years, 1,812 (more than half) had in-door employments. Among my own out-patients, the numbers of those who ply their trade in close, ill-ventilated rooms, and during long hours, are very great: clerks, compositors, tailors, shoemakers, among men; and milliners, dressmakers, among women, are attacked at an early age.

Want of proper food acts by impoverishing the blood and lymph, whether the fault lies in the quality or quantity of food. If healthy pabulum be not supplied for nutrition of tissue, it is impossible for it to retain its normal standard; it starves, and the pabulum not good enough for the tissue will go to form morbid material.

predisposing cause can be seen in the children who attend at the Brompton Hospital, in whom a very slight exciting cause brings on the consumptive disease.

Typhus and typhoid fevers.—Of these, typhus is the least powerful cause, though it exercises some influence; but many cases of consumption are to be traced to an attack of typhoid or pythogenic fever. Dr. Murchison says, 'an attack of pythogenic fever is often followed by tubercular deposit in the lungs.' And again, 'in my experience, acute tuberculosis of the lungs is a far more common complication or sequela of pythogenic fever than of typhus; and it is intelligible why this is the case, when we recollect the more protracted duration of the former malady, and the greater emaciation it entails. Louis records four fatal cases of pythogenic fever, in which the lungs were found studded with recent tubercles. Bartlett also observes, that consumption is a common sequela of this fever in America.' [1]

It is worthy of notice, that the organs so commonly affected in typhoid fever—viz. the solitary glands, Peyer's patches, and the mesenteric glands—are also frequently the seat of tubercular disease. The wasting, too, which accompanies both these diseases seems to be connected with a disordered state of the lymphatic system, particularly of the lacteals. We know that the organs attacked by typhoid fever and the intestinal forms of consumption are portions of the lymphatic system, and the recent researches of Sanderson [2] and Wilson Fox [3] have shown in some of the pulmonary lesions in artificial tuberculosis, too, that the lymphatics are the seat of the disease, and that the principal morbid changes take place in and around them.

Scarlatina and Measles are very common causes of

[1] Treatise on Continued Fevers, p. 503.   [2] Op. cit.   [3] Op. cit.

K

consumption, chiefly in children. Acting generally, they exhaust the patient, and leave him an easy prey to the first exciting cause that comes. Acting locally on the lungs, by their sequelæ, bronchitis, and inflammation, they embarrass them with consolidations more or less prone to caseation. (See pp. 101, 104.)

The *cessation of habitual discharges*, as those from fistulæ in ano and old ulcers, will sometimes give rise to symptoms of consumption, which often diminish on the discharge being re-established. In fistula this is so marked, that many physicians refuse to sanction, and many surgeons to perform, operations for fistula on patients who have shown evidence of consumptive disease of the lungs.

Miscarriages, bad confinements, and over lactation, are fertile causes of phthisis among the poor, chiefly through the great exhaustion consequent on them ; but we must not overlook, in the case of the two former, the highly fibrinous state of the blood, which predisposes to the production of material of a phthino-plastic kind.

Mental depression.—Some doubts have been expressed by authors as to this exerting any influence in the causation of consumption. When mental depression arises from any great loss, whether of relatives, friends, or property, it is often followed by irregular habits. Food is not taken regularly, nor in sufficient quantity ; and, on the other hand, stimulants are often taken too freely. In these cases, it is doubtful whether we ought to assign as the cause the mental depression, or the irregular living accompanying it. Laennec gives an interesting instance of the effect of mental depression.

'I had under my own eyes,' says he, ' during a period of ten years, a striking example of the effect of the depressing passions in producing phthisis, in the case of a religious association of women of recent foundation, and which never obtained from the

..... authorities any other than a provisional toleration, on account of the extreme severity of its rules. The diet of these persons was certainly very austere, yet it was by no means beyond what nature could bear; but the ascetic spirit which regulated their minds was such as to give rise to consequences no less serious than surprising. Not only was the attention of these women habitually fixed on the most terrible truths of religion, but it was the constant practice to try them by every kind o contrariety and opposition, in order to bring them, as soon as possible, to an entire renouncement of their own proper will. The consequences of this discipline were the same in all : after being one or two months in the establishment, the catamenia became suppressed, and in the course of one or two months thereafter phthisis declared itself! . . . . During the ten years that I was physician of this association, I witnessed its entire renovation two or three different times; owing to the successive loss of all its members, with the exception of a small number, consisting chiefly of the superior, the grate-keeper, and the sisters who had charge of the garden, kitchen, and infirmary. It will be observed that these individuals were those who had the most constant distractions from their religious tasks, and that they also went out pretty often into the city on business connected with the establishment.[1]

Damp.—A damp atmosphere may be generated either by moisture brought to the locality through the prevalence of certain winds, or by the impermeable nature of the soil underlying it, causing the accumulation of moisture on the surface. Whether a damp atmosphere generated in the first-mentioned way gives rise to consumption, there is as yet no decided proof; but of its origin in the last-mentioned way, viz. from a damp soil, the investigations of Drs. Buchanan and Bowditch leave no room to doubt. Dr. Buchanan was appointed by the Privy Council to investigate the effects on the public health produced by the improvements lately made in the drainage, water-supply, &c. of certain towns. He found, with regard to

[1] *Diseases of the Chest*, Sir John Forbes's translation, p. 334.

phthisis mortality, that its diminution or non-diminution
depended on whether the sanitary improvements of the
place had or had not included any considerable drying of
the soil.   In fifteen large towns where a diminution had
taken place after the improvements, the death-rates from
phthisis had fallen some 11 to 20 per cent.; in others, 20
to 30 per cent.; and others again, 30 to 49 per cent.; and
in many towns this diminution of deaths from phthisis
formed the principal sanitary amendment.   'This,' as
Mr. Simon [1] says, 'is extremely interesting and significant,
when it is remembered that works of sewerage by which
the drying of the soil is effected must always precede, and
do indeed sometimes precede by years, the accomplish-
ment of other objects—house-drainage, abolition of cess-
pools, and so forth—on which the cessation of various
other diseases is dependent.'

These results naturally directed attention to the influence of the soil in the distribution of consumption, and
led Dr. Buchanan to institute a farther inquiry on this
point.   By a careful comparison of the geological formations of the registration districts of the counties of Surrey
Kent, and Sussex with the death-rates from phthisis in
these districts, and by an elimination of all probable chances
of error, he arrived at the important conclusion, that *wet-
ness of soil is a cause of phthisis to the population living
on it.*   This conclusion was supported by the evidence of the
Registrar-General of Scotland with regard to that country; and by that of Dr. Bowditch of Boston, U.S.A., who in
1862 had drawn attention to the inequality of the distribution of phthisis in the state of Massachusetts, and to
the connection of this inequality with differences of moisture of soil.   He cited the written statements of medical
men resident in 183 towns, which tended to prove the
existence of a law in the development of consumption in

[1] *Report of the Medical Officer of the Privy Council for* 1867.

. . . . that dampness of the soil of any township . . . locality is intimately connected, and probably as cause and effect, with the prevalence of consumption in that township or locality; and be also adduced particular instances as demonstrating that even some houses may become the foci of consumption, when others but slightly removed from them, but on a drier soil, almost wholly escape. The following instance of this law came under my notice, one of the family being for some years under my care.

The rector of a parish in Essex resides on a clay soil, and has a large pond immediately in the neighbourhood of his rectory. He and his wife have always enjoyed good health, and there is no hereditary disease traceable, either in his own family or his wife's. Of their twelve children, eight were born at the rectory, and four in a neighbouring parish; but all spent childhood and youth at their father's house. The eldest, if alive, would now be 36; the youngest is 19. Six have died; four of consumption, one of scrofulous disease of the spine, and one of hooping-cough at the age of 5. Of the six alive, three are healthy, one is delicate, but I have not heard from what cause; two have scrofulous disease of the spine. The three healthy ones have spent but little time at home since they have grown up, and one spends much time in travelling. So that out of twelve children, there are no less than four cases of consumption, and three of scrofula.

This seems to me a fair instance of phthisis arising from endemic causes; the social position of the family, who are rich, precluding many other causes, which we have been discussing, from entering into consideration. We may therefore conclude that dampness of soil is an undoubted cause of consumption; and in our preventive treatment of the disease we should aim at either the drainage of the soil, or removal of the inhabitants to a drier locality.

Of the *local* causes of consumption, the most important have already been considered, and it only remains for us to notice :—

Trades and occupations giving rise to a dusty or gritty atmosphere.—A life pursued in an atmosphere abounding in small particles of flint, or iron, or coal, or cotton, or flax, or straw, as is the case with stonemasons, potters, fork-grinders, needle-grinders, cotton-carders, and chaff-cutters, is shown by Dr. Greenhow and others to be a short one : and the cause of death was generally found to be tubercular phthisis, induced by constant inhalation of the irritating particles. These have been detected chemically and microscopically in the lungs. They seem to set up irritation in the larger bronchi, causing thickening ; and also in the lung-tissue, causing induration and consolidation. It was at first doubted whether these lesions were tuberculous ; but the presence of both gray and yellow tubercle, and the tendency of the consolidations to soften and form cavities, sufficiently demonstrate their consumptive nature. Dr. Greenhow calculated that 45,000 deaths occurred from these causes in England and Wales ; and he clearly showed that the whole of this mortality was preventible by the introduction of better methods of ventilation and working. Since his reports, Acts of Parliament have been passed which, if carried out, ought totally to abolish this cause of phthisis ; and it is is to be hoped that ere long we may no longer be able to number ' *dusty occupations* ' among our *causes* of consumption.

It may be well, before closing this chapter, to allude to the position occupied by consumption with reference to *infection*—a subject of very great importance to the community. The idea of the disease being infectious is an

aid me, and has always held its ground in Italy. Recently in this country it has been supported by Dr. William Budd,[1] who holds that tubercle is a true zymotic disease in the same sense as typhoïd, scarlet, and typhus fevers, never originating spontaneously, but perpetuated according to the law of continuous succession; and that the tuberculous matter itself is, or includes, the specific morbid matter of the disease, and constitutes the material by which phthisis is propagated from one person to another and disseminated through society. Among the grounds on which Dr. Budd supports this theory, are (1), the prevalence of both zymotic fevers and phthisis in very crowded communities, and in prisons, convents, and barracks; (2), the geographical distribution of phthisis in past and present times, and its great fatality in countries which when first discovered by Europeans were known to be entirely free from it; (3), instances in which there was evidence to show that the disease was communicated from one person to another.

As regards the first ground, it may be observed that the coincidence of the diseases may be explained by the coexistence of common causes, independent of infection, such as impure air and water, bad food, &c.; and as to the second statement, if it be well authenticated, it is hardly fair to overlook the change in the habits of natives which contact with Europeans generally entails. This change, as we know well, is generally for the worse; and to a more domesticated life and the abuse of spirituous liquors, much may be ascribed, which Dr. Budd would assign to infection. With reference to the third reason, we must admit that recent experiments on the artificial inoculation of tubercle have given a fresh aspect to the subject of the contagion of phthisis, and have rendered it possible that the caseous and purulent material might infect those

[1] *Lancet*, October 1867.

brought into close contact with consumptive patients.
The instances of a wife of a consumptive husband, and the
sister of a consumptive woman, who had been sleeping
with, or attending closely on her, being attacked with the
disease, are those which most readily occur to the mind;
but we must remember that the close confinement which
occurs in these cases must be taken into account; and
moreover, if the above experiments point to a possible
inoculation from tuberculous material, they point also to
the same result arising from the inoculation of various other
noxious matters, as pus, putrid matter, &c. (See p. 98.)
We see, therefore, that if phthisis can be engendered in
this manner, it does not arise from any specific poison,
but it can be produced in the dissecting-room, or in the
surgical wards, as well as, and probably better, than in a
hospital for consumption. Dr. Cotton [1] justly remarks:—
'If Dr. Budd's views be correct, this (the Brompton)
hospital, as well as every like institution, must be nothing
more nor less than a pest-house, and must afford sad and
repeated proofs of its banefulness.' Now, what do facts
say on this subject? The statistics [2] of the Brompton
Hospital, as furnished by Dr. Cotton and Mr. Virtue
Edwards, directly negative any idea of infection. The
occurrence of phthisis among the physicians, resident
medical officers, chaplains, matrons, secretaries, nurses,
porters, and servants, and others closely connected with
the hospital since its foundation in 1846, has been very
rare, and the deaths very few. One assistant physician
and one clinical assistant (a member of a consumptive
family) have died, and three more of the clinical assistants
are said to be consumptive, out of a total of between
sixty and seventy. Of the numerous nurses and servants
who have been or are connected with the institution, only
one nurse and one servant have died of phthisis; and in

[1] *Lancet*, November 1867.   [2] *Lancet*.

■■■■■■■■ seems to have been contracted after ■■■■■■■■ the service of the hospital. None of the chaplains, matrons, secretaries, or porters have been attacked, and the last-mentioned, be it remembered, have to remove the dead from the wards, and subsequently from the dead-house. Two dispensers have died of consumption, but in the case of one it was doubtful if he had the disease when attached to the institution. This is surely a small mortality from phthisis in twenty-one years! Dr. Cotton says that his experience of one of the largest metropolitan hospitals during the same period, as regards the frequency of phthisis among its official staff, is decidedly in favour of the Hospital for Consumption. He states:—'In the same number of years, I have known, at the former institution, one physician, one surgeon, one chaplain, two house-surgeons, and four or five former dressers or clinical assistants, succumb to this fatal disorder.'

We need hardly add that a comparison of the number of cases of phthisis among the Brompton staff with the number occurring from zymotic fever among the staff of any fever hospital, will at once annihilate any hypothesis of similar contagion.[1]

---

[1] Although I concur in the opinion that we have no evidence that pulmonary consumption is infectious, like small-pox, scarlatina, or typhus, or that it depends on a specific poison, yet I think that both reason and experience indicate that a noxious influence may pass from a patient in advanced consumption to a healthy person in close communication, and may produce the same disease; just as foul pus or putrid muscle will produce tubercles in an inoculated animal. (See Chap. xiv.) I therefore always recommend such patients to sleep alone, and to use measures for increasing the purity of the air.—C. J. B. W.

CHAPTER XVI.

HÆMOPTYSIS AND THE HÆMORRHAGIC VARIETY OF CONSUMPTION.

By Dr. C. Theodore Williams.

Hæmoptysis—Its significance—Views of Louis, Laennec, Andral, Watson —Niemeyer's Explanation of large Hæmoptysis — His Comparison of Bronchial Hæmorrhage with Epistaxis inappropriate.—Differences in the Bronchial and Nasal Tracts—Niemeyer's Views of the Relation of Hæmoptysis to Phthisis discussed—Origin of Phthisis from Hæmoptysis improbable and unproved—Author's Experience—Hæmorrhage of Early Phthisis explained by Fatty Degeneration of Vessels— Of later Stages by Pulmonary Aneurism—Varieties and Pathology of latter—Hæmoptysis from Congestion—Influence of Age and Sex in Hæmoptysis—Influence of Stage— Illustrative Cases—Influence of Form of Disease—Hæmorrhagic Phthisis— Its characteristic Symptoms and exciting Causes—Examples—Effects of Hæmoptysis in Phthisis—General and local Pneumonia—When and why set up—Results—Illustrative Cases—Influence of Hæmoptysis on Duration of life.

So many cases of phthisis are accompanied by hæmoptysis in some part or another of their course, most commonly in the early stages, that spitting of blood, or 'bursting a blood vessel,' as it is popularly called, has long been considered by the public, and to some extent by the profession, as an indication of consumption. The connexion of hæmoptysis and phthisis, though simple in the stages of softening and excavation, is by no means always so in the early stages of the disease, and especially in cases where large hæmoptysis takes place, and but slight if any physical signs are detected at the time of its occurrence. Here the existence of consumptive disease is often denied ; and when at a later date it developes itself more clearly, its cause is referred by some writers to the blood

...fused into the bronchi during hæmoptysis, which is considered to have given rise to inflammation and destruction of the lung substance. We propose in this chapter to examine the views held by various writers on the relation of hæmoptysis to phthisis, and to state the conclusions which our own experience has led us to adopt on the subject.

What then do authorities say as to the significance of hæmoptysis? Louis states, that excluding cases of amenorrhœa and mechanical injuries to the chest, he did not find a single instance of hæmoptysis among 1,200 cases, unconnected with tuberculous disease of the lung. Laennec holds much the same opinion; and Andral states, that of persons who have had hæmoptysis, one-fifth have not tubercles in the lungs; but he does not state whether any cardiac or other lesion existed to account for the hæmorrhage. Sir Thomas Watson[1] says, 'If a person spits blood who has received no injury to the chest, in whom the uterine functions are healthy and right, and who has no disease of the heart, the odds that there are tubercles in the lungs of that person are fearfully high.'

On the other hand, Niemeyer, after stating that bronchial hæmorrhage is the 'most frequent cause of hæmoptysis, explains that it 'proceeds from rupture of the capillaries, caused either by over-distension, or else by a morbid delicacy of the walls, a result of perverted nutrition.' He remarks very justly, that 'trifling capillary hæmorrhage, such as occur in bronchial catarrh, violent irritation of air-passages, and in the circulatory disorders attending organic disease of the heart, proceed from the first of these

---

[1] *Practice of Physic*, vol. ii. 200.

Hand-Book of Practical Medicine, vol. i. p. 141. Although we cannot subscribe to all Niemeyer's views, we deeply lament the loss which Clinical Medicine has sustained in the recent death of so careful and accomplished

causes, but that in most hæmorrhages in which large quantities of blood are poured into bronchi to be ejected by
hæmoptysis, they are due to the latter condition.' It is
much to be regretted that Niemeyer uses such vague
terms as 'morbid delicacy' of walls of vessels; but as far
as we understand him, in regarding the vascular walls as
the seat of disease, and their fragility the cause of large
hæmoptysis, we agree with him. Why he should assign
such hæmorrhage to the bronchial trunks and capillaries,
we are at a loss to understand, as he gives no fact to support his statement, and we know that as yet simple bronchial hæmorrhage has never been demonstrated by post-
mortem examination. The comparison with the large
hæmorrhage from the nasal mucous membrane, which occurs in profuse epistaxis, does not hold good, as may be
shown by structural differences in the two tracts. The
Schneiderian membrane in parts, as on the septum nasi
and over the spongy bones, is very thick, partly through
the presence of glands, but chiefly as Todd and Bowman[1]
say, 'from the presence of ample and capacious submucous plexuses of both arteries and veins, of which the
latter are by far the more large and tortuous. These
serve to explain the tendency of hæmorrhage in case of
general or local plethora.' The bronchial mucous membrane, though undoubtedly vascular, cannot be said to
present in its structure any explanation of copious
hæmorrhage like that of the nasal tract.

Niemeyer[2] sums up his views on the relation of hæmoptysis to phthisis in the following paragraphs:—

'1. Bronchial hæmorrhage occurs oftener than is generally believed in persons who are not consumptive at the
time of the bleeding, and who never become so.

'2. Copious bronchial hæmorrhage frequently precedes
consumption, there being, however, no relation of cause

[1] *Physiological Anatomy*, vol. ii. p. 3.   [2] *Op. cit.* p. 144.

.... the hæmorrhage and pulmonary .... Here both events spring from the same source —from a common predisposition, on the part of the patient, both to consumption and bleeding.

'3. Bronchial bleeding may precede the development of consumption as its cause, the hæmorrhage leading to chronic inflammation and destruction of the lung.

'4. Hæmorrhage from the bronchi occurs in the course of established consumption more frequently than it precedes it. It sometimes, although rarely, appears when the disease is yet latent.

'5. When bronchial hæmorrhage takes place during the course of consumption, it may accelerate the fatal issue of the disease, by causing chronic destructive inflammation.'

With regard to the first class, Niemeyer states that hæmoptysis occurs, though rarely, in young persons in blooming health and of vigorous constitution, and that there is absolutely no explanation of the disorder, which is often followed by such sad results. Here we question the facts, both of the hæmorrhage being really bronchial, for the reasons we have given above, and of the health of these persons being really sound. In few such cases have we failed to find signs of disease, limited, it is true, and generally confined to the inter-scapular regions of the chest. Niemeyer admits that exceptional instances occur in which tubercles and inflammatory processes form in the lungs in a manner so latent that no tokens of disease are manifested by the individual affected, until he is suddenly attacked by a fit of hæmorrhage; but he denies that this is the case in the great majority of instances, where the first attack of hæmoptysis has not been preceded by cough, dyspnœa, or other sign of pulmonary disease. How he distinguishes between these two classes, on what grounds he supposed that they are separate

classes, does not appear; but he continues, ' that bronchial
hæmorrhage is by no means so rare an event where there
is no grave disease of the lungs, is shown, moreover, by
the tolerably numerous cases in which persons, after suffering one or more attacks of pneumorrhagia, regain their
health completely, and indeed often live to an advanced
age, and after death present no discoverable traces of
extinct tuberculosis in their lungs.   Unfortunately, none
of these ' tolerably numerous cases ' is given to support
this statement, which can hardly therefore be considered
to be supported by satisfactory evidence.

Our own experience is exactly the reverse; and we have
generally been able to detect signs of disease during life
in the lungs of all those patients who have had extensive
hæmoptysis, unconnected with heart disease, injury to the
chest, or disorder of the menstruation.

Niemeyer also finds ' a strong tendency to profuse
capillary hæmorrhage from the bronchi in young persons
between fifteen and twenty-five, whose parents have died
of consumption, and who have suffered in infancy from
rickets or scrofula, have often bled at the nose, and grown
rapidly tall.   He is tempted to refer the remarkable frequency to a deficiency of vital material which has been
immoderately expanded in the maladies of childhood or
in the process of growth; and therefore does not leave
sufficient to maintain the normal nutrition of the capillary walls.   He remarks that this does not explain why
the seat of the hæmorrhage should be, first in the nose,
and secondly in the bronchi, &c.   Now we would ask our
readers, could a case for probable consumptive origin of
hæmoptysis be more clearly made out than it is here by
Niemeyer himself?   The family history, predisposing influences and diseases, and structural features are complete.
Some exciting cause, like catarrh, only is wanting to determine the outbreak of disease in the lung, and those

will run the course of phthisis. We do not wish to state absolutely that hæmoptysis does arise in these cases from tubercular disease, but that the fragile state of the vessels is connected with consumptive disease we entertain no doubt. Again, Niemeyer seems to forget that there is a common tendency in childhood to coryza and epistaxis which may continue in youth, if disease in the vessels of the lung do not cause a diversion. We are quite ready to confirm the accuracy of Niemeyer's fifth paragraph, and can cite many cases illustrating the destructive effects on the lung, of large hæmorrhage during the progress of phthisis. Such inflammation and consequent destruction of the pulmonary tissue is more likely to occur at the base of the lungs to which the blood gravitates, than at the apex, and in our own cases it has always been found there.

We notice, however, that in one of Niemeyer's cases (Dr. N.)[1] and also in one of his translators, Dr. Baümler's,[2] the physical signs gave evidence of disease of the *apex* of one lung. This is surely a strong argument against a hæmorrhagic origin for the disease; for we know no reason why the blood effused from the bronchial mucous membrane should be exempted from the laws of gravity, directing it to the lower portions of the lung, and should flow upwards towards the apex, the portion of all others, it may be remembered, most prone to tubercular attack.

Whether the presence of the coagula in the bronchi is the cause of the inflammatory changes is open to question. It does not appear why blood coagula should irritate more than mucous or croupous matter, which cause collapse of the lung and not inflammation; but it is probable that in these cases of pneumonia after hæmorrhage, some laceration or congestion of the lung has taken place, and in this way is started the inflammatory process which, in a

---

[1] _____ on Phthisis, p. 86.   [2] *Clinical Transactions*, vol. ii. p. 86.

warning, and often in
have been attacked by p
who, without rallying, ha
a phthisis florida, or " ga
me that such patients s
monary tuberculosis in i
usually die of a form of
thought of, and of which
immediate cause.'

We must confess we ha
tice, or in consulting the
posal, met with a case of
simple hæmoptysis, though
moptysis, accompanying v
come . under our notice, a
pyæmic symptoms.   We
out the symptoms of lun
of blood and recover, with
patients were generally
arcus senilis, from which
fatty degeneration may h
the pulmonary vessels, as w
have caused their brittlene
is the rule in

...bronchial plugging, exist, there follow increased
...and fever, and the lung passes rapidly through its
... of destruction. Again, looking at Niemeyer's view
... the aspect of probability, if persons have been really
... health, without any previous disease of the
... or of their vessels, why should they, without warn-
... suddenly spit up quantities of blood and go into
... consumption, when really healthy persons may be
subjected to all sorts of violent exertion without such
results?

Having discussed Niemeyer's views, we will state that
our experience of many thousand cases has led us to conclude, that hæmoptysis to the extent of more than a drachm,
in a person, free from the hæmorrhagic diathesis, from
cancerous disease of the lung,[1] injury of the chest, disease
of the heart, and from disorder of the uterus—is indicative of a fragile state of the vessels of the lungs, closely
connected with, and generally arising out of, consumptive
... of these organs. What are the changes which
... been traced in the blood-vessels to account for their
... fragility? Two causes have at present been ob-
... but in a disease which embraces, as phthisis does,
... forms of degeneration of tissue, it is probable that
... will in time be discovered.

... fatty degeneration has been demonstrated, by
... Radcliffe Hall, to exist in the small blood-vessels.
... series of careful observations 'On the varieties and
... morphoses of tubercle,' well illustrated with plates,
... the reader is referred,[2] Dr. Hall records having
... fatty degeneration of the blood-vessels in phthisis
... instances, ' near to, but not mixed up with tubercle

... cases of fatal hæmoptysis from cancer of the lung are related,
... Thompson, in *Pathological Transactions*, vols. vii. and

... and *Foreign Medico-Chirurgical Review*, April–October, 1855.

received considerable attention from pathologists, and great light has been thrown on the various steps of the process. We believe that Dr. Peacock,[1] and Mr. Fearn of Derby, were the first to record instances of pulmonary aneurism in this country.

Rokitansky gave an excellent account of it in his 'Pathological Anatomy;' and of late years numerous cases have been described by Drs. Cotton,[2] Quain,[3] Moxon,[4] Douglas Powell,[5] and others. Dr. Rasmüssen,[6] of Norway, has treated very fully of the modes of formation and bursting in these vascular expansions, as exemplified by nine cases, carefully investigated by himself. From the accounts of the above-mentioned observers, and from several cases we have witnessed ourselves, the course of events appears to run thus : When the processes of softening and excavation are going on in the lungs, branches of the pulmonary artery are laid bare, and are to be occasionally seen, as yet undilated, in the walls of cavities in phthisical patients who die from other causes than pulmonary hæmorrhage. This state of the vessels, if there is much obstruction to circulation in the lungs, does not last long ; either a rupture takes place, as occurred in one of Dr. Powell's cases, or the want of support causes the vascular wall to dilate on the side towards the cavity, and a protuberance varying in size and shape according to that of the unsupported portion of vessel, takes place. The slightest form of aneurism is that denominated *ectasia*, by Dr. Rasmüssen, where the vessel touches the cavity for for only a limited extent, and a small oblong dilatation is formed, due partly to the expansion of the bore of the vessel, and partly to the wall growing thicker. The burst-

[1] *London and Edinburgh Monthly Journal*, 1843, p. 383.
[2] *Lancet*, 1841. [3] Vol. iv. p. 117.
[4] *Medical Times and Gazette*, Jan. 13 and Oct. 20, 1866.
[5] *Path. Trans.*, vols. xvii. xviii. xxii.
[6] *Beale's Reports, for* 1869.

ing takes place on the boundaries between the vessel and
the wall of the cavity, and the point of the lid always
lies in the direction of the blood current.' A very good
example of ectasias was recorded by Dr. Quain, where in
one cavity two small branches of the pulmonary artery
exhibited several varicose dilations, one of which had
burst, causing fatal hæmoptysis. The other form of
aneurism is sacculated, and varies in size from a pea to a
small orange, being sometimes large enough to nearly fill
a small cavity; a larger amount of the vessel is exposed
than in the ectasias, and the pouch contains sometimes
clots of blood, sometimes laminated fibrin; the perforation, according to Dr. Rasmüssen, being found on the
most protruding portion of the dilatation. Several
aneurisms or ectasias are sometimes found in the same
lung, though their presence is always confined to cavities.
The cause of the formation of these aneurisms does not
always lie in any general diseased condition of the pulmonary vessels, for these, except at the points of dilatation,
have been hitherto found to be healthy, but it owes its existence principally to the want of support of the wall of the
vessel turned towards the cavity, and partly to heightened
intervascular pressure, from a strong tendency of blood
to fill the vacuum caused by the contraction of the lung,
especially about the cavities, and also from the obliteration of so many branches of the pulmonary artery. That
pulmonary aneurism is a very common cause of fatal
hæmoptysis in phthisis is proved by Dr. R. D. Powell's
table of 15 cases of fatal hæmoptysis occurring at the
Brompton Hospital in the last few years, in all of which
cavities of various sizes existed. In all but two, a ruptured vessel was discovered; in one there was rupture
without dilatation of a vessel; and in 12 ruptured aneurisms were found. The hæmoptysis from this source is
frequently fatal, although the first attack is not necessarily

so, for in eight of the Brompton Hospital cases, there had
been copious hæmoptysis on more than one occasion, previously to the attack which terminated life. Having thus
pointed out the pathology of large hæmoptysis in phthisis,
we may state that the expectoration of small quantities
of blood is probably due to congestion or inflammation of
one or other of the two systems of vessels existing in the
lung, similar to what occurs in heart disease or in pneumonia. For such slight oozings of blood it is not necessary that there should be any rupture of vessels, as it has
been ascertained that the red corpuscles can, like the
white corpuscles, migrate through the vascular walls and
pass into the surrounding tissues, but it is extremely improbable that any considerable hæmorrhage can take place
in this way.

It will be useful now to consider certain other points
connected with hæmoptysis, such as

(1). The influence that age and sex exercises on its occurrence.

(2). The stage and form of the disease in which it is
most marked.

(3). What effect it exerts locally and generally on the
course of the disease—what complications it gives rise to.

(4). Whether or not it curtails the duration of life.

The influence of sex, according to the first Brompton
Report,[1] is very trifling, the females showing excess over
the males of only 3 per cent. In 1000 cases tabulated
from private practice, the majority of whom have been
under observation for many years, we arrived at a different
result. The total number of cases of hæmoptysis in both
sexes was 569, or about 57 per cent.; but among the
males the percentage was 63, and among the females 47,
giving an excess to the males of 16 per cent.

Again, in 283 cases where the amount of blood expec-

[1] p. 28.

torated at any one time exceeded an ounce, the liability of males was still more marked.   Large hæmorrhage was found to occur in 34·76 per cent. of the males, and in only 17·67 per cent. of the females, this greater liability of males to spit blood in large quantities being amply confirmed by Dr. Pollock and the second Brompton Report.

Age cannot be said to exercise a very marked influence, except that, according to the first Brompton Report, in the case of females, hæmoptysis occurred more frequently under 35 years of age than between 35 and 70.

The influence of the *stage* of the disease is of much greater account; and here the first Report demonstrated, from observations on 696 cases, that hæmoptysis is more frequent (as 3 to 1) before softening than after that process has taken place.   Our own observations amply confirm this; and with a view of carrying these investigations farther, we have classified our 286 cases of profuse hæmoptysis into stages, annexing the number of deaths from this cause to each stage :—

Stage.	No. of Cases.	Deaths.	Per centage.
1st	187	26	13·95
2nd	65	16	24·61
3rd	31	21	67·74
	283	63	

The figures demonstrate most convincingly the significance of large hæmoptysis in the third stage of phthisis, and its comparative slighter importance in the first stage; but a few cases to illustrate these points may not prove unacceptable. The first three are instances of hæmoptysis in the third stage.

CASE 14.—Sarah B., a single woman, aged 26, was admitted into the Brompton Hospital, under the care of Dr. Quain, Nov. 21, 1870.   She had lost a brother and sister from consumption, but gave no history of illness previous to two months before admission, when she was attacked with cough, streaky expectoration, followed by great wasting, feverishness, and night sweats.

Whereas, her cough was constant, with muco-purulent expectoration, and she had some dyspnœa. Tongue furred; bowels active; appetite good; catamenia regular till last period, but scanty, now absent about two weeks. Pulse 120.

On examination of the chest, *cavernous gurgle was audible over right side of chest, front and back, and some crepitation over the left side.*

A few days later I saw this patient, and, in Dr. Quain's absence, had charge of the case. She became worse, losing flesh, in spite of taking oil and nourishment, and about January 12, was attacked with hæmoptysis, which was checked by styptics, but recurred again on 16th, and she brought up large quantities, *i.e.* more than a pint at a time, for several days, the hæmorrhage being only slightly influenced by treatment. She died suddenly on the 21st, after bringing up a large quantity of blood. The temperature during the last few days of her life, was, according to Mr. Giffard, the clinical assistant's, observations, as follows:—

	Morn.	Even.
January 17, .	99·3	102
„ 18, .	99	101·2
„ 19, .	99	100
„ 20, ..	99	

On post-mortem examination by Dr. R. Douglas Powell,[1] the left lung appeared highly emphysematous. The right was firmly adherent at its base, and the pleura thickened and gelatinous. The base of the lung was consolidated, and contained a cavity, projecting into which was the pulmonary aneurism which gave rise to the fatal hæmorrhage. The aneurism was situated on a vessel which originally crossed the cavity, and at the time of death projected into it about an inch, having, at this point, broken across in the progress of the disease. The arterial channel was preserved to the end of the truncated vessel, where it was dilated into a bulbous extremity. One side of this channel was formed by the brittle degenerated wall of the vessel, and presented a longitudinal rod-shaped deposit of lymph, the opposite side being made up of a considerable thickness of laminated coagula, filling up the sac of an aneurismal dilatation. Another cavity was found in the upper portion of the lung containing clots of blood, and an aneurismal dilation of a small pulmonary vessel which had burst.

In this case the rapid breaking down of the lung tissue had led to the failure of the vessel from loss of support and degeneration; but it is strange that the same process should have taken place in two cavities at nearly the same time.

Case 14.—A young gentleman, aged 16, was seen by Dr. Williams, in consultation with Mr. W. Jones, on May 5, 1853. Had suffered from cough for six

---

I am indebted for some of the notes of the *post-mortem* examination to months, and during the last month from pain in the left shoulder, and considerable loss of flesh and strength. *Dulness, and crepitation, fine and coarse, in upper left chest.*—Ordered oil, acid tonic, and counter-irritation.

November 28.—Vastly improved, and has gained 14 lbs. Walks eight miles, and for the last three months has been shooting in the country. *Dulness and tubular sounds in upper left chest as low as third rib.*—Ordered oil in sulphuric acid tonic.

May 17, 1854.—Wintered well, with only slight cough and expectoration and short breath. Has been riding a good deal, and a week ago was caught in the rain, and rode home in wet clothes. Has since had pain in the left side, with night-sweats, and diarrhœa. *Increase of dulness and moist coarse crepitation in upper left chest.*—Ordered a blister, and mercurial and chalk powder, with effervescing saline; afterwards to return to oil, which had been discontinued for six months.

August 9.—Has been taking oil in the country, and is improved; but has cough and yellowish expectoration, occasionally tinged with blood. *Liquid cavernulous sounds below left clavicle.*

The patient continued better; but in September, after having been out shooting for five hours, was attacked with hæmoptysis to the amount of two pints. This recurred again and again, and he died in a week.

On examination after death there were found only a few miliary tubercles at the apex of the left lung, and a cavity of the size of a walnut, lined with a thick membrane, deficient at one point, where the hæmorrhage had come from. The rest of the lung was congested. The right lung was healthy. But for his imprudent exertion, this patient would probably have avoided this fatal hæmoptysis, and might have completely recovered.

CASE 16.—Robert S., æt. 34, brewer's drayman, admitted into University College Hospital, under Dr. Williams, May 30, 1840.—Stout-built. Is habit of drinking much porter. Has had cough six months, but no illness till last February, in bed brought up, without cough or vomiting, a large quantity of blood. He was bled and, after taking medicines some days, returned to work. A week ago, while stooping, again brought up a quantity of blood. Was again bled, and took medicine; but has brought up considerable quantities daily—to-day nearly a pint, frothy and florid. Breath, very short: pulse, hard and frequent; skin, hot; face, flushed. Has not lost flesh till the last week. Bowels open. No sleep for three nights. *Flattening below left clavicle, dulness and cavernous sounds, with gurgling, above left scapula. Some dulness and tubular sounds below right clavicle.* Was bled to twenty-four ounces, which made him faintish. Three grains acet. lead, three times a day.

May 31.—Continues spitting large quantities of blood, with much cough. Pulse 104, jerking; skin, hot and dry.

June 2.—At 3 a.m. suddenly threw up blood copiously, and died in a few minutes.

Subcutem, 19 hours.—Body little emaciated. Blood generally fluid. External jugulars distended with it.

Left lung adherent by dense membrane at posterior part of apex, and in separating it a cavity was torn open of size of hen's egg, containing frothy blood, and a few dark clots, one of which partially plugged an opening into a large blood-vessel. Walls of cavity irregular, with broken grey matter, and several large veins containing fluid blood. Anterior part of lung pretty healthy, but a few grey solid masses below the cavity, and a few tubercles scattered through both lungs. A larger mass at the right apex, in some points opaque and softening, in others, intersected by dense bands. Bronchi contained much frothy blood and bloody mucus. Bronchial glands much enlarged, with pinkish and grey deposit. Blood-vessels of the lung very large: the veins more than double the size of their accompanying bronchi. Heart rather large, without increased thickness of walls. Aorta somewhat dilated.

Kidneys large and much congested. Liver very much enlarged, rather pale; substance fragile.

Although considerable disease must have existed before the hæmorrhage, it had not attracted much attention. There was no material loss of flesh, and he continued his work, and probably his habit of drinking freely of porter. This filled the blood-vessels, and led to the hæmorrhage, which in the post-mortem was traced to ruptured vessels.

The following is an example of hæmoptysis occurring during the second stage :—

Case 17.—A medical man, aged 45, was seen by Dr. Williams, June 2, 1863. He had been long in India, where he had suffered from fever and dysentery ; and during last winter a cough had come on, which had often been hard. In the last few days he had brought up a quantity (according to his own computation) of blood.

Dulness, obstruction and crepitation sounds in upper right chest, crepitation coarse in parts. Under doses of bitartrate of potash and gallic acid followed by occasional draughts of sulphate of magnesia and sulphate soda, the hæmoptysis was checked, and the cough lessened, but the bleedings recurred several times.

December 29, 1865.—Wintered at Bournemouth, but was confined to house, and had hæmoptysis to the amount of several ounces several times. Cough troublesome, and expectoration increased, but patient is by no means thin, and looks well.

Dulness and crepitation in upper right chest, most marked in the front. Dulness and tubular sounds audible above left scapula. This patient was, the spring of 1868, having lived nearly 6½ years after his first

The following is a good example of hæmoptysis accompanying the first stage, in which the patient remained well for many years, though eventually excavation of the lung took place :—

CASE 18.—A gentleman, aged 36, of strong, large frame, consulted Dr. Williams first on June 19, 1850. Had been in good health, with no cough; but after much exertion in May he expectorated half a pint of blood, and yesterday about the same quantity. Had been bled and leeched on the right chest, with diminution of the dulness; signs of congestion were found in the right lung. Pulse quiet; no cough; bowels confined.—Ordered gallic and nitric acids, and digitalis; an aperient of sulphate of magnesia with sulphuric acid.

June 24.—Hæmorrhage returned slightly next day, but not since. *Dulness and tubular sounds in the upper right front and back.*—A blister to the scapula; nitric and hydrocyanic acid mixture.

July 20.—No return of hæmorrhage; cough slight. Has taken cod-liver oil with acid mixture a fortnight. *Less dulness, but still large tubular expiration in the upper right front and back.*

September 26.—At Norwood. Taking oil, &c., regularly. Much improved in flesh and strength. Cough and expectoration slight. *Dulness and tubular expiration less marked.*

June 21, 1851.—Wintered in Madeira. Well, but frequent colds from damp weather. Continued oil and acids till the last three months. *Breath harsh and loud below right clavicle; little dulness and less tubular sounds in right back.*

September 25, 1852.—Has continued well.

November 24, 1853.—Passed last winter with only one attack of cold and cough, when the sputa were discoloured. Has been pretty well since; but has had an occasional feeling of oppression in the right lung, and three weeks ago, after much exertion of voice, brought up four ounces of blood, and some on the following days, when it was checked by gallic acid. Still much cough and wheezing. Urine scanty, red, and turbid. *General wheezing rhonchi in right lung; little dulness or tubular sounds.*—Ordered iodide of potassium, carbonate of potash, squills, stramonium, and liquorice, and a croton-oil liniment.

Under this treatment he soon got the better of this illness, and continued in good health, except occasional attacks of the same kind; more wheezy and asthmatic than phthisical. He continued active in business, and often gave lectures and spoke at public meetings, although warned against doing so.

February 13, 1863.—Three months before had coughed up four ounces of blood, and about the same quantity three days ago. Breath had been shorter since, with more expectoration. Feels the cold more, but voice and

.... Urine often thick.—*Dulness and tubular sound at* .... right scapula; *moist crepitus and mucous rhonchus above and* ....—To take oil, with sulphuric acid, calumba, &c.; saline at night.

June ..—Several times hæmoptysis this year; now about half an ounce ....., five days. Physical signs the same.

December 27, 1864.—Hæmoptysis recurred every two or three weeks till ...., when he went to Bournemouth; none since. Has regained some .... and strength. *More extensive dulness, obstruction, and coarse crepitus* *over greater part of right lung; cavernous sounds in scapular region; dulness* *and loud bronchophony now also at and above left scapula.* These signs have been increasing during the last twelve months, with more constant cough, copious opaque flocculent expectoration, pulse 100, and loss of flesh and strength.

A few months later the cavernous sound in the right lung became amphoric, with signs of increase in the left also. In the autumn of 1865 he went to Madeira, and died on the voyage back, early in 1866.

From 1853 to 1863 the disease was so much arrested that he resumed active habits, and ceased to regard himself an invalid. The disease in consequence recommenced its activity, and ran its destructive course.

While hæmoptysis may accompany all stages of consumption, and may vary considerably in amount, it may also be entirely absent throughout the whole course of the disease. In the acute forms, and particularly in acute tuberculosis, hæmoptysis rarely occurs, and the relief in the more chronic varieties of the malady often derived from a copious hæmorrhage has led some physicians to think that the great congestion noticeable in acute cases might be relieved by local or general blood-letting.

Whilst the most rapid cases of phthisis are nearly free from hæmoptysis, there is a class of patients already alluded to in whom the amount of the disease is small, and large and repeated hæmorrhage the principal feature. We described a few of these cases three years ago under the term of the hæmorrhagic variety of consumption,[1] and it is no small satisfaction to us that so careful an observer as Dr. Peacock also recognised in them a sepa-

[1] *Lancet*, June, 1868.

is no measure of the danger resulting to the patient, as in this form of the disease a large amount of blood may be brought up without fatal or even pernicious results.

Our 1,000 tabulated cases furnish 72 instances of this form of phthisis, of whom 60 were males and 12 females, a proportion of 5 to 1 of the former to the latter, which forms a contrast to the proportionate numbers of the two sexes in all forms of consumption, which was as 2 to 1. Thus we see that males are far more liable than females to the hæmorrhagic form of phthisis, and this for a reason that will presently appear. The patients were attacked rather later in life than the generality of consumptives. The average age of attack for the males being 30 and for the females 27. Family predisposition was not usually present, appearing in only 25 instances, and perhaps this may account for the later age of attack. In 42 cases the hæmoptysis was preceded for a shorter or longer time by cough, but in the rest hæmorrhage was the first symptom. In 45 no exciting cause was recorded. In 27 an explanation was to be found either (1) in the patient having been subjected to some great bodily exertion, as preaching, lecturing, acting on the stage, rowing, climbing, or running; or (2) in his having been inhaling an atmosphere either mechanically or chemically irritating to the lungs, as that of a laboratory or workshop; or (3) in his having been exposed to decidedly lowering conditions, as chills from getting wet through, great mental worry, fasting, too close application to a sedentary occupation, severe attacks of certain lowering diseases, as dysentery, measles, and syphilis, the latter being in one case followed by mercurialization.

We see, therefore, that in a large number of these cases the attack of hæmoptysis did not occur, without, as Dr. Peacock expresses it, some more or less decided excess, and it is probable that had great attention

... dulness; moist crepitation, with slight tubular sounds below left ... apex ... above; slight dulness and tubular voice in right inter- ... region.—Ordered oil in a tonic of nitric and hydrocyanic acids, with the tinctures of hop and orange, and a liniment of acetum can- tharidis.

September 16.—Much improved, under the oil, in flesh, strength, and breath, and able to walk fast and up-hill. Came from Hastings to-day, and after much talking, on lying down at night, expectorated blood to the amount of two ounces, with irritating cough. Is in too much tremor from fear to bear examination; pulse 90. Ordered gallic acid, with syrup of poppy, followed by an aperient draught of sulphate of magnesia and sul- phuric acid.

21.—No return of hæmorrhage; dulness, with crepitus above left scapula.

30.—Hæmoptysis to a pint and a half in last two days, and cough still troublesome. Ordered a blister and a morphia linctus, together with the gallic acid.

April 17, 1851.—Has wintered at Hastings, taking oil regularly, and gradually recovered from a state of great weakness; moderate cough and only slight expectoration. Has so much improved that now he can walk for five or six hours daily. Physical signs diminished.

May 4, 1854.—Has taken oil regularly, and been quite well all the win- ter, without cough or expectoration; but has lately had neuralgia of the eye and occasional flushes of blood to the head; urine thick, with lithates; very little dulness or tubular sounds, but breath obscure above left, scapula, and whiffy in left scapular region; tubular voice above right scapula.— Ordered oil in nitric acid and tincture of orange, and an occasional effer- vescing saline.

January 21, 1858.—Has done duty well since. Only occasional cough, but always some mucous expectoration. Is strong and active, although of late has been much worried by a lawsuit. Signs diminished.

May 18, 1860.—Active and well till a month ago, when cough returned, with opaque expectoration, which has since improved. Still some dul- ness and tubular breath in both scapular regions, chiefly in left, and in left ...

September 26, 1866.—Wonderfully well, and generally does duty. ... and expectoration very slight. Weighs twelve stone—heavier than ever.

This patient was alive and well in January, 1871, more than twenty years after his first visit, and more than twenty-one since his first symptoms; and for the last thirteen years has done duty regularly.

CASE VII.—A gentleman, aged 32, consulted Dr. Williams, Aug. 9, 1854. ... he had hæmoptysis to the amount of half a pint, and afterwards ... some months he continued to bring up a smaller amount, till June,

.... was attacked in 1866 with similar symptoms and signs, and .... large quantities of blood repeatedly, requiring gallic acid in .... He has been more careful of himself, has implicitly followed his instructions, and has been restored to health, unbroken when last heard of, 1870.

CASE 21.—An officer in the army, aged 20, was first seen by Dr. Williams March 11, 1860, and gave the following history:—He had been subject to cough in winter, but otherwise enjoyed good health till the previous September, when he had a chancre, followed in December by sore throat, and an eruption on the legs. Four weeks ago cough came on, and a week later he had hæmoptysis to the amount of three drachms. Feels much weakened. *Slight dulness; tubular sounds in upper part of right chest.*—Oil was ordered in a tonic of nitric acid; iodide of potassium and tincture of orange, and a night draught of iodide of potassium and bicarbonate of potash.

June 8.—Has been at Pau since. The cough is better; but he has had occasional hæmoptysis to the amount of a drachm; and he still has syphilitic eruption and pains. Submaxillary glands swollen.

November 12.—Has been living in Ireland, and was better till he caught cold in the camp, and fresh cough came on, with increased expectoration, and occasional hæmoptysis to the amount of several ounces. *Dulness and tubular breath and voice above right scapula. Crepitation, and obstruction sounds in the upper third of left chest.*—To continue oil in acid tonic, and winter at Torquay.

September 18, 1861.—Wintered well at Torquay till April, when he brought up 4 ounces of blood, and continued spitting some blood for 10 days. He remained well till 18 days ago, when hæmoptysis recurred to the amount of four ounces, and he discovered he had recent syphilitic symptoms. *Dulness and deficient breathing and some croaky sounds in upper left chest.*

July, 1862.—Wintered in Madeira, and remained well, and married there; but after some exertion he brought up an ounce of blood, and some slight amount since. There is still *dulness, with rough breath in upper left chest, harsh behind. Dulness increased above right scapula.*

October 2, 1863.—Passed winter travelling in Italy, Sicily, Spain, and Egypt, with little cough, and only hæmorrhage to amount of half an ounce. Took oil pretty regularly. In the summer went to Turkey and Malta, and enjoyed the heat. Still *dulness above right scapula, and croak on deep breath.*

December 26, 1864.—Was last winter at Bonchurch, and able to walk 12 miles a day, and lost cough. Lately has been in Edinburgh, and tolerably well except occasional colds and pain in the side. Oil omitted from May till November. *Weak breath, and some friction sounds in left back.*

June 2, 1868.—Remained well, living in Hampshire till last summer. When in Paris spit half an ounce of blood, and in November brought up

cough; and once had hæmoptysis,
later half an ounce. Has suffer
Weak breath and whiffy sounds a

June, 1870.—In the spring fol
lowed by pneumonia of right lung
and is now stronger than before the
breathing at left apex.

The lung affection in this case pr
which were perceptible in several p

CASE 24.— A gentleman, aged 35, w
He had lived freely, but had been f
sional giddiness before the end of
chilled. Hæmoptysis came on, and
and was much reduced.

Three months before the attack
minished, but had not quite disappea
expectoration. At present his breath
and has been taking cod-liver oil and
voice and breath in left interscapula
spine of right scapula.

January 17, 1866.—Remained qu
after fifty-four miles hunting, brough
and soon recovered. At present has
signs—still *bronchophony can be detec*

Let us now consider the
general and local, on the cou
plications it gives rise to.
attack may cause imm

greatly to be influenced by treatment; but it will be useful to notice the effects on the system generally, and on
the lung locally, of moderate hæmorrhage. To many
patients its occurrence seems beneficial rather than otherwise, for the congestion is thus relieved, and the system
not materially weakened by the loss of blood. The
effusion of blood into the smallest bronchi and air-cells
does not necessarily cause any general irritation; for after
hæmoptysis the presence of blood in the air-vessels may
often be detected by physical signs; but these may dis-
appear in a few hours or days, and no results follow. On
the other hand, in some instances its presence irritates
the lung considerably, giving rise to bronchitis and even
catarrhal pneumonia. A rise takes place in the temperature; and sometimes while the hæmoptysis is going on, the
pulse becomes more frequent, the breathing more rapid,
and the cough more troublesome. Crepitation is heard in
the lower lobes of one or both lungs, intermingled with a
good deal of sibilant rhonchus, and the case becomes one
of pneumonia. Fresh consolidation of the lung may even
arise in this way, but according to our experience it is
seldom permanent, being reabsorbed. Why the effusion
of blood into the smaller bronchi should be in some cases
followed by bronchitis and pneumonia, and should give
rise to no symptoms whatever in others, it is difficult to
say, but we are inclined to ascribe the inflammatory consequences to a previous congestion, not sufficiently relieved
by the hæmorrhage, rather than to the mechanical irritation caused by the blood-clots in the bronchi, which is the
cause assigned by Niemeyer. The occurrence of hæmorrhage is generally preceded by violent exertion, sudden
change of temperature, or something which produces
pulmonary congestion. If the hæmorrhage removes this
congestion, no inflammation follows; but if not, the injury
of the ruptured vessels, and the reaction, after the

19th.—Worse. Aspect blanched; breathing embarrassed. *Crepitation audible in lower left lung as well as in right.* Pulse 108; temperature 101·5; respiration 32. A blister was applied to the left side.

20th.—Blister rose well, and patient was relieved as to breathing and cough; but, after severe fit of coughing, slight hæmoptysis came on, and now cough and other symptoms are worse. Pulse 108; temperature 101·2; respiration 36.—Ordered oil again.

22nd.—Slight hæmoptysis, and cough has increased. Pulse 100; temperature 101·1; respiration 28.

March 3rd.—Patient was very restless, cough very troublesome, and breath very short till a few days ago, when he expectorated largely of thick mucopurulent matter and some frothy mucus, and since then his aspect is much brighter. *Crepitation in lower left chest. Rhonchus and crepitation (uttered) over whole right side.*—Quinine, in two-grain doses twice a day, was ordered to be combined with the oil, and patient took it for two days, and then refused to take any more.

6th.—Worse; much paler; tongue, which has been generally slightly furred, is now glossy and red. Pulse 120; temperature 100; respiration 32.—Ordered sulphurous acid with tincture of orange, to be taken with the oil.

9th.—Aspect much brighter; tongue cleaner and moister; appetite improved; and patient gets up for some hours in the day. Cough only at night and in the morning, and expectoration frothy. *Crepitation in right lung has diminished.* Pulse 100; temperature 99·2; respiration 28.

March 28th.—Has steadily improved in the last three weeks, and gaining in flesh and strength. Oil and sulphurous acid have been taken the whole time. Breath remains short. *Some dulness above the right scapula, with increased vocal fremitus, and slight crepitation in the upper front; some crepitation at the posterior base of both lungs. Harsh tubular expiration throughout the left lung.* Pulse 96; temperature 98·1; respiration 28.—Ordered oil, with diluted nitro-hydrochloric acid.

April 21st.—Now walks about, though finds breath rather short. Cough only in fits. Has taken oil regularly. Pulse 80; temperature 98·4; respiration 24. *In right chest slight dulness and crepitation to third rib. Some scattered crepitus behind. In left chest crepitation has quite disappeared, but harsh tubular sounds are audible in parts.*

In this case hæmoptysis occurred several times without giving rise to any inflammatory symptoms; but at length after an attack, pneumonia was set up, which was happily ended in resolution.

The following is a remarkable instance of hæmoptysis, ending in fatal suppuration.

Case 26.—A nobleman, aged 48, of a gouty family, first consulted Dr. Williams, July 18, 1855. He had suffered from gout more or less for years,

similarly extensive hæmoptysis, the average was 8 years
3·23 months—about the same as that of the living cases
generally. These facts certainly do not indicate that
hæmoptysis exercises any curtailing influence over phthisis
viewed as a whole. When, however, we classify the deaths
according to the stages the patients were in when the
hæmorrhage took place, we perceive the significance
which attaches to the state of lung at the time of its
occurrence :—

Stage.	No. of Deaths.	Average Duration.	
		Yrs.	Mths.
1	26	9	2·11
2	16	7	4·62
3	21	7	1·42

We here see that hæmoptysis occurring in the second
or third stages is more likely to curtail the duration of
the disease than in the first; and in the first, as in phthisical cases generally, it is comparatively unimportant.

CHAPTER XVII.

OUTLINE OF PHYSICAL SIGNS OF VARIETIES AND STAGES OF PULMONARY CONSUMPTION.

Signs of Phthisis originating in Bronchitis—Of Pneumonia passing into Phthisis—Suppuration—Signs of Congestion leading to Phthisis or Emphysema—Signs of miliary Tubercles—Signs of increasing Disease—Softening—Excavation—Corruption—Signs of Cure, and arrest of Consumption—Complete—Partial—Residuary Lesions and Signs—Calcareous Expectoration.

THERE has been so much said on the pathology and clinical history of consumptive diseases, that we cannot afford space for a complete separate description of their signs and symptoms. It must suffice to sketch the most common and remarkable physical signs which attend the development and progress of phthisis in its chief varieties.

When a common cough or bronchial cold turns to consumption, there will generally be an increase of the signs of bronchitis in particular spots, especially in the upper portions of the lungs. Below a clavicle, or at or above a scapula, a persistent sonorous or sibilant rhonchus, or still more any degree of crepitus, is suspicious; and the more so, if these signs are confined to these parts. In general capillary bronchitis there is also crepitus; but, then, it is more in the lower than in the upper regions. All fine crepitus may be taken as a sign of the parenchyma being either congested or inflamed; and the finer, the sharper, and closer to the ear—the more purely vesicular, like the crepitation of pneumonia. But the crepitus of early phthisis is not like this; it is more subcrepitant, crump-

ling, or mere roughening, of inspiratory sound, and often
accompanies the expiratory, which the crepitation of pneumonia never does.   The natural vesicular breath-sound is
impaired, or superseded, by the crepitation, except when
it is so slight as only to roughen it.   Fine crepitus, with
or instead of the breath-sound, signifies some intermitting
or vibrating obstruction to the entry of air into the lung
tissue, such as may be produced by swelling and increased
secretion of the bronchioles and air-cells.   Now, wherever
these sounds of crepitating obstruction are heard, it may
be inferred that some plastic or histotrophic change is
going on—sarcophytes are at work, proliferating and
migrating, whether for euplastic or for phthino-plastic
results: therefore does the sign at its first appearance
demand attention.

Soon other signs follow, indicating the partial consolidation of the lung.   The sound on percussion becomes
duller, very slightly it may be at first, but still perceptible on careful manipulation, and on comparison of the
two sides of the chest.   Then may come also the tubular
sounds, usually inaudible through the ill-conducting lung
texture, but now transmitted through its becoming more
solid.   These are hardly distinct where and whilst the
crepitation prevails; but as this diminishes with increased
obstruction, in situations overlying considerable bronchi,
below the clavicle, above, within, and at the scapulæ, and
in the axillary and middle dorsal regions, the sound of air
passing into and out of the tubes is heard, having more
or less of a whiffing or sharper blowing quality, which
contrasts well with the soft diffused character of vesicular
breath-sound.   Often too, but not always, the morbid
sound differs in an increase in loudness and duration of
the expiratory sound, which is hardly audible in natural
breath.   This is not one and the same thing as tubular
breath-sound, for although this commonly includes it, yet

sound, transmitted from the large tubes, expiration may be made audible and prolonged by any resistance to the escape of air through the small tubes, short of producing a rhonchus or wheeze (which is a totally different sound), and such a resistance may be caused by tubercles or other solids outside these tubes. So likewise the expiratory part of tubular breath-sound is increased in intensity, by partial obstructions in the large bronchi, as at the root of the lungs, from pressure of enlarged bronchial glands; in the trachea, from goitre or aneurism; in the larynx, from constricted glottis; and even in the throat by enlarged tonsils. Exaggerated tubular sounds of this kind may sometimes be heard through every part of the lungs, where there is no disease, but then may readily be traced back to their source. Excluding such extreme cases, tubular sounds near the root of the lung, especially the right, heard above and within the scapulæ, are among the earliest and most common signs of disease in the lungs; and it is rare to find a case with mischief in other parts of the lung of any duration, without this becoming manifest. But I have before explained that it may arise from an enlargement of the bronchial glands, without involving the lung tissue; and whilst we recognise its significance, as proving an infection of part of the lymphatic system, we must not accept it as an indication of the consolidation reaching into the lung, without the additional evidence of dulness on percussion, bronchophony, or impaired, or crepitating vesicular sound in the part.

Bronchophony, or tubular voice, does not always accompany tubular breath-sound. It generally requires more consolidation to transmit it, and a greater freedom of the tubes from constriction and secretion. It is most heard in vicinity of large tubes, like tubular breath ; and its combination with this forms the snuffling or whispering bronchophony so ominous under a clavicle, or above a scapula. Over smaller tubes it has often a reedy quality, as in the mammary and subscapular regions.

If phthisical tendency prevails, soon signs of softening and excavation follow, in increase of crepitation in one or more spots, looser and coarser, or of more croaking character, generally with diminished breath-sound, and small crepitation around. These spots, soon becoming cavities, form little islands of cavernous voice and breath-sound, first mixed with coarse crepitus or gurgling; afterwards, more croaky and dry, with the characteristic pectoriloquy, and the occasional concomitant, cracked-pot, or chinking percussion. When the cavities become large, the souffle voilée, or cavernous puff with the cough ; the amphoric resonance or metallic tinkling, which I long ago explained as an echo from the walls of the cavity, give decisive information of the ravages of the consuming disease in the lung.

Thus, in bronchitis passing into phthisis, there is a gradual transition of the signs of the former into those of the latter. In the variety when the phthino-plasms are peribronchial, there is a longer persistence of bronchial rhonchi, sonorous, sibilant and mucous, giving the disease a wheezy or asthmatic character, until softening ensues and cavities form, which relieve the constrictions.

Acute pneumonia passing into phthisis, from the hepatisation being a plastic or of cheesy nature, is marked by the persistent dulness and by the same loud[1] tubular

---

[1] The remarkable loudness of the tubular sounds of a completely hepatised lung has not to my knowledge been satisfactorily explained. The 'consonance' of Skoda is not applicable, inasmuch as it would require a certain relation between the sound of the voice and the size of the tube, as

sounds, and other signs of consolidation giving place to coarse liquid crackling or gurgling, commonly in the central or superior portions of the lung, and the signs of one large or of several small cavities soon follow, to announce the rapid destruction in this form of galloping consumption.

The signs of suppuration of the lung, or abscess ending in phthisis, are those of one or more cavities forming and extending; and of tubercles or other phthinoplasms forming in other parts—such as crepitus, dulness, and tubular sounds at or near the apex of the opposite lung, which may have been previously sound.

The more common mode in which pneumonia or pleuropneumonia terminates in phthisis, is through the chronic consolidation, which they leave behind them, instead of dispersing, becoming *phthinoplasms* — that is, degenerating into fibroid and caseous matter, the one dwindling and contracting—the other softening and disintegrating—the affected tissues of the lung. The course

in the case of the reciprocating notes of tubes or chords. But I believe the true explanation to lie in the fact that, whereas the lungs are naturally constructed to destroy the vocal sound by the tubes ending in a spongy texture, which thoroughly damps or chokes all sonorous vibration—so sooner is this spongy tissue made solid than the tubes become reflecting cavities, capable of reverberating the voice with all the loudness which it has in the trachea, and the vocal vibrations are not only heard, but may be felt by the hand applied over the part. Thus the voice is not only better conducted, as supposed by Laennec, but it is also greatly intensified, by the solidification of the lung. There is yet another acoustic effect developed in the tubes of a consolidated lung, which explains the loudness and almost musical tone of its tubular breath-sound. Naturally the air passes to and fro in the tubes and air-cells, and although its passage causes the breath-sound, and any accidental rhonchus in the tubes, yet this prevents any longitudinal vibrations in the whole tube. But when the tubes are stopped at their ventricular end by consolidation, the air breathed no longer passes through them, but passing across their open ends, in its way to and from the still pervious lung, it may cause a hollow whistling sound like that produced by blowing across the open mouth of a panpipe. The same principles are applicable to some sounds heard in cavities in the lungs.

phthinoplasms is marked by the signs of extensive dulness, absence of vesicular breath-sound and motion,
and exaggeration of tubular sounds of breath and voice,
persisting for months or even years; the collapse and
slight dull sound of the walls of the chest of the contracting portions; the irregular and sometimes cracked or
chinking dulness over the parts undergoing caseation and
excavation, which also yield their signs of crepitation and
gradually increasing cavernous sounds; whilst, in other
portions of the lung, the breath-sound may be puerile, or
mixed with crackling, from emphysematous over-distension,
which is also seen in the protrusion of the intercostal or
supraclavicular spaces on coughing. These and other variations in the signs of post-inflammatory phthisis have been
already noticed, and will be found exemplified in the
related cases, therefore it is unnecessary to enter into
further details here.

There is another mode in which phthinoplasms, both
contractile and caseating, may form and induce consumption, without any distinct inflammatory attack; without
pain or fever; with little cough and expectoration; but
generally with shortness of breath and weakness. A peculiar crumpling crepitus invades a considerable portion of
one or ‚both lungs, superseding the breath-sound in the
part—in some cases gradually inducing dulness and
tubular sounds; in others becoming mixed with wheezing
rhonchi and the clear stroke-sound of emphysema. The
primary condition seems to be one of congestion rather
than inflammation—hence the absence of active symptoms, and the slow rate at which phthisical processes
follow. In fact, they sometimes do not follow; but that
portion of the lung becomes partially emphysematous,
and the tendency to further deposit is thereby restrained.
This is a common result of those long-continued congestions at the base of the lungs, resulting from organic

Our lamented colleague, the late Dr. Theophilus Thompson, and others, have laid much stress on the wavy or jerking respiration (*respiration saccadée, entrecoupée*) as an early sign of phthisis; but no one seems to have traced it to its true cause. It is nothing more than the respiratory sound modified or divided by the successive pulsations of the heart. These, on the left side especially, slightly impede the passage of air in part of the lung, and thus give its sound a jerking or interrupted character. The presence of tubercles in the lung increases this effect by transmitting the heart's pressure further, and by narrowing the area of the passing air. Hence, too, this kind of respiration is observed most in females, with a narrow chest, and a palpitating heart; and in such I have frequently heard the wavy breathing, without any evidence of the existence of disease of the lung at all. With this understanding of the true nature of the sign, we can better estimate its value as indicative of disease in the lung.

The same remark may be applied to the subclavian arterial murmur which was mentioned by Dr. Stokes as a sign of incipient phthisis. It is caused by pressure of the apex of the lung on the artery, and although such pressure is more readily produced when the lung is partially condensed, yet it does occur in some subjects without any disease of the lung.

With the advance of the tubercles to caseation and the infection of new parts of the lung, the various degrees of crepitus, click, and croak become developed, and are the more striking in lymphatic or infected tuberculosis, from not being preceded by the rhonchi or crepitus of inflammation. And the signs which follow—increased dulness, tubular sounds, cavernous croak and gurgle, pectoriloquy, hollow puff or souffle with cough, &c.—commonly have a more remarkable character of isolation in this than in

As we do not profess to give a complete history of consumptive disease in its worst as well as in its more tractable form, it is not necessary to dwell on the *symptoms* which mark this last stage of decay. They indicate not only rapid degeneration and waste, but often corruption and decomposition, in which septic parasites, vibrios, bacteria, and aphthous fungi, lend their destructive aid. Thus φθίσις passes into φθορά. It is not to be forgotten, in connection with the subject of this worst form of decay, the putrefactive, that it sometimes occurs at an earlier stage in the form of gangrene and gangrenous abscess, and the fœtor is a physical sign of its presence. The secretion of dilated bronchi is sometimes also very offensive, from being long retained, in consequence of the mechanical difficulty in expectorating it.

The signs of the cure of phthisis might be expected to be the complete disappearance of those of the disease, but it is rare that the disease and its effects are so completely removed as to leave no trace behind. We can record a few cases of incipient disease, chiefly of inflammatory origin, and of decidedly consumptive character, in which crepitation, dulness, and tubular sounds, have been entirely removed, and the patients have been restored to complete health.

But the commoner degree of what may still be called a cure, is where the general health is recovered, cough, and expectoration, and other symptoms, have ceased; yet the physical signs, whilst showing a cessation of all active disease, still indicate traces of its effects on the lungs and their coverings. Thus, a collapse under a clavicle; a flattening of the upper or lateral walls of the chest; slight variations in the sound on percussion, and in the respiratory movements; a weakness or a mere roughness of the in-breath-sound in the former seat of disease; a remnant of tubular sound, especially above a scapula, in trifling changes left by former diseases, but not materially interfering with function or structure, and therefore productive of no further disorder than perhaps slight shortness of breath, and disposition to cough on exertion and on changes of temperature.

If the disease has lasted long, and especially if its phthinoplasms have passed into caseation and softening, more permanent injury is done to the lung textures; and although even these, if limited, may be checked and repaired, there remains more or less injury to the organ, producing various characteristic signs. Some of these have been already noticed in the pathological history of of the disease (pages 38, 63), and will be further exemplified in the abstracts of cases.

In the acute forms of phthisis, the first step towards arrest or cure is by the disease becoming chronic; the high temperature and other febrile symptoms subsiding, the pulse losing its frequency, and some abatement taking place in cough, oppression, pain, and other local symptoms. The physical signs, although more tardily, also show a change; the crepitus becoming less liquid, and more croaking or crumpling, and small degrees of it (subcrepitation) being heard in parts previously quite obstructed; and the dulness on percussion diminishes, in parts at least, and often is replaced by patches of unusual clearness (emphysema). If excavations exist, their cavernous sounds become more croaking and dry, and albeit often louder, yet more limited in extent; and the crepitus around them and in other parts of the lung diminishes or disappears.

A consideration of the more conservative and reparatory properties of the less decaying phthinoplasms will supply a key to a knowledge of some remarkable physical signs developed in cases of arrested phthisis. The forma-

tissue of fibroid, or scar-tissue, checks the progress of decay
and disintegration; but being itself a shrinking and
dwindling material, it causes contraction and puckering
of parts of the lung texture, and consequently either collapse of the corresponding chest-wall, or the emphysematous distension of neighbouring air-cells. Therefore
in chronic phthisis, where the disease is arrested or retarded in its progress, we often see partial sinking or
flattening of the walls of the chest, especially below and
above the clavicles, whilst near or even at the same spots,
a cough or forcible expiration will cause a protrusion of
emphysematous lung in the intercostal and supraclavian
spaces. And we have before pointed out (p. 65) that
in a considerable number of cases, this substitution of
emphysema for lung decay eventually converts phthisis
into habitual asthma, with its signs of tympanitic stroke-
sound, and wheezy dyspnœa and cough, and its symptoms
of limited respiration and circulation, and consequent
reptile scale of life.

In more partial forms of arrested phthisis, signs of
emphysema are common in the vicinity of old cavities or
cicatrices; namely, clear stroke-sound, dry whiffy breath-
sound, and sometimes more or less of a permanent dry
crepitus, generally in the middle or lower regions.

Among the cases will be found examples of permanent
recovery with signs of a cavity still persistent in the lung.
A few also are recorded of pneumothorax, with its unequivocal signs, terminating in complete recovery. Instances of calcareous expectoration are more numerous,
and may be referred to here, as affording a kind of physical
evidence of the arrest of phthisis by its decaying matter
passing into a state of mineral obsolescence. But some
of these examples show that even petrified phthinoplasm
may excite fresh symptoms; and it is commonly thrown
off in consequence of some new attack.

CHAPTER XVIII.

ABSTRACTS OF CASES ILLUSTRATING THE NATURE, VARIETIES, AND TREATMENT OF PULMONARY CONSUMPTION.

Large number of Cases—Grounds of Selection—Division into Groups—First Group—Phthisis originating in Inflammation—Acute Inflammation—Chronic Induration—Fibroid with Contraction—With Cavities—Purulent Phthisis.

DURING a period of upwards of thirty years I have been in the habit of keeping notes of every case of any gravity in which I have been consulted in private practice. I find that I have 256 little volumes of these notes, containing on an average 100 cases in each, amounting to 25,600 altogether. As it is difficult to deal with such large numbers, it has been judged advisable to make selections, both for statistical purposes and for illustration. The grounds of selections for statistics will be stated in the chapter on that subject. The selections of cases now made for illustration are intended to bear on the views on the pathology and treatment of pulmonary consumption as explained in this work : in truth, these cases are samples of the facts on which those views are founded. Where the facts are so numerous, there is much difficulty in dealing with them, in choosing the most instructive and representative cases, and in confining these within reasonable limits; and I am not at all sure that I have succeeded in either of these points. In the endeavour to abridge and condense details, I have been obliged to sacrifice elegance of diction and minuteness of description; but I hope that the histories will be sufficiently intelligible for practical purposes. It has been my practice in taking notes to confine them to the *positive* facts, or points of essential importance, and not to lengthen the description by *negations*, except in special instances. If a symptom is not described, its absence may be inferred, without the necessity of expressing 'no this' or 'no that.'

In thus professing a preference for brevity as essential in a practical work of this kind, I would not disparage the importance of accuracy and minuteness of description in clinical medicine generally; and students and young practitioners especially, should beware of slighting it. But from those sketching the results of large experience, a few bold outlines, drawn with a master's hand, may be as truthful and characteristic as a finished portrait, and are the best substitute where fulness of detail is inadmissible.

The value of numerous facts is much increased by their being accurately counted and calculated. Unfortunately, I have neither taste nor talent for figures, and it is the more satisfactory to me that my son has undertaken and worked diligently at the statistical parts of this book, and with results which appear to be of great importance. Judging from general impressions, when I delivered the Lumleian Lectures at the College of Physicians, I announced that in my experience the duration of life in pulmonary consumption had increased from two years to five. It will be seen in the chapter on that subject that, on numerically calculating the results in 1000 cases, the average duration was nearly eight years.

The cases will be distributed in groups, corresponding in some measure with the varieties indicated by the Table (p. 60), and described in the following chapters. The general head of Phthisis from Inflammation will form the first group, including these varieties:—*The Fibroid*, Chap. IV. and VIII.; *the Suppurative*, Chap. IX.; *the Chronic Pneumonic*, Chap. X.; *the Scrofulous Pneumonic*, Chap. XI.; and *the Catarrhal, Albuminous, and*

Hæmorrhagic, Chap. XII. This large group will also include other varieties originating in inflammation, but more mixed in their results. and in their course assuming more or less of the form of constitutional phthisis. See Chap. IV.

The second group comprehends phthisis of *Constitutional Origin*, which we have identified with the lymphatic system, Chap. V. This includes *Acute Tuberculosis*, *Chronic Tuberculosis*, and *Scrofulous Consumption*. Chap. XIV.

In some respects it must be admitted that this division is arbitrary, and I am by no means sure that the cases are all rightly distributed; but be it remembered, that the division is attempted to distinguish *varieties* only of *one common disease*; and although the recognition of these varieties may be useful to elucidate the forms which this disease may assume, yet it must not exclude the fact, that the disease is one and the same, and that the varieties are not always distinct, but may pass easily and variously into one another.

A group of miscellaneous cases is added; which will be found interesting in many particulars in both their nature and results.

CASES OF PHTHISIS ORIGINATING IN INFLAMMATION.

CASE 27.—*Pleuro-pneumonia. Acute Phthisis.*

E. J., aged 36, admitted into U. C. Hospital, December 19, 1840.—Carpenter; lived in London.—Quite well till four months ago; was attacked with pain in left mammary region, with cough and expectoration. Has continued to suffer ever since, with much loss of flesh and breath. Still frequent cough, with viscid, opaque expectoration. Pulse quick and weak. Sweats at night. Appetite bad.—*Imperfect expansion of the lungs on both sides; complete dulness in lower portion of left chest, with little breath sound, except in the mammary region, above which it was bronchial, but no vocal vibration. Dulness below right clavicle, with puerile breath-sound, and crepitus at end of each inspiration. Tubular sounds in right scapular region.*

One small bleeding; repeated blisters, and a variety of remedies were prescribed, but with very little benefit. He became rapidly worse with more laboured and very frequent breathing, rapid pulse, lividity of surface, and died December 29.

Six or eight ounces of serum in left pleura, and some loose masses of yellow lymph, with harder granules scattered through them. The whole left pleura, costal and pulmonary, very red and vascular, and studded with yellow granular tubercles, and with patches of lymph of the same color and density. The more diffused patches were between the lobes, and at their margins, here forming a layer a quarter of an inch thick; but they did not differ in color or density from the small granules, and there were gradations in size between these and the patches.

The left lung was partially consolidated by rounded tuberculous masses, some grey, some opaque yellow, without softening. The latter in color and consistence perfectly resembled the masses of lymph on the pleura.

Right lung partially adherent to the chest, the false membranes being dense, but not tuberculated. The lower lobes were almost completely consolidated by opaque yellow deposit, the masses of which appeared prominent through the pleura. When cut open, one large mass in the lower lobe was quite yellow opaque, and tough like the lymph on the left pleura. In other parts there was a mottling of the red and black of the lung tissue, like the appearance of Castile soap. The upper lobe of this lung was in he first stage of inflammation; very red, fragile, exuding frothy serum; and a few granular tubercles were scattered through it. Weight of lungs: right, 2lb. 15oz.; left, 1lb. 14oz.

Mucous membrane of larynx very vascular, with a few tubercles.

Mesenteric glands enlarged; and some contained yellow tuberculous matter, crude and soft.

CASE 28.—*Pleuritis. Phthisis.*

John B., admitted February 4, 1840; robust laborer. Mother died of phthisis. Quite well till three weeks ago; when had chills, cough, and short breath, with great weakness, which have continued, with much loss of flesh. Sputa viscid and greenish; pulse frequent; skin hot; urine scanty,

Right side of chest at lower part measures 1¼ *inch more than left. Complete dulness and absence of breath-sound in lower two-thirds of right chest. About fourth and fifth ribs at side friction sound with respiration. Stroke clear above third rib in front; clear stroke and puerile breath-sound on left side.*

Bled to 15oz. Twenty leeches to right side. Calomel and opium night and morning. Saline antimonial, ter die.

February 6.—Breath and cough much relieved. Pulse 104, sharp.

February 8.—Further relieved by blister, &c. Pulse 84; urine more copious.

February 18.—Continued better, with little complaint of breath or cough. Pulse 85. Gums sore from calomel. *Less dulness and more breath heard in right chest, with loud friction sound.*

February 27.—Breath has been getting ~~shorter, and cough more troublesome~~,[^] some, although he has been again blistered. Pulse 84. *More dulness in right chest, and loud leather-creak at the side.*

May 2.—Condition gradually become worse. Breath and cough always troublesome; only temporarily relieved by repeated blistering, &c. Pulse risen to 90. Expectoration now mucopurulent, sometimes rusty.

June 20.—Occasional sweats, and diarrhœa. Pulse 100. Losing flesh rapidly. Sputa viscid, purulent, sometimes streaked. *Dulness of right chest increased; and now cavernous sounds heard above left mammilla.*

Throat became aphthous, and died July 5.

Sectio 34 horis post mortem.

Body much emaciated.

Right pleura at posterior, contained a pint of turbid serum. Both pleuræ strongly adherent to upper, front, and back walls of chest, and in many parts thickened by red tough false membrane, thickest on right side, behind and laterally.

Right lung large, dense to the feel, scarcely at all crepitant. On cutting into it the substance is found pervaded by solid matter in grey opaque masses of roundish shape, from size of walnut to that of cherry-stone; these in many points presented opaque yellowish specks; and in some parts small cavities; these were chiefly in upper part of lung; towards the base the lung was more generally red and tough. The same appearances to less extent in left lung; the lower lobe most free; with dilated marginal air-cells. At apex of left lung was a cavity of size of hen's egg; the walls composed of dense tissue, studded with soft yellow tubercle; superiorly quite thin, consisting chiefly of pleura, which was quarter of an inch thick at this spot. Bronchial glands, enlarged and soft.

Pericardium contains ʒii yellow serum.

Heart pale, large and flabby, containing fluid blood, staining lining membrane; mitral valve thickened at free margins, by dense deposit under serous lining; attachments of aortic valves also thickened, and a little corrugated.

Several patches of ulceration, with raised edges, in mucous membrane of colon and rectum; no increased redness. Mesenteric glands slightly enlarged in several parts. Liver large; substance fragile.

CASE 29.—*Phthisis after Pleuro-pneumonia.*

Anne S., aged 42; admitted January 5, 1844. Tall, and has been very stout till the last four years. Has not been well fed in the last year. No serious illness till eighteen months ago, when she had severe pain in the side, which was called inflammation of the liver. Was ill for many weeks, and was bled, cupped, and blistered. There was tickling of throat, but not much cough till some time after, and it became much worse in November; lately with much opaque expectoration, and diarrhœa, and has become very

.... No return of catamenia since November. Pulse frequent; .... Extensive dulness in right chest, with loud cavernous sounds in ...... regions, front and back. Loud puerile breath in left lung.

Pills, with ⅛ grain sulphate of copper, opium, and creasote, three times a day, moderated the diarrhœa, but the cough became worse. Pyroxylic spirit was tried, but discontinued, as the purging returned, and continued till her death, which was preceded by an aphthous state of the mouth and inability to take food. The diagnosis given was extensive excavation and consolidation of right lung. Partial tubercles in left lung; tuberculous ulceration of intestines. Died February 5.

Body much emaciated. Five ounces turbid serum in left pleura, which posteriorly was patched with red and granular lymph. A few clusters of tubercles in the upper lobe of left lung, and some miliary granulations scattered below. Posterior parts of left lung red and congested, but lower part of upper lobe in state of soft grey consolidation, with a few small cavities. The right lung was generally and firmly adherent by dense cartilaginous deposit, which extended also between the lobes. The whole right lung was in a state of dense grey consolidation, speckled with yellow spots, and the upper lobes riddled with numerous cavities, freely communicating. Liver healthy, but small; weighed 2 lb. 8 oz. Several tuberculous ulcers in the ileum, and much inflammatory ...... through the small and large intestines.

Remarks.—In all probability this phthisis originated in the attack of pleuro-pneumonia which began the fatal illness, and ended in general consolidation of the right lung, the universal adhesions and dense thickening of the pleura between the lobes proving its inflammatory origin. Subsequently this lung caseated and softened, and miliary tubercles formed in the other lung.

CASE 30.—*Chronic Pleurisy. Phthisis.*

John B., aged 37; admitted July 26, 1844. Tailor. In good health till twelve months ago, after frequent exposure and often getting wet had cough and pains in limbs, with much weakness. Was out-patient of a hospital, with some relief; but in last two months has suffered with short breath, pain of right side, and temporary swelling of the legs. He also expectorated a quantity of dark stuff. Has lost much flesh, orthopnœa; urine very scanty; mouth aphthous. *Chest movements imperfect, especially over right side, which is altogether dull, except above the second rib, where stroke is tubular, and breath and voice sounds are tubular, and also above the scapula. No vesicular sound, but ægophony also below scapula. In left ...... puerile and stroke clear, but some dulness and tubular sound ...... crepitus below clavicle. Friction sound in left lower lateral and ...... regions. Heart pushed to below the mammilla. Liver reaches to*

A blister was applied, and he was given blue pill, squill. and digitalis, with decoction of Iceland moss, acetate potass. and borax. *ter die.*

July 27.—Breath not better; urine still scanty, albuminous, specific gravity, 1019. *Less friction sound in left back.* Pills omitted, and 4 grains calomel and ½ grain hydrochlorate morphia given at bed-time. No relief followed, and he died on the 29th.

Sectio 2 horis post mortem.—There were 10 pints of purulent serum in right pleura, with flakes of curdy lymph floating in it. Right lung compressed against mediastinum and spine, and middle dorsal ribs. Much tough opaque lymph over the surface of the lung in granules and in patches. On inflating the lung it became partly expanded, but was chiefly bound down by the deposits on the pleura. Texture of the lung flaccid, dry, dark purplish in colour, sinking in water; several small tubercles scattered through it, and a cluster of tubercles near the root, all dark grey-coloured and gritty—some near surface paler. Left lung covered with recent false membrane, forming a series of rough ridges of granular texture. Several grey tubercles in this lung, chiefly in upper lobe. Lower lobe heavy and congested. Yellow cheesy matter in bronchial glands. Weight of lungs: left, 2 lb. 9 oz.; right, 10 oz. Pericardium strongly adherent to whole heart; adhesions dense, especially over right ventricle. Heart, with pericardium, weighed 14 oz. Liver weight, 3 lb. 2 oz. Some granular irregularity of surface, with predominance of pale matter, and texture coarse. A few white tubercles scattered through it. Both kidneys much congested: texture soft: on surface of right one cyst and one white tubercle: weight, 5½ oz.: left, 5 oz. A few pale tubercles in spleen.

CASE 31.—*Chronic Pneumonia. Phthisis.*

Mary D., aged 57, admitted January 27, 1843; married, one child. Generally good health till winter 1840, when she had a severe cold, followed by cough and loss of flesh and strength. Lost cough in summer, but did not recover her strength; and in the following winter the cough returned, and has continued ever since with increasing expectoration, shortness of breath, and loss of flesh. Much worse in last six months; often suffering from severe spasms of the stomach and chest, and failure of appetite. Profuse night sweats. Pulse 100. Sputa copious, in separate opaque clots. *Dulness on percussion in both upper regions, most under right clavicle, where gurgling and cavernous breath.*—Ordered mixture diluted nitric acid, tincture of henbane and hop, three times a day.

February 4.—Cough easier, but the expectoration very purulent, and weakness increases. Wine and full diet. Two grains sulph. quinine to be added to each dose of mixture.

7th.—Getting weaker. Expectorates with difficulty darker matter. Pulse thready, irregular. Dozes much, and is incoherent.

... there was some rallying, but she gradually sank, and ... the 16th.

... 68 hours post mortem; body much emaciated. Right lung extensively and firmly adherent at apex by very tough old false membranes: ... and more recent adhesions posteriorly; middle and lower lobes covered by opaque rugous membrane, in parts shreddy and hardly organised. At posterior part of apex was a cavity, size of hen's egg; its walls little more than the thickened corrugated pleura; it contained purulent and curdy matter; its internal walls very red, pretty smooth, with shreds of opaque lymph. The middle and posterior portions of this lung were firmly consolidated, and dark red on section, with mottled grey and opaque yellow patches. Another small empty cavity in the anterior of upper lobe. Anterior portions of middle and lower lobes were pale, distended with air, and very flaccid and thin to touch, with general dilatation of air-cells. Left lung partially adherent at apex, in which also was a cavity, rather smaller than that in right lung, containing a little opaque liquid, and quite loose, an irregular calcareous nodule of the size of a horse-bean. Texture below this cavity much puckered, indurated, and mottled with perfectly black nodules for an inch downwards. A few clusters of very hard miliary tubercles were scattered through lower lobe of this lung; but the greater part was light, very pale, porous, and flaccid, with generally dilated air-cells (flaccid emphysema). Liver and kidneys small, and somewhat granular in ...

CASE 32.—*Chronic Pleuro-pneumonia. Fibroid Phthisis.*

A barrister, aged 45; March 18, 1843. Always delicate, with bilious ... Has been more ailing since losing his wife in consumption last autumn. In November in Cheshire, and after getting chilled, he had what was called rheumatic influenza. On return to town he found his breath short, and perceived that he was breathing with one side only. He consulted several physicians, and got almost as many different opinions; and was blistered and physicked in various ways without much benefit. He persisted, however, in going to chambers till the last three weeks, when the breathing has become much shorter, with dry cough and rapid ... Pulse 100, easily quickened; tongue furred. Urine scanty, ...

... *quite dull and rather contracted in lower two-thirds, and without ... or motion; upper third clear on percussion, with loud harsh ...; loose crepitus in mammary region. Right chest dull in lower half, ... or voice: above, loud reedy vocal resonance. Heart pulsation ... Liver dulness extended, with tenderness.*

... After treatment with repeated blisters, and at first mercurial ... and subsequently iodide potass. and sarza., great improvement took ... and strength, although he is still wasting and the breath ... No cough.

Signs on the left side unchanged. On the right there is less dulness, with some breath-sound with crepitus down to the lower third, and less bronchophony above.

He afterwards went to Sandgate, where his strength further improved; but the breath remained very short, with a little cough. The medical attendant then concluded that there was a cavity in the left lung. He died October 2, after a few days' illness with sickness, slight jaundice, and delirium.

On examination both pleuræ were found firmly adherent at diaphragm, and anterior and upper walls. Several ounces of serum in lower and posterior part of both pleuræ. Lower and posterior parts of both lungs (but most left) in a state of tough, red consolidation, or carnification; with crepitant tissue only on anterior surface. No trace of tubercle or cavity in either lung. Liver much congested and enlarged. Gall bladder contained a quantity of very dark bile.

CASE 33.—*Chronic Peripneumonia. Fibroid Phthisis.*

A proctor in Doctors' Commons, æt. 39, February 18, 1845. Sedentary, and much occupied in writing; but lives well. In last two years breath has been getting shorter, with slight cough, worse in winter. Losing flesh and strength; but face red with acne. Thinks he strained himself two years ago by running, which brought on severe pain in chest. Lately pain in right hypochondrium. Pulse quiet. Urine, scanty, dark. *Dulness with wheezing in upper third right back; crepitus with weak breath-sound at both bases.*

Under regulated diet, diminished stimulants, and a course of iodide potass. with carbonate potass. and sarza., and occasional mercurial aperient, considerable improvement took place: but the breath was still short, and *crepitus still in the back.*

July 31.—A week ago, after exposure to cold, a pain came on in the right side, which has been only partially relieved by a mercurial dose. Is chilly, and feels ill.—*Crepitus increased in both lower dorsal regions, which now are dull. Liver large and tender.*—C.C. lat. dextro, ad ʒviij. Pil. Hydrarg. scillæ et digitalis, bis die. Haustus sennæ o. m.

September 9.—Was relieved of the pain, and afterwards improved on a mixture of nitric acid, taraxacum and chiretta. Lately pain in right side has returned, with loss of flesh and breath.—*Dulness, with contraction, in right interscapular region, and in both lower dorsal, with crepitus.*

April, 1846.—Has had several attacks of low inflammation, affecting successively both lungs, with cough, mucopurulent expectoration, and much loss of flesh and strength. Has been repeatedly blistered, and had blue pill, squill, and digitalis, which gave temporary relief. In June some improvement took place, under iodide potass. and nitric acid three weeks. *Increased dulness and contraction with crepitus in lower half of right lung, and lower third of left.*

.... he moved to Brighton, and gradually declined, with the ordinary .... of consumption, constant cough, and opaque expectoration, and .... loss of flesh, strength, and breath. More than usual œdema .... his death, which took place at the end of 1848.

His usual attendant, Mr. Ridout, informed me that, on examination after death, both lungs were found universally and firmly adherent, and their lower lobes in a state of dense, tough, reddish-grey consolidation. No cavities or tubercles.

These two cases are remarkable exceptions to the general degenerating tendency of phthinoplasms. The fibroid induration persisted without either caseation or tubercular formation. But the wasting process was still there, the decaying matter passing off in the purulent expectoration.

Case 34.—*Fibroid Phthisis after Pleurisy. Cavities.*

Mrs. M., aged 20, seen October 18, 1842. Two and a-half years ago she had pleurisy of left side; since then has had slight cough, and breath has been short. In last year has had several recurrences of pain and cough, and is now much worse, after exposure to cold outside a coach three weeks ago. The cough is suffocating, with copious purulent expectoration, sweats, and extreme dyspnœa. *Moist cavernous sounds under both clavicles. Extended dulness in region of liver.*

The patient died the same night. On *post-mortem* examination the left lung was found to be closely adherent to the back and side of the chest wall. It was much shrunk, nearly the whole front being occupied by the heart. Texture of left lung was of dark colour, and very dense, with a few cavities. Right lung not condensed, but with several tubercles and cavities, chiefly in upper lobe. Liver large and fatty, floating in water.

Case 35.—*Phthisis after Pneumonia.*

Mr. C., aged 30, February 12, 1856.—Four years ago had inflammation of the right lung, and ever since has had cough, with yellow expectoration, and lost much flesh and strength. Taken oil for two years. *Dulness; defined and obstructed breath-sounds throughout the right chest. Large .... sounds and crepitation in upper portions.* To continue the oil, with a .... of nitric acid. hop. &c., and occasionally use acetum lyttæ.

.... 25, 1857.—Has taken oil on and off ever since, but always in the .... Is wonderfully improved in all respects, but never quite free from .... with expectoration, which has lately been worse, and accompanied by .... the right side. Bowels costive. Suffers from piles. Has several .... expectorated calcareous matter. *Dulness and tubular sounds above .... ; ne crepitus, and chest clear elsewhere.*—To continue oil and .... confection with sulphate of potass.

.... 1870.—Pretty well, and attending to business. Flesh and strength good ; but always some cough with yellow expectoration, and flatulent coryza. Sometimes bilious, and liver now tender.—*Dulness, and during inspiration and long expiration at and below right scapula.*—To take a blue pill occasionally, and the oil once daily.

CASE 36.—*Pleurisy ending in Phthisis.*

Master H., aged 10, June 26, 1863.—Delicate, but pretty well till, a fortnight ago, fainted at church ; after which slight pain of chest, and cough, but not laid up till last two days with increasing shortness of breath and swelling of left breast. *Whole left side quite dull and motionless. Dulness extends to right of sternum and spine, and heart displaced to right of sternum. Intercostal spaces bulge, especially near left mammilla.* A mixture of citrate and nitrate of potass was prescribed, but arrangements were made for tapping the chest next day. On the morrow, however, the dyspnœa was less, and the swelling less prominent ; so a blister was applied, and the saline continued. He gradually recovered, the fluid dispersing, and weak breath-sound and resonance returning to the left side ; but considerable dulness and contraction remained in August. Cod-oil with tonic, iodine tincture externally, and country air were prescribed. This treatment was carefully pursued, and in 1865 he was considered quite well, having nearly outgrown the contraction of the left chest, which was, however, still apparent.

August 3rd, 1867.—Has been well, and is now at Harrow. Three weeks ago caught cold, and has since had pain in left side, wheezing, and cough. Looks ill. Pulse 100.

Deficient motion and percussion, and croaky rhonchi through left lung.—To resume the oil and have iodine painted.

February 17, 1869.—Improved, and lost cough soon. Has been pretty well since, but grows fast, and requires care. In the last three weeks has again had cough and short breath, and appetite has been failing.

Dulness and tubular sounds now at and above right scapula.—Left lung more free.

June 26, 1869.—Improved with constant treatment and care ; but there is still some cough, and lately a little blood has appeared in the expectoration. Bowels not free ; and he has been taking quinine pills as well as the oil and mixture.

Dulness and tubular sounds at right scapula, rhonchi at left.—Oil to be taken with phosphoric acid and hypophosphite of soda. Bowels to be carefully regulated, and iodine regularly used.

July 29, 1869.—Much better, cough gone, and *signs diminished.*—Continue same.

November 2, 1869.—Continued better till return to Harrow, when cough again, with pain in chest and increasing weakness. To go to Ventnor.

Croaky crepitus at and above left scapula. Tubular sounds above right.

April 18, 1870.—At Ventnor, taking oil, &c., and better till January 7,

..... worse, and spit 2 oz. of blood; since expec-
...... appetite bad, bowels costive.—Oil has been left off three
..... and in her taken iron.

*Much dulness and creaky obstruction through left lung; tubular or caver-
nous in upper part.*—To resume oil, with phosphoric acid and strychnia
mixture. Bowels to be kept regular. Tinct. iodine to be regularly applied.

June 7, 1871.—Continued pretty well during the summer, and in December went to Madeira, and, as advised, steadily persevered with the oil
and tonic, and rode regularly up the hills; so he kept fairly well. On voyage home, a fortnight ago, encountered cold winds, and cough much increased, with yellow expectoration. *Left chest rather contracted. Heart
beats at fifth rib. Moderate dulness, and crumpling subcrepitus through
left lung. No cavernous sounds, but tubular above scapula.*

CASE 37.—*Fibroid Phthisis, with cavity, arrested 15 years.
Emphysema.*

A merchant, aged 45, first consulted Dr. Williams July 13, 1855. Was
well till eight months ago, when he caught a severe cold, with cough and
yellow expectoration, which have continued, with much loss of flesh, and
lately with very short breath. Took oil in the winter, but soon sickened of
it. *Extreme dulness on left side of chest, mostly in upper front, where there
are large tubular sounds, and some liquid rhonchus, almost gurgling. Less dulness behind, but tubular sounds and mucous rhonchus.*—Ordered oil in a
basis of nitric and hydrocyanic acids and strychnia, and counter-irritation
with acetum cantharidis.

April 19th, 1856.—Wintered at Hastings, and very much improved under
the above treatment. Now walks six miles. *Still marked hard dulness
and obstructed breath in left front; but voice less tubular. Coarse crepitation in parts.*

November 28th, 1856.—Passed summer well, but six weeks ago brought
up half a pint of blood, and was largely leeched. Has taken oil regularly,
except during six weeks, and is quite stout. Breath still short, Cough
has increased in last ten days. *Physical signs the same, except the addition
of loud tubular breath above right scapula.*—To continue oil, but in tonic of
nitric and hydrocyanic acids, with iodide of potassium and tincture of

April 26th, 1857.—Continues well, and fatter than ever. Breath short,
but walks six miles. Just now has headache and increase of cough.

December 7, 1859.—Passed last winter at Hull, and pretty well; but
breath short, and had morning expectoration. No oil for one year. Has
lately had more cough and slight hæmoptysis. *Dulness, cavernous croaking in upper left chest.*

February 21, 1861.—Has taken oil, but was shut up at Hull all the
winter. Lost flesh, and lately appetite and strength. Cough increased,

and occasionally streaked expectoration. *More ... . left, front and back.*—Ordered strychnia, with oil.

March 29, 1862.—At Hull through the winter, and not ... . house; but breath shorter, and losing flesh since August. Three weeks ago had pain in left side, increase of cough and expectoration, which was more opaque. Symptoms relieved by blisters, and patient has resumed the oil and strychnia since. *Large tubular sounds and crepitation in upper left front and back. Cavernous sounds below clavicle.*

March 24, 1864.—Again recovered, and has been generally well. Has little cough, but breath very short. Weighs twelve stone. Attends to business. No oil for one year. *Less dulness, no cavernous sounds, but breath weak and subcrepitant. Tubular voice, and little breath at and within left scapula. Large tubular sounds above right scapula.*—Ordered nitric acid, tincture of nux vomica, and glycerine.

March 7, 1865.—Fatter, and pretty well; but breath always short. Six weeks ago had hemiplegia of left side, and confused state of mind; but, after leeching and blistering, was relieved. *Moderate dulness, crepitation, and croaky sounds over whole left chest. No large tubular sounds, except above right scapula.*

June 1, 1866.—Pretty well; but lately palpitation, and pain in left arm. *Breath-sounds feebly audible throughout left lung, only tubular in back.*

April 15, 1868.—Was pretty well; but during last year breath has become shorter, and palpitation has increased. Has little cough, with only transparent expectoration. No oil for two years and a half, and has spent the last winter at Hull. *More dulness in left front, and upper back, and large tubular or carvernous sounds above left scapula and immediately below left clavicle; dulness and obstruction sounds in lower part of left lung, with some sibilus; more tubular sounds in upper right chest. Heart's apex drawn up, and beating at left mamilla; action weak.*

March 4, 1869.—Wintered at Hull pretty well, with little cough, but breath very short on exertion, and some palpitation. *Still moderate dulness and defective breath and motion throughout left chest, but no carvernous sounds, and tubular only at and above scapula. Heart-sound and impulse, high and feeble.*—To take three drops of liquor arsenicalis and two grains of hypophosphite of soda in a gentian and glycerine mixture, twice a day.

February 26, 1870.—Improved much in strength, and somewhat in breath during the summer, complaining only of his breath. Lately has suffered from fluttering at heart. Four months ago, for three days, had difficulty of articulation, but it passed off; only he complains of his memory failing. Lately closely confined to the house, and has indigestion, and become paler. Urine high coloured and scanty. *Physical signs much the same. Liver rather full and tender.*—To take iodide of potassium and digitalis, with tincture of calumba, and a few mercurial pills.

May 26, 1870.—Health and appetite better; but breath very short, and

...when he leaves off medicine. About three months ...well; and he died suddenly in a faint.

...degree of dulness in the left chest found on first exami-... it probable that the disease was inflammatory, causing a hard ...deposit. This was afterwards partly softened and excavated, ...absorbed and contracted. The general inference from several examinations (some of which for want of space have not been given) was, that emphysematous dilatation of the air-cells took place in the consolidated front of the left lung, rendering the stroke-sound more clear, whilst the breath and voice were obscured; but the signs of old cavity and consolida-tion were still heard in the scapular region. In the last two years the lung disease was stationary, and there was neither cough nor expectoration; but the heart showed signs of weakness, and death is to be referred to this ...Post-mortem examination not permitted. More than fifteen years elapsed since the first attack.

Case 38.—*Chronic Induration after Inflammation.*

A builder, aged 37, first consulted Dr. W. January 13, 1842. Has lost a child from tuberculous disease of the lung. Twenty years ago had inflammation of the chest, for which he was bled, and was very ill for six months. Remained very weak till two years after, when he went to Venice, where he improved sufficiently to resume his occupation, but was always short-breathed, with more or less cough. Five years ago, after much exertion, was attacked with pain in the chest and dyspnœa, lasting six weeks, and has had cough every winter since. Symptoms worse since September after exposure, with loss of strength and flesh. *Dulness under both clavicles; deficient breath under left; and bronchophony, almost amount-ing to pectoriloquy, under humeral end of right clavicle.* Expectoration scanty, sometimes tinged with blood.—Ordered iodide of potassium, sar-saparilla, and liquor potassæ; also counter-irritation.

December, 1842.—Much improved in flesh and strength; little or no cough; dulness diminished; tubular sounds almost gone.

June, 1845.—Heard from Dr. Martin that he was quite well, and busy at work in the Isle of Wight.

Well and active in 1869, *twenty-seven years after his first visit, and forty-seven after his first attack of inflammation of the chest.*

It is by no means clear that the disease in this case ever assumed a de-cidedly tuberculous character; but it may be considered one of phthino-plastic deposit resulting from inflammation, and capable of degenerating. It is a significant fact that one of his children has died of tubercles in the lungs.

CASE 39.—*Fibroid after Inflammation.*

A gentleman, aged 32, who had lost a brother and sister from consumption, first consulted Dr. W. January 25, 1855, and stated that a year ago he suffered from pleurisy of the left side, and since that time from weakness and short breath. No cough or expectoration, but lately had pain below the left clavicle. *Extreme dulness over the whole of the left side of chest, with only weak breath in upper portion ; expiration and voice tubular ; heart close to chest-wall, and felt over a large space.* Arcus senilis well marked ; urine scanty. Has taken cod-liver oil, but it purges.—Ordered oil combined with tannic acid and infusion of orange ; iodide liniment to be rubbed on chest.

May 23.—Oil agreed well. Much improved in flesh, but still weak ; urine still thick ; appetite bad. *Left side a little less dull, but no more breath-sound or motion.*—To take iodide of potassium, liquor potassae, and sarsaparilla.

August 13.—Has been at Ems, where the waters proved strongly diuretic. Breath and strength improved, but has now slight cough. *Still dulness, although less, and weak breath in left chest.*

May 6, 1856.—Continues pretty well ; but often pain in left chest, and urine turbid, unless when taking the iodide and potass mixture, which has been continued at times. *Some further diminution of dulness, and slight return of breath-sound, chiefly in upper parts.*

October 23.—Pretty well, till five weeks ago, large boils appeared on the cheek and throat. *Chest continues to improve.*—Ordered chlorate of potass, with nitric acid and quinine.

March 17, 1857.—No more boils, but lately is thinner and weaker. *Still defective breath and dulness in lower left chest.*—To take oil in quinine mixture.

June 4.—Better in flesh and breath ; *also in chest sounds.*

October 14.—Lately has slight cough and more pains in chest. Has lost flesh. No oil or medicine lately.

April 21, 1858.—Well through winter, but in last two weeks cough and yellow expectoration. *Signs the same.*—Oil and acid tonic to be resumed.

July 14.—Took oil and tonic six weeks, and lost cough. In last month large boil on neck, now discharging.—To take syrup of iodide of iron, tincture of calumba, and glycerine.

March 5, 1859.—Passed winter pretty well, but continues thin. In last week cough and expectoration. *Breath still weak, and limited motion in lower chest, but sound on percussion clearer. In left scapular region stroke-sound is tubular.*

This patient has not been seen since 1861, when he was reported to be well and improving in breath, and may be presumed to have recovered.

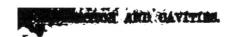

Case 48.—Phthisis after Inflammation.—Post-mortem.

A lady, aged 35, was first seen December 14, 1841. Had three children and four miscarriages. Had suffered from phlegmasia dolens, mammary abscess, and other puerperal complaints. Twelve years ago had right pleurisy; and ever since breath has been short, with some cough. Suffered lately from pain and tightness of the chest. Occasional hæmoptysis to the amount of several ounces. Has been often bled for the tightness of the chest, and with much relief; but has lately become very pale and weak. Cough has increased, and is occasionally accompanied with profuse muco-purulent expectoration and night-sweats; aphonia; pulse 120. *Dulness throughout right chest, especially in the lowest parts, where there is little motion. Tubular breath in middle, front and back. Cavernous sounds in lower back. Subcrepitus under left clavicle; breathing puerile below, throughout left chest. Heart beating under sternum. Liver enlarged.*—Ordered iodide of iron with tincture of hops, and aconite ointment for neuralgic pain.

March 8, 1842.—In the country, and improved in breath and colour, but lost flesh, and in last few days had pain and œdema of left leg. Cough better, with expectoration more mucous and slightly tinged with blood. *Breath and voice loudly amphoric in lower right back; obscurely vesicular above, but shortened. Right front very resonant, with loud cough and tubular breath. Tubular sounds under left clavicle.* Dyspnœa and weakness increased, with extensive œdema in both legs up to the abdomen; and she died on June 11.

On post-mortem examination the left lung was found to contain scattered grey tubercles in the upper lobe, and a small cavity, with broken-down walls, at apex, where the lung was adherent to the chest. The right lung was adherent on all sides, except in front; adhesions being tough and firm, especially that connecting the lung to the diaphragm. The tissue of the lower lobe was solid, tough, and of a dark-grey colour; the bronchi greatly dilated, even to their ends. In the posterior portion was a well-lined cavity, of the size of a large egg, containing purulent fluid and communicating by three round openings with dilated bronchi; a smaller cavity at the base of this lobe. The middle lobe was very emphysematous and flaccid in front, but consolidated behind, and contained nodules of grey tubercle. In the upper lobe was a cavity of the size of an orange, with grey irregular walls, containing broken-down tubercle. The rest of the lung was in a state of grey consolidation, which in some parts had become yellow and softened. The large bronchi were very red.

In this case the contractile consolidation of the lung, resulting from inflammation twelve years before, eventually went into tuberculous degeneration. This case occurred before the use of cod-liver oil was well known, and may be contrasted with the following examples.

... ...
... ...

Night sweats.—... ... pretty well ... ... with taking ... ... before around at times. ... ... agree ... ... quiet ...

... 2?.—Pretty well. Little dry ... cough and throat. ... ... with ... and quinine.

March 17, 1877.—No worse ... but little better ... bowels and did less to ... ... mixture.

June 4.—Better in flesh and breath ... ...

October 14.—Lately has slight cough at ... flesh ... or medium. Lately ...

April 21, 1878.—Well ... ... winter and yellow expectoration. ... ... resumed ...

July 14.—Took cold and took six weeks ... ... That

A lady, aged 35, was first seen December ?, 184?. Had three
children and four miscarriages. Had suffered from ?????????
mammary abscess, and other puerperal complaints. Twelve years ago
had right pleurisy; and ever since found her very much out of
cough. Suffered lately from pain and tightness of the chest. Had raised
hæmoptysis to the amount of several ounces. Has been three days in
tightness of the chest, and with much relief, but has only been some
pale and weak. Cough has returned, and is ?????????????????? with
profuse muco-purulent expectoration, and expectoration affords ???? ??
*Inhales throughout right chest, especially in the lower part, where has a
little motion. Tubular sound is audible, but the ????, ???????? sound*
in lower back. Subcrepitus rale of ????? throughout ????, ??
throughout left chest. Heart beating over ?????. Liver ???????
Ordered iodide of iron with tincture of hops and ?????? mixture for
neuralgic pain.

March 8, 1842.—In the country, and ??????? ?? much attention, is
but fresh, and in last few days had some alteration of ?????. ?????
better, with expectoration now ????? of ????? ???? ?? ????
Breath and ???? ????? ???????? a ???? ???? ???, ??????? ?? ?????
close, but shortened. Right front ???????? ???? ?? ?? ?? ??
breath. Tubular sounds under left ??????. ???????? ?? ??????? in-
creased, with extensive ????? in ????? ????? ?? the ?????? and she
died on June 11.

On post-mortem examination he ?? ??? ???? ???????
grey tubercles in the upper side and a small ??????? ?? ?? the
walls, at apex, where the lung was ??????? ???????. The ??? ??
was adherent on all sides, except a few ?????? ?? ?? ???, and at ????
especially that concerning the lung at the ?????. In ???? of the
lower lobe was solid, tough, and ???? ???? ?? ??? ??? ??? were ????
dilated, even to their exit. In the ????? were ??? ?? ?? ????
cavity, of the size of a large ??? ??????? ????? ???? ????????
cating by three round openings ??? ???? ???? ?? ?? ?????? ??
the base of this lobe. The ???? ???? ?? ?? ???????? and ??
flaccid in front, but somewhat ???? ???? ?? ?? ???? ?? ????
tubercle. In the upper lobe ??? ?? ?? ???? ?? ?? ???? ????
irregular walls, containing ?? ???? ???? ?? ?? ???? ?? ????
in a state of grey ?????? ?? ?? ?? ?? ?? ?? ????
and softened. The lung ?? ?? ?? ????

In this ?? ?? ?? ????
??????? ?? ??

Case 42.—Fibroid Phthisis after Inflammation.

Mr. ——, aged 39. Grandmother died of phthisis.

September 15, 1856.—Two months ago, after much exertion, he had a fever which was called gastric, but it was accompanied with cough and expectoration, once bloody, and the cough has continued, with opaque sputa; and although he has regained some strength, he has not recovered flesh, and sweats much at night. *Defective motion, and extensive hard dulness over the whole right chest—most in upper parts, where there are large loud tubular sounds, and strong vocal vibration. Some crepitus in the lower parts, but no vesicular breath-sound.*—He had been taking cod-liver oil, a dessert-spoonful twice a day; to be increased to a table-spoonful, and taken in infusion of orange-peel with sulphuric acid.

October 13.—Cough less, and improved in strength. He passed the next winter at Rome, with little improvement, the emaciation, cough, and expectoration continuing, and the state of the lung much the same—extensive consolidation, but no decided softening or excavation. The winter of 1857-8 was spent at Nice, and during this year a gradual improvement took place in flesh; the patient gained 9 lbs., and the cough and expectoration ceased. *Still much dulness, and tubular sounds in right back and front, but more motion and breath.*

October 4, 1859.—Last winter in Rome, with more strength and activity. Is much less thin. Has been lately at Spa, and suffered from rheumatism of the back and sweats. *Motion and sound on percussion much improved in right chest, but there are still some dulness and large tubular sounds at and above right scapula.*—To take mixture of iodide of potassium and quinine, with nitric acid.

December 6, 1860.—Has been generally well, except occasional pain in right chest, and perspiration on exertion. *Movement and stroke-sound of the right side still not equal to those of the left, and some tubular sounds remain in the scapular region; but there is good vesicular breath-sound elsewhere.*

1866.—Quite well in health. *Still some tubular sounds and dulness in upper right.*

1871.—Continues well.

Case 43.—*Phthisis with Cavity after Pleurisy.*

A married lady, aged 31, consulted Dr. Williams on February 12, 1857. After having suckled her child for nine months, she had right pleurisy in July last, and cough and expectoration had continued ever since. The symptoms had increased in the last two months, and had been accompanied by great loss of flesh. *Dulness; deficient breath throughout whole right side, and marked in the lower portion.*—Oil was ordered in nitric and hydrocyanic

████████ ██████ tolerably well at Torquay in winter, but expectoration ████ ███ ████ lately. Amphoric cavernous sounds over two-███ ██ ████ ████. ████ crepitus at right apex. Takes iron and quinine ███ ███.

September, 1863,—Whitered tolerably well at Torquay; but in June suffered much from palpitation and costiveness, left off oil, and has been getting weaker, with increasing breathlessness. Died in October.

Case 45.—Phthisis—Contractile Induration of Lung.—Ascites.

Robert B., aged 26, admitted September 3, 1839. Father died of diseased lungs. Fifteen months ago caught cold, and suffered from cough, pain in left side, and shortness of breath, which have continued, and seven weeks ago abdomen began to swell, and soon after his legs. Has lost much flesh and strength. Abdomen much distended, and suffers from distress after food. Bowels regular; urine scanty; sputa mucopurulent. *Extensive dulness over whole left side; gurgling, pectoriloquy, and cracked-pot stroke below left clavicle. No breath behind. Heart's apex between third and fourth ribs above nipple.*

Was tapped in abdomen on the 4th, and much relieved. The fluid rapidly increased again, although the kidneys acted freely under blue pill, squill, and digitalis. Again tapped on September 23rd, and twenty-three pints drawn, with much relief. Tartrate of iron was then tried, but increased cough and difficulty of breathing caused its disuse. In spite of various diuretic and soothing remedies, the symptoms became worse, and the abdomen became as large as ever. On October 24th, twenty more pints of straw-coloured serum were drawn off, with relief to the breath, but much weakness followed. *Loud pectoriloquy and cavernous respiration below left scapula.*

Died October 30th.

Examined October 31st.—Moderate emaciation. Left pleura and external pericardium closely adhering to walls of chest, except near axilla and at anterior part of diaphragm, where was 1½ pint of clear serum. Heart lay with apex at upper margin of fourth rib, and its base under midsternum. Diaphragm two inches higher in the left chest than on right side. Left lung consolidated throughout and much contracted, of dark leaden colour, and substance generally hard and tough, but in parts, especially upper and posterior, there were softer patches, some yellow tubercles, and several cavities. One large cavity occupied the posterior lobe, and communicated freely with bronchi. Anteriorly some bronchi were enlarged to the length of two or three inches, with saccular ends. Right lung partially adherent, unequal yellow tuberculous masses, softened in parts, and at apex a cavity the size of nutmeg, with hard walls, and puckering of the pleura over it. Marked hypertrophy of right ventricle of heart; left ventricle rather small.

... the patient improved in general health, and
... several attacks of bronchitis during the cold weather.
... became much more troublesome; the breath shorter
... was accompanied by pain in the right shoulder. The
... was mucous and transparent, and often contained streaks of
blood. At the end of the mouth the blood was quite florid; the patient had
orthopnœa, and the physical signs increased. *Dulness and loud superficial
cavernous sounds, accompanied by crackle, were detected above the right
scapula and below the clavicle.* Under styptics the blood disappeared, and the
expectoration was viscid, but never opaque. Mucous rattle was almost
constant in the trachea and right bronchus, causing perpetual annoyance;
the breathing became more laborious and shorter; appetite and strength
failed, with increasing distress and orthopnœa, and the patient died April 5.

On examination twelve hours after death the body was moderately
emaciated, with patches of ecchymosis on the posterior portions of trunk
and thighs. The heart was healthy, but the aorta was atheromatous, and
the ascending portion contained some osseous material, a spicula of which
protruded from the wall, and had probably caused the systolic murmur
mentioned in the history. The liver and spleen were enlarged and somewhat granular; the kidneys were healthy.

The left lung was highly emphysematous, but free from consolidation.
The right lung, to the extent of its upper third, was firmly adherent to the
posterior walls of the chest, and to the spinal column, and could not be
separated without considerable laceration. At the apex was an oblong
ragged cavity, about an inch and a half in length, the walls of which were
torn open in the removal of the lung. The upper third of the lung was in
colour dark grey, in texture hard and fibrous; and along its posterior
border and around the root there were light-coloured portions of harder
fibrous material, having on the outside, and also passing through them,
white bands. These, in some cases, were connected with the pleura, which
at the apex was much thickened.

The bronchial glands were enlarged and hard. The right bronchial tube
was contracted to less than half its usual size; as also the right pulmonary
vessels: both appearing to be compressed by the dense fibrous material
surrounding them.

The rest of the lung contained a few patches of consolidation, which,
under the microscope, proved to be pneumonic, which was free from the
fibrous tissue which pervaded the upper portion.

The cervical, axillary, and mesenteric glands, and the pancreas, were
healthy. Sections of the upper part of the lung were examined, under the
microscope, by Dr. Burdon Sanderson, Dr. Payne, and Dr. Theodore Williams.
The septa between the alveoli were greatly thickened; the connective tissue
of the lung considerably increased in amount, and contained fresh nucleated
... with a stroma of delicate filaments, called by Dr. Sanderson ' adenoid
... The alveoli were much compressed, and in parts nearly obliterated,

... in intervals most free from cough and oppression, ... crepitus, and obstruction in the middle parts of ... but always cranky or cavernous sounds at the base.

The patient was not seen by Dr. Williams after the last date; but it was reported that he continued to use the same remedies, and lived in a tolerable state till the autumn of 1868, when he was carried off by an attack when Dr. W. was out of town.

The case probably originated in abscess at the base of the right lung, the deep position of which prevented its being emptied and healed, and favored the continual accumulation of offensive decomposing matter. In such cases the fingers become clubbed more than in ordinary phthisis.

CASE 49.—*Purulent Phthisis after Inflammation.—Recovery.*

Mr. ——, aged 30, florid.—September 4, 1841. Was sent to Dr. W. for an opinion as to prognosis. Three years ago had inflammation of the chest, and last spring two years was sent by Sir J. Clark to Ventnor, where he was very ill, expectorating large quantities of matter and blood. He was leeched and kept very low, and was said to have much disease of the lungs. Returned to London in a very weak state, and was sent for the next winter to Madeira. Not improving there, in June he went on to Brazil, where he improved rapidly, and returned in May apparently well, and has continued so ever since. Breath and strength good. *Deficient breath in upper right front, and tubular sounds. Slight dulness at and below left clavicle.*

February 22, 1845.—Continues well. Signs the same.

October 30, 1845.—Been generally quite well, except occasional head-ache and indigestion.

Physical signs the same, but slighter; prognosis favourable.

Alive and well in 1868, twenty-seven years from first illness.

CASE 50.—*Bronchitis and Induration of Lung.—Recovery.*

Mr. R., aged 50—December 10, 1862. Brother and sister died of phthisis. Twelve months ago had cold and cough, which has continued more or less ever since, with loss of taste and smell, much snuffling, coryza, and transparent expectoration. Urine often thick. Much given to field sports engaged thereon. *Only bronchial rhonchi in various parts.* carbonate potass. squill, hemlock, and liquorice mixture.

——— 28, 1863.—Living in Yorkshire, he has not abstained from his amusements. Therefore he has had cough all the winter, and two weeks ago had inflammation of the lung, with pain in right chest, low ... some gout after. Had profuse sweats, and was much reduced in ... strength; but has since taken oil and improved. Still cough and

... had been pronounced hopeless by an eminent ... in a fortnight she was free from cough and fever, ... flesh and strength that she was considered well, and ... by Dr. W. till September 15, 1849, when she had become very anæmic in the previous six weeks, having only once menstruated. *The right lung had recovered its permeability in the lower parts, but there were still dulness and tubular sounds in the scapular region.*

January 7, 1852.—Under long-continued use of iodide of iron regained colour and strength, and catamenia returned, but tardily, and had to continue iron, sometimes with oil, several years. Had no return of cough, became quite well, and has been married several years; 1870.

CASE 52.—*Induration and Cavity after Inflammation.—Recovery.*

A young gentleman, aged 14, first seen by Dr. W. on August 3, 1843. Three years had inflammation of the chest, for which the patient was bled five times and otherwise severely treated, and suffered much from faintness and palpitation for several months afterwards. A similar attack occurred half a year later; and since then he has had occasional cough, which during the last six months has become constant, and is accompanied by abundant green expectoration, sometimes fœtid. Did lose ... flesh and strength; but he has lately regained them, and his colour is good. *Dulness and deficient motion in upper right front. Tubular sounds and loud mucous or sonorous rhonchus in the mammary region on deep breath. Some dulness and obscurity of breath in upper left. Right side ... quarters of an inch larger in circumference than left.*—Ordered iodide ... potassium and sarsaparilla, with an iodine liniment, also a linctus containing stramonium.

December 15.—Expectoration diminished, and now opaque white, not ... Flesh and strength good, and face blooming. *Less rhonchus, but ... below right clavicle. Tubular breath below left clavicle.* Ordered a tonic of nitro-hydrochloric acid and sarsaparilla. To winter in Madeira.

July 1, 1845.—Lost cough and expectoration soon after his arrival in Madeira, and has remained well since, except short breath and occasional ... *Collapse and dulness in right upper chest; loud tubular sounds ... clavicle; breath free on left side.* Ordered a liniment of camphor ... iodide.

Nov. 16, 1846.—Wintered again in Madeira without cough, except ... a month. Well grown and active, but thinner. *Still collapse of right chest, with tubular sounds, but more vesicular breath. Left side ... slowly and fully than the right.*

... 31, 1848.—Has wintered successively in Ventnor, Devonshire, and ... . Walks several miles, and breath improved. Has only occa-

sional cough, with copious expectoration. ~~Some signs~~ ~~...~~
scapula, and marked tubular sounds ~~below right clavicle, but other~~
sounds audible everywhere, with fair motion of the chest. ~~Upper inter~~
spaces protrude on cough (partial emphysema). Took oil ~~afterwards got~~
quite well, and has required no advice since.

Was heard of as quite well in 1864—*twenty-one years* after the first ~~visit~~,
and *twenty-three* after the first attack of inflammation of the chest.

CASE 53.—*Induration of Lung after Empyema.*—*Recovery.*

Mr. K., æt. 37, April 11, 1864.—Had a slight cough since croup
in childhood, but was in good health till 14 years ago, when he had right
pleurisy, followed by empyema and very offensive expectoration. A deep
incision was made in right dorsal region of chest, and half a pint of very
fœtid pus was discharged, after which the cough and expectoration ceased.
The wound discharged for several months. The side contracted considerably, the ribs being drawn together, and he was restored to fair health.
He married (has now eight children) and lived an easy country life, but
was never quite free from cough. Four years ago he took the command of
a Volunteer Corps, after which had more cough, and breath was shorter.
He paid no attention to these symptoms till they increased, with some pain
and expectoration and considerable loss of flesh, then he took oil and iron,
and used counter-irritation. *Defective motion of right chest, most lower half,
dulness only on deep percussion. Breath-sound weak, especially below: above
right scapula, stroke clearer than on left (emphysema)*—To take oil in nitric
acid mixture, and use croton oil liniment on the side.

October 11th.—Much improved in flesh, breath, and strength. Still
cough and morning expectoration, chiefly mucus, with opaque streaks.
*Still defective and irregular breath in right lung, chiefly below. Tubular
sounds at and within left scapula.*

December 2nd.—Continued better till last week, more cough and expectoration. *More obstruction in right lower lobe.* To go to Pau.

May 29, 1865.—Not much out at Pau on account of weather. Has still
cough and expectoration, and short breath. Took Cauterêt's waters three
weeks. Has lost 14 lb. in weight. *Signs not altered.*—To resume oil and
tonic. Saline at night.

October 5.—Much improved, and has gained 14 lb. Cough and expectoration much diminished, he thinks by the application of turpentine to his
moustaches. *Sounds of right lung clearer.*

1871.—Favourable reports. No examination.

CASE 54.—*Gangrenous Abscess of Lung.*—*Recovery.*

Mr. H., æt. 56, consulted Dr. Williams, January 21, 1844.—He had been
well, except being subject to winter cough, and five months ago had been

the lymph ... Was chilled at the end of November, and attacked ... cough, rusty sputa, and feverish symptoms, for which he was largely ..., with considerable relief, but is now extremely weak, and oppressed. The expectoration became opaque and offensive, and is now abundant, ... to from six to eight ounces a day. Cough violent, especially so ... the expectoration is most fœtid. Pulse 70. *Dulness throughout right lung, most marked in the lower portions, where coarse crepitation and friction ... are heard. Tubular sounds in upper portion.*—Was ordered quinine ... nitro-hydrochloric acid, good living and wine.

April 16, 1846.—Cough and expectoration gradually diminished in three ..., and the patient improved in flesh and strength. Only occasional ... of pain in right side. *Dulness, obscure breathing, and slight sub-... through right chest, dulness being most marked at apex.* Was ... mixture of nitric acid, iodide of potassium and sarsaparilla, twice ..., and a blister to right side.

May 1st.—Quite well. *Sounds in right lung almost natural.*

1871.—Has enjoyed good health ever since, and · is now a hale old man

nd gained flesh and colour; but lately pale, and
everal asthmatic attacks, and breath is very short...,
bular sounds above right scapula; dry whiffy sounds

Sputa of two kinds: some opaque, yellow, and
nd transparent.—Ordered to continue taking oil,

gh and tight breathing became worse after taking
acid and quassia were substituted, and a pill of
nonium given at night. Patient found that the
n at Ascot, better at St. John's Wood, but best at
been seven weeks, and gained strength, but not
pitation sounds in upper left chest.
re in the autumn of 1868, suffering much from
ough.

crackling and croaky sounds at the left apex,
e purulent character of part of the expectoration,
t small cavities had formed between the emphy-
lung. The cough and occasional fits of dyspnœa
emaciation and aspect of the patient were con-

—*Asthma passing into Phthisis.*

, August 7, 1860. He had been subject for seven
chial asthma, which were much relieved by iodide
onium, prescribed by Dr. Williams in 1856; but
er more severely, and were accompanied by more

P

..., but the patient is losing flesh and strength. Patches ... again on his arms for the last nine months. *Dulness ... tubular sounds in upper part of right chest, chiefly above scapula. Slight bronchophony above left scapula.*—Was ordered oil, with mixture containing iodide of potassium; stramonium at night, in case of asthma returning.

June 22, 1862.—Has been to Madeira; and improved for six weeks. Then had severe asthma for one month; then returned to England, and has been improving under stramonium and oil. Lately has been taking beer and wine, and has had long sittings in Convocation, and the eczema is increased. —Arsenic solution in gentian mixture was prescribed.

September 20, 1866.—Has been much better in skin and breath, suffering rarely, and attacks slight, till last January, when he had an attack of cough, with fever, which was treated by stimulants. Since then the cough has been very bad, with purulent expectoration and night-sweats. A great loss of flesh. *Increased dulness, and large tubular sounds in upper right chest. Some obstruction sounds in upper left, in addition to the usual bronchial rhonchi.* Under oil and hypophosphite of soda and phosphoric acid he improved much in flesh and strength, and the cough and expectoration abated.

July, 1867.—Wintered at Cannes, and continued to improve. Has lately increased in weight one stone. In the last fortnight has had fresh cold; cough moderate. Strength good, and regularly does duty. Expectoration still purulent. Physical signs greatly improved.

February 27, 1869.—Spent the following winter at Cannes, and was quite well, able to be much in the open air; but no medicines were taken. In the spring, however, the legs became œdematous (no albumen in urine), and remained so more or less up to the present time. In October cough came on, with copious expectoration, first bloody, since very thick and opaque, accompanied by feverish symptoms and much loss of flesh, but the patient has been better lately. No albumen can be detected in the urine. *More dulness, and large tubular or cavernous sounds in right upper chest, chiefly below clavicle. Breath not clear at left apex. Dry whiffy emphysematous breathing below.*—To resume oil, with phosphoric acid and strychnia, and paint the chest with tincture of iodine.

August 9, 1870.—Improved much again during the summer, gaining weight and strength, and losing œdema. Remained at home during winter, being quite equal to public duties. In the last month some return of cough, with opaque expectoration, streaked with blood. Patches of eczema have also appeared. Had left off medicine for several months. *Dulness in upper right diminished, but occasional click with the tubular sounds.*—Oil ... to be resumed.

August 14, 1871.—Pretty well through last winter; but always opaque expectoration and dulness in upper right. Has lately lost a daughter, ... 15, from acute tuberculosis.

below right clavicle. Same signs, but less, on left side. Blister, mixt. of ipecac. squill. and stramonium ordered. No relief followed, and he died on the 6th. Sectio 6 horis post mortem. Emaciation moderate. On opening chest, anterior surface of both lungs presented a remarkable puffy appearance of emphysema, with numerous cells projecting beneath the pleura, of various sizes, from a pin's head to small pea. Left lung, weight 16 oz. Volume large, with dilated cells in every part, especially at margins, which were very thin and flaccid. A large cell, of the size of a marble, projected from the root. A small consolidation at apex, with a deep dimpled depression on the surface, to which a tough old membrane adhered. Right lung weighed 14½ oz. Several old pleural adhesions. Upper lobe covered with tough opaque false membrane, thickest at apex, with one small patch of consolidation of lung-texture to depth of half an inch, quite grey and opaque. A tough opaque membrane also covered much of the middle lobe, and similar opaque tissue appeared around the blood-vessels and bronchi near the root. The texture of the lung generally showed general dilatation of the air-cells, and only here and there small gritty solid black particles of consolidation. The lower lobe, like that of the left lung, was in extreme state of atrophied emphysema, at the margins feeling like a single thin membrane, which contrasted remarkably with the texture near the root, which was much more dense and resisting. Bronchial mucous membrane very red, and circular fibres very conspicuous. Walls of large bronchi near root much thickened. Heart weighed 12½ oz.: an oblique valvular opening of foramen ovale. On the liver were many patches of deposit, and marked depressions on its surface, corresponding with the ribs which had pressed against it. Texture adhered firmly to capsule. There were other evidences of granular induration, with increase of fat globules; weight 3 lbs. Kidneys also had adherent capsules, and much fine granular matter in the tubules.

This case illustrates the origin of general emphysema of the lungs from contractile consolidation at their roots.

CASE 60.—*Phthisis arrested. Asthma long after.*

A gentleman, aged 58, whose brother was phthisical, saw Dr. Williams, July 28, 1858. He stated that in 1832 he had had a cough and expectorated blood and calcareous matter; he was considered consumptive, was ordered to Madeira. He returned much improved, and gradually recovered, being able to lead an active life, and even to hunt.

He remained free from cough till the last four or five years, and then it recurred in fits of some violence, occasionally causing stupor; and last winter he had a convulsive cough, with long back draught, and wheezy breath and expectoration, referred to the left lung. Pretty stout and strong, and is actively engaged in heavy business. Arcus senilis. *Some dulness and tubular sounds with prolonged wheeze in left upper front and right back. Emphysematous clearness below.*—Was ordered a mixture of iodide of potassium, bicarbonate of potash with squills, stramonium and hops, and to winter in a warm climate.

MAY 7, 1859.—Was unable to go away for his health or to diminish his business, and has become weaker and his breathing more oppressive ; but his cough is less. *Stroke-sound clear, but more obstruction and wheezy sounds audible in several parts of the lung, especially the left.*

CASE 61.—*Suppurative Bronchitis and Emphysema originating in Inflammation.*

· Mr. N., aged 34, December 31, 1848. Eighteen years ago had severe inflammation of the lungs, from which he slowly recovered ; but in the following year had an attack of hæmoptysis (several ounces) ; and this recurred several winters, followed by cough and purulent expectoration, lasting from six to twelve weeks, leaving him pretty well during the summer. Has spent several winters in the south of Europe with benefit. The last two have been passed at home, and there have been several attacks, lasting six or seven weeks. During the last summer was in Wales, able to walk several miles and to climb mountains. A fortnight ago was attacked with rigors and oppression, and coughed up a quantity of dark blood, and has been suffering from cough and dyspnœa ever since. Expectoration now purulent. Is much alarmed by his physician telling him that it was from an abscess in the lung. Pulse 120. Skin cool. Urine clear. Lips rather livid. Sweats at night. Is taking bark in the day and half a grain of morphia every night. No appetite. *Chest distorted by spinal curvature ; anterior upper regions project, stroke-sound clear, with harsh puerile breath-sound ; irregular dulness and loud tubular sounds at and above both scapulæ, with coarse crepitus below, with lessening breath-sound downwards ; only obscure short clicks at left base, which is rather duller than the right.* The chest was freely blistered with acetum cantharidis ; a mixture of nitric acid and decoction of Iceland moss with tincture of hop, given three times a day ; and a weak opium linctus for the cough at night. The cough, expectoration and dyspnœa soon diminished, and the appetite returned. Cod-liver oil was then given in an acid tonic, and in six weeks the patient was free from the attack, and had nearly recovered his usual state.

The crepitus and obstruction had cleared from the greater part of the right lung ; leaving still some at the base and the lower third of the left lung ; breath-sound above harsh, and either tubular or cavernous at and above both scapulæ.

Notes have not been kept of the subsequent history, which ended in death about 1863, but this is the summary :—He gained considerably in health and strength during the intervals of the attacks, but having always slight cough and opaque expectoration, and being wheezy on exertion. The attacks came on generally two or three times during the winter, sometimes with symptoms of bronchitis and coryza, and sometimes with oppres-

... and sometimes hæmoptysis; but all with ... cough ending in profuse purulent expectoration; ... *the slight wheezy obstruction in the lungs was replaced by coarse liquid respiration.* A colliquative stage of great wasting and weakness followed; but this was successfully combated for several years by generous diet and the sustaining measures. Eventually the lungs became more emphysematous, and the dyspnœa more permanent, and death was preceded by anasarca. This case, originating in inflammatory consolidation, may be considered as occupying an intermediate position between consumption and asthma.

CASE 62.—*Phthisis going into Asthma.*

Mr. T., aged 35; May 7, 1842.—Six years ago spit a little blood, which much alarmed him, being very nervous; but no other symptom occurred till two months ago, when he again coughed up blood, and slight cough has continued since, with opaque expectoration in mornings. Pulse 84, jerking. Breath shorter, and has lost some flesh. *Some irregular dulness in upper regions of both sides, in right interscapular and left subclavian. Bronchophony, almost pectoriloquy, below right clavicle.*—Nitric acid and sarsaparilla. Iodine Liniment.

Dec. 16th.—Cough and expectoration has been slight. General health improved; but now more cough, disturbing sleep. *Still dulness with cavernous sounds in right subclavian and mammary regions; below, tubular expiration.*

April 17, 1843.—Wintered at Hastings. Cough moderate. In the last few days has been expectorating blood. *Breath-sound weak below left clavicle. Still loud cavernous aspiration below right clavicle.*

September 20th.—Has remained in the neighbourhood of town, much in open air, taking the acid and sarza. No cough or hæmorrhage. *Sounds only tubular below right clavicle.*

April, 1844.—Has wintered in Italy. Free from chest symptoms, but weak. *Same signs.*

November 1, 1845.—Has continued well till a few days ago, when having caught cold, he spit some dark blood, without cough. *Still a little dulness, and tubular sound in upper right. Expires 180 cubic inches. Height 5 feet 8½ inches.*

1860.—Lived in Italy for some years, and subsequently in the West of England; generally in good health, but breath rather short, and subject to occasional attacks of asthmatic bronchitis, from one of which he was now suffering. No obvious dulness or tubular sound, only wheezy breathing in upper part of chest.

From the imperfect notes kept of this case, it can hardly be decided whether there was a cavity or merely consolidation of the apex; but, in either case, the original lesion seems to have disappeared, and left a somewhat emphysematous state of that portion of the lung, with asthmatic rather than consumptive tendency.

CHAPTER XX.

CASES OF SCROFULOUS PNEUMONIA AND ACUTE TUBERCULOSIS.

Scrofulous Pneumonia—Acute or Chronic—Acute Cases; two fatal, with post-mortem—Acute Cases arrested, five—Acute Tuberculosis—Rapid Phthisis—Six fatal Cases with post-mortem—Origin from various Causes—Caseous Glands—Abscess—Measles combined with Tuberculous Arachnitis—Post-mortem Characters of Acute Tubercle.

THE following group, which might be easily enlarged, include those cases of acute phthisis in which the disease has been so much localised as to resemble those of inflammation more than those of scattered tubercle. But they have proceeded so rapidly to excavation, and so early declared their phthisical character, that their place seems to belong to consumption rather than to common inflammation; and this corresponds with the designation, Scrofulous or Caseous Pneumonia described in Chap. XI.

Their acute and very consumptive character approximates them to those of Acute Tuberculosis which follow: but the disseminated and adenoid distribution of the miliary tubercles in the latter strongly marks them as a distinct variety of consumptive disease.

CASE 63.—*Phthisis. Acute Caseous Pneumonia.*

S. N., aged 18; admitted into University College Hospital, November 23, 1839. Cellarman. Always weakly. In last six months overworked in wine-cellars, damp and draughty, and kept up at night at the bar. Three weeks ago became suddenly weak, with loss of appetite, thirst, and violent cough, and mucous expectoration. Ten days ago came on pain of left side, and been since confined to bed. Has lost much flesh and strength. Expctoration was streaked; now viscid and opaque. Pulse 84; respiration 57. Urine high coloured. *Dulness in upper left, most front. Cracked pat-strokes under clavicle, and loud tubular sounds. Breath-sound bronchial, with some dulness in left back, except the base, which is quite dull, and aegophony is heard in mid-region. Breath puerile in right lung.*—18 leeches to the right chest, calomel, James's powder, and opium every night. Senna draught in morning; nitrate and tartrate of potass., in camphor mixture, three times a day.

November 26.—Much relieved in breathing and pain, especially since blister on the 23rd. Still much cough and expectoration, but less viscid, and no blood. Pulse 120. *Less dulness in left back, and more breath-sounds.*

December 5.—In last week cough relieved by eruption on side, produced by tartar emetic ointment. *Left front of chest still dull and collapsed. Pulse 96.*

December 17.—Cough easier; but weakness increasing.—Ordered iod. potass. in infus. cascarillæ.

December 24.—Cough increased, with rusty sputa, and pains on both sides, with increasing weakness. *More crepitus and dulness in posterior regions.*—Ordered antimony and henbane mixture, instead of cascarilla, &c.

December 31.—Has been better in every respect, and feels stronger. Cough and expectoration diminished, but the latter still rusty. Squills substituted for antimony.

January 14.—In last few days more cough, rusty expectoration, and increasing weakness. *Loud amphoric breathing, pectoriloquy and gurgling in left front.* Pulse 120. Occasional night-sweats.

Continued to get weaker, with harassing cough and copious yellowish ditty expectoration, and died on March 11.

Examination 48 hours after death.—Great emaciation. Left pleura firmly adherent throughout. A large cavity in anterior part of left lung capable of holding half a pint of fluid. Its anterior walls were little more than the adherent pleura; in other parts the surface was irregular, with some bands stretching across, and contained muco-purulent matter. The upper and posterior part of this lung was in a state of grey consolidation, here and there mottled, and with small excavations communicating with the large cavity. The base of the lung was firmly adherent to the diaphragm by a large mass of organised lymph, which contained in its interior opaque patches of yellowish-white colour, some tough and some softened (yellow tubercle). Right lung in first stage of pneumonia, with several patches of yellow tubercle, some crude, some soft. No adhesions in right lung. Mesenteric glands much enlarged in parts, with patches of crude grey tubercle. Mucous membrane of larynx and trachea rough, red, and partly thickened with numerous isolated pits, apparently ulcerated some; and several were found also in the bronchi of the left lung.

CASE 64.—*Phthisis. Acute Caseous Pneumonia.*

Fred. R., aged 38, tailor, admitted March 20, 1840. In good health till last five months, when he was out of employment and living badly. He then began to cough, and soon to expectorate, and lose flesh and strength. A fortnight ago the cough became much worse, and he brought up about a tablespoonful of blood, which has recurred nearly every morning. There is also pain in left side; thirst and increasing weakness. Pulse frequent. *Whole left side more or less dull, and with crepitus super-seding breath-sound. Crepitation also in upper right.* Was cupped ten ounces, and ordered tart. antimony.

April 2, 1840.—Pain and cough better. Vomited several times after medicine. Sweats at night. Pulse 108. Ipecac. wine and tinct. camph. co. substituted for tartar. emetic.

April 7, 1840.—Cough has again become severe, and breath more tight. Has been blistered and again put on antimonial treatment. *Left side dull (except at apex), with mixed crepitus and bronchophony. Dulness and coarse crepitus at right apex.*

April 21, 1840.—Has continued to get worse in spite of all remedies; breath very short, cough urgent, and now the sputa have become partially rusty. Pulse 120. Veins much distended. Distress great. To be bled to six ounces. Ammonia and wine.

Some relief from the bleeding, but weakness increased, with inability to expectorate.

Died on the 25th.

Percussing the chest below the left clavicle elicited the cracked pot-sound, which could be traced to the mouth of the subject, showing that it was caused by the succussion in the cavity communicated to the air in the trachea.

Both lungs adherent to the ribs and diaphragm, most firmly posteriorly and below; but some recent lymph was found at left base. In the substance of both lungs were consolidations of various sizes—those in the left pervading many lobules, and of the density of liver; some small as miliary tubercles, harder than the others. Parts of the general consolidation were yellow opaque, and softened at points. At the summit of the left lung was a cavity of the size of a small orange, and some smaller ones below. At the summit of the right lung were several solid grey masses, with small yellow patches of softening in some. The lung tissue between the masses was generally red and congested, and in parts hepatised. Bronchial membrane generally much injected. Many dilated air-cells in marginal lobes.

The consolidations of the lungs in this case presented every gradation between recent acute hepatisation and the grey nodules commonly called tubercular, and the change to the opaque state (caseation) was seen in parts of both.

The case is an example of acute phthisis arising from inflammation degraded by malnutrition.

Case 36.—Scrofulous Pneumonia. Cavity. Death from
Hæmoptysis.

Mr. J. V., aged 28, April 9, 1867.—A brother had hæmoptysis. Devoted
tropical horticulture; has travelled in Australia and China. Cervical
ids occasionally swollen. In the end of February caught severe cold
i cough, which has been increasing with tinged expectoration, pain in
left chest, high fever, and extreme weakness and wasting. Pulse 120;
hot, 104°. *Dulness, deficient breath, crepitation on deep breath, in*
le left, except apex. Ready bronchophony in mammary and scapular
mus. Blister to left side; nitric acid, calumba, and glycerine morning
mid-day; effervescing saline with opiate, evening and night.

lay 31.—Fever, hard cough, and viscid expectoration continued a fort-
t, requiring repeated blistering and continued saline. Then expectora-
became purulent, cough looser, and temperature lowered. Cod-liver
was then added to the morning doses, and improvement soon followed.
rreous sounds in mammary region. Some breath above.

rtober 15.—Has steadily continued the oil with phosphoric acid and
ophosphite of soda; quinine and iron being added at times. Fever and
its have long since subsided; the cough and expectoration are much
erated; appetite is good; 10lbs. have been gained in weight, and he can
t a mile. *Dulness and collapse of left front, with croaky cavernous*
nds, most marked in mammary region. Moderate dulness and sub-crepi-
with obscure breath posteriorly and above. Tubular sounds above right
nds.

une 2, 1868.—Wintered at Hyères. Able to be much in the open air,
steadily improving the whole time, taking oil with phosphoric acid
hypophosphite of soda, and sometimes quinine. Weight has increased
a 9st. 9lbs. in October, to 10st. 7lbs. in April. Cough and expectoration
hily diminished; and have been trifling in last three months.
llapse and dulness with cavernous sounds in left front, most marked at
h, and 5th ribs. Clearer, with a little breath above and in upper dorsal
n; more dull and obstructed below. Tubular still in upper right.

eptember 23, 1868.—Quite well through summer, except shortness of
th and slight cough with opake expectoration. *Cavernous sounds are*
br higher up, and heard in the scapular region also, but less. Heart drawn
bove an inch. Rather less obstruction in lower dorsal region.

lay 5, 1869.—Again wintered at Hyères, regularly taking oil and acid
ophosphite. Weight has risen to 11st, 1lb., and has walked four or five
a daily.

une 25.—On his return home he attended to business in nursery
nds and hothouses, and lived more freely, and at end of May coughed
oz. of blood, and less for three days, with pain in right side, fever and
d expectoration. *Fine crepitation in lower two-thirds right lung.* After a

blister and a few days with antimonial saline, this attack of pneumonia sub sided, leaving him weak, with loss of 13lbs. weight. *Now breath pretty good through right lung, but large tubular sounds above right scapula. Cavernous sounds on left side are still further drawn upwards and backwards, and heart occupies the front up to the third rib.*

August 25.—Has gradually improved, having lost all pain and hardness of cough, and has regained some strength and flesh. *Signs in left chest much the same. There has been some crepitus at right apex, but that is no longer heard.* Is bilious, and requires occasional omission of oil, and a dose of blue pill, &c.

October 11.—Has been distressed, and called into exertion by the death of his father. More cough, expectoration, and weakness. Has re quired blistering with acetum cantharidis. *More crepitus in left lung, but no extension of cavity.*

May 31, 1870.—Wintered again at Hyères, taking oil with strychnia and phosphoric acid and hypophosphite mixture; and has gradually im proved, gaining twelve pounds in weight, and some breath and strength, but not up to the point of this time last year. *Dulness and collapse of left front as before, but the cavernous sounds are more croaky and muffled. A little crepitus also above right scapula.*—Still occasionally bilious, so on. Treatment accordingly.

August 1.—Has had a slight recurrence of hæmorrhage, the bowels being confined at the time. Since has frequently taken acid sulphate of magnesia in mornings, and has improved, and breath and cough are better. *More breath-sound at left apex. Cavernous sounds croaky and dry in scapular region. Crumpling crepitus below. No crepitus at right apex, but breath sounds are loud there.*

In the following week, during Dr. Williams's absence from town, hæmor rhage came on, became profuse, and death followed in two days.

This case at first appeared to be a hopeless one of galloping con sumption, and was pronounced to be so by a physician who had been consulted. The great and continued improvement afterwards was very remarkable, and might have been more permanent, but for the patient's too early return to active business and his subsequent heavy trial. Although at first the disease appeared to be scrofulous pneumonia, the subsequent affection of the apex of the right lung was probably tubercular.

CASE 66.—*Scrofulous Pneumonia. Cavity. Arrested.*

Mr. F. W., aged 24, January 14, 1867. Mother scrofulous. Is re ported to have been quite well till October, when he caught a severe cold, followed by pain in left side, cough, and expectoration, which lately has become very clotty and opaque. Has lost much flesh and become ex tremely weak, with fever and profuse sweats at night; much annoyed with piles. Pulse 110.

Dulness and obstructed breath through whole left chest. Large tubular

... in mammary region, and less above. *Tubular* ... ... —To take oil with phosphoric acid and strychnia. ... with the tincture of iodine. Morphia linctus at night.

... Has vastly improved in all respects. Gained 21 lbs. in ... Has long lost fever and sweats. Cough and expectoration ... In last two months quinine has been added to tonic. *Still* ... dulness and obstruction in left chest ; but no crepitation. Dry cavern- ... sounds in left mammary region. Tubular above.

... 10.—Except a bilious attack, requiring a few doses of aperient ... the suspension of the oil &c. for a week, improvement has been con- ... Gained 8 lbs. more. Has lately suffered from bleeding piles. *Cavernous sounds in left front and upper back. Breath still obstructed* ...—To take electuary of senna with sulphate and bitart. potass. Con- ... oil and tonic.

... 30, 1868.—Has wintered at Hyères, and generally well, having ... regularly out for exercise. Had gained 8 lbs. up to January. Then ... from piles, and left off the oil for five weeks, and lost 9 lbs. in ... Now has a fistula. Cough and expectoration still, but moderate. *... dulness and obstruction in left side. Cavernous sounds obscurely ... in mammary and subclavian regions. More tubular above scapula, ... breath below.*

... 30.—More cough expectoration and tightness of breath since in- ... exertion and exposure in an excursion to Germany. *Signs much* ...

... 13.—Has been well and active and gained 6 lbs. Cough ceased ... weeks in August. Fistula still open. *Cavernous sounds heard ... in deep breath, which causes a 'squash,' and some crepitus posteriorly.* ... oil once daily.

... 24, 1869.—At Hyères, and out all the winter, though often wet. ... 1½ lbs. and much strength. No cough, except in mornings, with a ... expectoration. Fistula has discharged more, till touched with ... *Obscure pectoriloquy with croak on deep breath in upper left. ... obstruction and dulness below. Tubular sounds above right scapula, ... good vesicular breath sound.* (Enlarged bronchial gland).

... 22, 1869.—Has been well and active in his business (builder), ... weeks ago; caught cold and has had more cough and expectoration, ... is now quite yellow. Has lost 3 lbs. *Signs much the same.*

... 31, 1870.—Wintered well at Hyères, although a bad season. ... three tablespoonfuls of oil with tonic once daily. Gained only ... *No material change in signs.*

... 1870.—Continues well ; about the same in flesh ; but stronger ... business. Pulse 72. Little cough or expectoration. *Cavity ... and with only crumpling crepitus around.*

... had all the aspect of acute phthisis from scrofulous pneumonia, ... by treatment. The fistula had probably a salutary in-

CASE 67.—*Scrofulous Pneumonia. Cavity. Arrested.*

A medical man, aged 30, whose paternal aunt had died of consumption, saw Dr. Williams on October 14, 1859. In 1856 he had a bad attack of scarlatina, and has not been strong since, but remained in laborious practice till March, 1858, when he was attacked with severe pneumonia of the right side, followed by copious purulent expectoration, sweats, emaciation, and other signs of acute consumption. Wintered at Malaga without amendment; suffering much from cough and expectoration. Occasional hæmoptysis to the amount of ʒiv. After a time he crossed to Tangier, and there improved a little, but remains very weak and thin, and lately suffering from nausea and hoarseness. 'Cannot take oil.' *Collapse, deficient motion, dulness, large tubular (cavernous?) sounds in right front; less dulness, some breath-sound audible but mixed with crepitus in back.*— Ordered oil in tonic of phosphoric acid, strychnia, and tincture of orange; the use of a cantharides liniment. To winter at Hyères.

October 24, 1863.—Wintered at Hyères, steadily continuing oil and tonic, and much in open air. Has improved so much in all respects that he has returned there every winter since, practising as physician. Passes summers in North Wales with further improvement in flesh and strength. Breath better, but still short on exertion, and has always had some cough, expectoration, and hoarseness. Last winter, after going out at night, had another attack of the right lung, which weakened him much; but he gradually recovered, and again gained much ground during the summer in North Wales, although the weather was wet. *Dulness, collapse, deficient motion and breath throughout right chest. Loud tubular or dry cavernous sounds above. Coarse crepitation below.*

June 2, 1867.—Still living at Hyères in winter, and in North Wales in summer. Has steadily improved; is stouter than he ever was, and has little cough or expectoration. Last winter expectorated some calcareous matter. Still collapse, deficiency of motion, dulness of whole right side of chest, but dulness diminished in anterior portion. Some breath sound, with subcrepitus is heard, especially under clavicle, at scapula, and in lateral region. Strong percussion gives a raised pitch note in upper half. Tubular and cavernous sounds to be heard nowhere, except tubular above the right scapula. Left lung quite healthy.

1871.—Remains very well in bodily health, although he has been much tried in mind and body of late. Oil has been taken at least once a day regularly. Had charge of an ambulance during the siege of Paris.

CASE 68.—*Scrofulous Pneumonia. Cavity. Arrested.*

Mr. E. J., æt. 21. January 2, 1863.—Lost an aunt in phthisis. Since cold taken two months ago, has coughed with much yellow expectoration, and lost much flesh. *Complete dulness, and loud, large tubular sounds in*

.... linear down, and above clavicle.—To take oil,
.... mild and calumba; morphia linctus at night, and to
...... the chest with acetum cantharidis.

............—Much better, and gaining flesh. Still cough and opaque ex-
.... Still dulness and creaky crepitus below right clavicle.

............—Continued improvement, but cough and expectoration, although much lessened, are not gone. Amphoric cavernous sounds below
right clavicle to third rib. Good breath below and behind.—Add sulphates
of iron and quinine (aa gr. j.) to tonic, with oil.

.. July 11th.—Hæmoptysis to one and half ounce. Bowels not free. An
...... pill every night. Substitute diluted sulphuric acid for phosphoric
with iron and quinine, with the oil.

September 10th.—Heard he was at Aberystwith; quite well, walking
several miles daily.

June 17, 1864.—Wintered at Aberystwith. Stouter than ever, without
cough or expectoration, but breath is still short on exertion. Defective
motion, moderate dulness, and large tubular sounds in upper third of right
chest, but vesicular breath heard there, and no cavity. Tubular sounds above
left scapula. The cavity was probably produced by caseating pneumonia.

CASE 69.—Scrofulous Pneumonia. Cavity. Arrested. Death from Heart Disease.

Miss P., aged 16.—Patient's aunt died of phthisis. Sister phthisical since.
.... 12, 1864.—In good health till last April, at school had cold
...... with pain in left side, but not attended to for three weeks, when
...... worse, with quick pulse, sweats, &c. Dr. — was consulted, who
...... the disease 'galloping consumption.' On oil and iron con-
...... improvement took place; but the breath is still very short,
...... cough continues with opaque expectoration: the catamenia have
...... since April. Extensive dulness in right chest with large moist
...... sounds in upper part, and obstruction and crepitus below. Coarse
...... also above right scapula.—Oil to be continued in mixture of
...... acid, calumba, and sulphate of iron. Tincture of iodine to the
......

.... 19th.—Great improvement. Catamenia have returned twice.
...... has appeared in the expectoration. Cavernous sounds drier. Large
...... sounds and no crepitus above right scapula.—Oil to be continued
...... sulphuric acid, instead of the phosphoric acid and iron.

...... 1, 1865.—Wintered at Cannes, pretty well; but by advice discon-
...... the oil several times, and has had more cough and lost flesh. Cata-
...... only twice. Large tympanitic cavity in upper left front. Breath
...... below. Crepitation above right scapula.—To resume the phosphoric
...... iron, with the oil.

.... 1866.—Improved much during last summer, and wintered at

Cannes much better, continuing oil and tonic steadily, until two months ago, when it was omitted for a time on account of diarrhœa. Was not confined to the house a day during the winter, but cough and moderate expectoration have continued. *Collapse and dry cavernous sounds in upper half of left chest. Some vesicular breath in back. Heart drawn upwards.*

May 7, 1867.—Was so well that she remained in Monmouthshire till February, but then cough was increasing, and she went again to Cannes, and again improved greatly, being much out, and almost losing cough and expectoration. Catamenia regular. *Percussion much clearer; and breath-sound vesicular, but coarse in great part of left front. Tubular sounds at and behind clavicle, and in whole scapular region, with obscure breath below.* It appears that the vesicular tissue below the cavity has become expanded, and pushed the condensed part with cavity backwards.

June 24, 1869.—Has passed last two winters at home. Quite well, except some cough and expectoration, and breath short on exertion; but can ride all day long, and has walked as much as twenty miles. Has taken oil and tonic pretty regularly, but is getting tired of it. Was urged to continue it with varied tonics, and cautioned against over-exertion. State of chest much as at last report. *Dulness and dry cavernous sounds confined to posterior region, with much vesicular breath in front. Heart impulse high and strong, drawn up by contraction of lung.*

January, 1871.—On his return from abroad, Dr. W. received an account of a new set of symptoms which had followed an attack of sore throat before Christmas. Strong and rapid action of the heart, with extreme breathlessness, preventing all exertion and disturbing sleep. No more cough or expectoration, and the body retained its plumpness; but colour was fading, and the legs began to swell.

February 9, 1871.—By a desperate resolve she was brought to London in a state of orthopnœa, with rapidly increasing anasarca, pulse 120, jerking; fresh cough and bloody expectoration. The heart was beating tumultuously, with a loud systolic murmur at the apex, above the fifth rib. Lower portion of left lung obstructed; superior and posterior cavernous as before. Breath in right puerile. A fatal prognosis was given from mitral valvular disease and embolism of left pulmonary vessels. She died the next day.

CASE 70.—*Acute Tuberculosis. Death in a month.*

Wm. H., aged 21, admitted December 8, 1840. Postilion. In good health till a month ago, after sleeping in a damp bed, was attacked with soreness of chest and cough, which have continued ever since, with viscid expectoration (once blood), and loss of flesh and breath; especially worse in the last week, with hoarseness and increased oppression. Pulse 108. Skin hot.

Bronchophony and whiffing breath under right clavicle, with long expiration. Dulness more at right scapula. Loud coarse crepitus and resonance

...below spine of left scapula.

... hyoscyami, syr. papav., ter die.

... slight relief, but since the breath has become ... cough more copious, and the sputa now quite purulent. Pulse 126. ... crepitation showing. themselves at both apices. A blister and other ... prescribed; but he continued to get worse, dyspnœa extreme, ... on the 31st.

... 18 hours post-mortem. Both lungs firmly adherent to chest. The false membrane on right lung dense, an eighth of an inch thick, and in ... parts studded with granular tubercles of the same colour and density ... membrane. Both lungs contained many tubercles, some granular ... scattered; more grouped in clusters; some grey, others opaque and yellowish white, and several softened and partly evacuated, the cavities being chiefly in the upper and middle portions of the lungs. The pulmonary texture between the tubercles was generally much congested, heavy, fragile, and exuding frothy serum. Bronchial lining very red, and filled with mucus. Much vascular redness in trachea and larynx, with some super-... ulcerations in parts. Weight of lungs:—Right, 2 lbs. 6 oss.; left, ... 4 oss.

... abdominal, intestinal, mesenteric, omental, hepatic, and ... matic, was closely agglutinated in most parts, and more or less ... studded with white granular tubercles; some in fine points not ... than pin-heads, others larger; and some flattened, forming dense ... The false membranes binding together the abdominal viscera ... the most part pale; and in some parts of glistening white, peeling into thin flakes; in parts they were thickened by granular masses, and ... could not be separated without tearing the peritoneum. Two or three crude ... tubercles in the liver.

CASE 71.—*Meningitis. Acute Tuberculosis. Death in 21 days.*

Robert I., aged 13, admitted January 13, 1848. A diminutive boy, four feet in height, employed in spinning tobacco. Quite well till sixteen days ago, after some failure of appetite, he began to suffer from pain in the head, which increased so much in two days that he was confined to bed, and screamed and moaned all night. Vomiting then came on, and has continued since, with obstinately costive bowels. Urine scanty and high ...—the day before admission had passed none for twenty-four hours. ... been repeatedly leeched, and has vomited all the medicine given. ... ; pupils dilated. Strabismus of right eye, said to be habi-... Head not very hot; but carotids pulsate more strongly than the ... arteries. Pulse 108. Slight twitching of arms.—Head to be shaved. ... to temples. Three grains of calomel every four hours; ten ... tincture of cantharides in a draught three times a day.

14th.—Blisters were applied to the nucha last night. He is conscious to-day, but is dull; moaning, and drivelling at mouth. Pulse 150, weak. No urine passed since admission. The catheter was passed, but none came. To be used again.

15th.—Catheter brought away three ounces urine, being the first for thirty-two hours: alkaline, phosphatic, not albuminous. More has since been passed in bed. More sensible, but moans much and takes hardly any food. Sordes on lips and teeth.

17th.—Almost unconscious, except when attempts are made to move him, when he screams.

18th.—Pupils now unequally dilated, right most. Pulse hardly percepti-ble. Very noisy in the night; and now talks incoherently. Right side slightly convulsed. Extremities cold.

Died on the 19th.

Post-mortem five hours. Body moderately emaciated. Dura mater vas-cular. Convolutions flattened. A good deal of serum escaped on removing the brain, and at the base, especially on the tuber annulare and crura cerebri, a considerable thickness of lymph infiltrated with serum. Opaque patches in the membrane between convolutions of cerebellum, not granu-lar. That at the base is partially so. Cineritious matter darker than usual, but few red points in the centrum ovale. Serum also in the lateral ventricles, the whole quantity of serum about two ounces. Lungs pale and light, weighing, right four and a half, left three and a half ounces. Small granu-lar tubercles were found scattered through both lungs. One caseous tubercle of the size of a pea in right, and the right bronchial also was enlarged with cheesy matter. Several tubercles in the spleen. Mesenteric glands simply enlarged.

This case is remarkable for the entire latency of the pulmonary tubercles which must have existed before the commencement of the fatal attack of meningitis.

CASE 72.—*Acute Tuberculosis.   Caseous bronchial glands.*

John B., 15, admitted April 22, 1843. Lived in ill-ventilated house, and unhealthy part of town. Father spits blood. Last winter had whooping-cough, and not well since. Two months ago had a rash, which some said was scarlatina. Three weeks ago suffered from pain in chest, cough, and short breath; hot skin and costive bowels. Has been very ill ever since.

Is now dull and heavy, sleeping much; skin very hot. Pulse 120. Bowels very costive; faeces very dark. Cough slight. Nose has bled several times lately. Pupils dilated. Much emaciated. Urine scanty, strong smelling. *Dulness and tubular sounds in both scapular regions, most on right.*—Head to be shaved, calomel and James's powder, ter die. Cras mane olei ricini 3ij.

24th.—Nose has bled again. Head still hot. Veins of neck full. Cough worse. Bowels open; faeces dark. A leech to each temple.

crying out with pain in head. Cold lotion.
moans in sleep. Heat less. Lips parched, and
with crusts. Pupils still much dilated. Takes no food, and
under him. Pulse 180 and more.
Died

Sectio 20 horis post mortem. Body much emaciated. Skin of back of neck and head suffused with blood. Both lungs studded throughout with miliary tubercles, mostly yellow and crude. Masses of yellow tubercle in bronchial glands. One at the root of the right lung much enlarged, with cheesy matter partially softened, and communicating with the right bronchus by an opening with vascular margin and elevated edges. A few tubercles under the pericardium covering the heart. One in the left ventricle and another in the septum. Liver studded with miliary tubercles, on the surface white and granular; in the substance larger, yellow, and seemed to enclose the ducts, some of which were enlarged, containing green bile. Peritoneum covering under surface of diaphragm patched with granular tubercles. Spleen more thickly studded than any other organ, of size of hemp-seeds. A few minute transparent granules on the surface of intestines, omentum, and meso-colon. A few pale tubercles in the kidneys.

Convolutions of brain much flattened on upper surface, and membranes very vascular. Granular tubercles on the right hemisphere, near the falx, collected in a patch posteriorly, and here the pia-mater adhered firmly to the brain. Carotid arteries and branches studded with granules. About three ounces of bloody serum at base of skull.

, **Case 73.—*Acute Tuberculosis from Vertebral Abscess.***

James S., aged 18; admitted March 11, 1843. Footman. Lived well, and enjoyed good health till last Christmas, when, for a short time, suffered from rheumatism in the hips. Two months ago, after a chill, began to cough, which increased, with pains in his limbs, head-ache, and rapid loss of flesh and strength. The pains have lately been bad in his back and hip, especially left side. Expectoration scanty in yellow clots; once brought up a mouthful of blood. Pulse frequent; skin hot; sweats at night; tongue furred; face pale, with slight flush on each cheek; moderate respiration. *Dulness and crepitus, fine and coarse, throughout left side; in the upper parts. Some crepitus also on right side.*—A blister to left side. Mixture containing antimony and hydrocyanic acid.

March 12.—Breath and cough somewhat better, but complains much of pain in left hip and back. Pulse 104. Heat great; very weak. Sputa cloudy opaque. Died next day.

Examination, eight hours after death.—Left lung very red and much engorged, with many clusters of miliary tubercles, most in the upper lobe. Lung was closely adherent to the posterior walls of the chest, and on removing it purulent matter was observed to pour out from an opening in the posterior mediastinum. This was traced to the body of the third dorsal vertebra, which was carious; the disease did not penetrate to the spinal canal, but there was a small abscess of the size of a pea outside the theca of the cord. The matter from the mediastinum also poured out from the posterior and lower part of the upper lobe of the lung, in which was an abscess about the size of a small egg. The right lung generally adherent. Its substance was partially consolidated by clusters of grey tubercles. At the apex were some opaque and partially excavated; and around each of these the lung texture was deep, red, and consolidated, but soft. Posterior portions of this lung all much congested. but crepitant. Liver large; weight, 3 lbs. 13 ozs.: much congested, as was also the spleen.

CASE 74.—*Acute Tuberculosis from Pyæmia. Purpura. Epistaxis.*

Richard H., aged 47 ; admitted October 28, 1843. Groom; of irregular habits; lately ill-fed. Lost a brother in phthisis. Has had three attacks of rheumatism; two in last four years. Six months ago attacked with severe pain in side, with difficult breathing; was bled to syncope, and relieved, but has been ailing ever since, attending at a dispensary. Has had a succession of abscesses in legs and thighs, which, after discharging, have healed. Is much reduced in flesh and strength. About a month ago began to cough, with night-sweats, and increasing shortness of breath, and weakness. Three weeks ago his nose began to bleed, and this has recurred several time since. Ankles are now œdematous, and there are a number of purpura spots on many parts of the body. Urine scanty; slightly albuminous. *General dulness and defective breath in left chest; most below clavicle. Abdomen enlarged, and some fluctuation over tympanitic intestines.*

Epistaxis recurred several times in the next week, greatly reducing his strength, whilst the skin became hot, with continued purpura spots, and more œdema of the legs. *Extreme depression ; more crepitus was heard in both posterior regions ;* and he died November 10.

Body much emaciated. All posterior parts of livid purple colour. Arms and legs œdematous. Several ecchymosed spots in costal pleura. The whole anterior surface of both lungs mottled with spots from ½ in. to ⅜ in. in diameter, of irregular rounded shape, having a pale yellow spot in the centre, and a deep red areola well defined around them. These spots were found to be miliary tubercles, with extreme congestion or ecchymosis in the texture, and similar nodules were found thickly scattered throughout the substance of both lungs, more in the left than the right, but not more at the apex than at the base. The tubercles were of a pale buff colour, but firm, though friable on hard pressure, and arranged in bud-like clusters. The interstitial parts of the lung were red, in front bright and containing air; but posteriorly of a very deep red, almost black, and on incision exuded frothy red fluid. Three pints of yellow serum in peritoneum, and a

.... Liver large, high in chest, and two inches below
.... Weight, 4 lbs. 2 oz. Surface coarsely mottled with pre-
.... of pale colour. Texture hard and tough, and capsule adherent.
.... large, weight, 2½ oz. Several yellow tubercles in its substance;
.... and, under the microscope, exhibited pus globules. Right
.... granular, and with several cysts containing lithic acid and urea.

CASE 75.—*Phthisis. Acute Tuberculosis.*

Edwin H. S., aged 32, admitted February 20, 1845. A painter; well-fed
and clothed, and no ailment till last winter, when he had slight cough and
short breath, but was well in summer. This winter the cough has returned, and in the last two months became severe, with great increase of
dyspnœa, and rapid loss of flesh and strength. Now respiration is very
frequent and laboured, and cannot lie down. Lips and cheeks livid. Expectoration mixed, purulent, scanty, and difficult.

*Left chest moves less and sounds duller than right. Little breath-sound,
but crepitus short and coarse. On right side much crepitus also, with a little
more breath. Same signs behind, but with more dulness at the base of the
lungs, and whiffy tubular near the roots.*

A blister was applied, and chlorate of potass. and carb. ammonia in effer-
vescence with nitric acid, given every three hours, and five grains of calomel;
two ounces wine.

February 21, 1845.—Lividity diminished, but dyspnœa not relieved.
Pulse 140. Blister rose well. Urine scanty, contains albumen and lithates.

Another blister between shoulders. Five grains calomel and half a
grain opium at night.

February 23, 1845.—Dyspnœa continued to increase, with more weakness and lividity; and he died this morning.

Examination 28 hours after death.

Body emaciated; veins of neck and arms much distended with blood.
Livid discoloration of all posterior parts of body. General adhesions of
the pleura on both sides; very dense posteriorly and laterally. Both
lungs much engorged with blood in parts unoccupied by tubercles, which
were found in various forms in every part. At the left apex was a large
cavity, with another mass below it containing a smaller cavity, and several
others in other parts. That at the apex contained cretaceous matter, and a
portion of size of a barleycorn was found loose in it. The walls were in
state of grey induration. Several tubercles were grey, others passing into
the yellow state with more or less softening. At apex of right lung was
a thick opaque false membrane, quarter of an inch thick, covering a cavity
which communicated with several large bronchi. In the outer part of this
lobe was another cavity lined with false membrane. Many tubercles,
singly and in clusters, were scattered through the other lobes, and their
...... margins were emphysematous. Bronchial glands enlarged, containing

Heart large, weighs 13½ ounces. Right ventricle somewhat thickened. Fibrinous coagula in both ventricles—that in right extending into pulmonary artery, and bearing impress of semilunar valves (therefore existed before death). Kidneys were healthy. Liver somewhat nutmegged, from hepatic venous congestion.

Case 76.—*Acute Tuberculosis. Measles.*

P. S., aged 23, admitted January 4, 1848.—Formerly farm labourer; lately policeman. Health good till 2½ years ago; had syphilis, for which he was salivated, and was quite well in a few months. Thirteen days ago was chilled whilst on duty, and began to cough and expectorate, and felt very weak. He vomited much dark green matter the day before admission, and that morning an eruption came out over the whole body. This rash, which is obviously measles, is now fully out, with suffused eyes, flushed face, and urgent cough and short breath. Pulse 88; tongue furred.—Ordered saline antimonial: calomel and haustus sennæ.

January 5.—Expectoration more viscid, partly opaque. Eruption was out in morning; now more faded. Pulse 100; soft, reduplicated.

Breath-sound obscure, especially in right back. Mucous rhonchus, most on left side.

Blister to chest.

January 6.—Breathing more embarrassed. Face much congested, almost livid. Expectoration in ragged opaque masses, floating in brownish liquid. *Left back dull; crepitation on both sides.* Cupped between shoulders to ℥iv., and later in the day, on right side to ℥viij.

January 8.—Breathing was much relieved yesterday, but to-day became as bad as ever; and this morning had ℥xi. blood drawn in full stream from the arm, with some relief, but he is very weak.

At the visit carb. ammonia and nitre mixture substituted for the antimonial. At night the dyspnœa increased, and a blister was applied.

January 11.—In the last two days breathing easier, and face less livid. Urine abundant; s. g. 1029, with plenty of lithates.

January 13.—Breathing easier in morning, but always worse at night, preventing sleep. Pulse frequent, jerking, sometimes irregular, and weak; urine 24oz.; s. g. 1021, contains a little albumen. *Breath-sound weaker on both sides, superseded by irregular crepitation. Tubular above right scapula.*

January 15.—Breathing more laboured, with pain in right side. Lividity increased. Pulse frequently irregular. *Crepitus rises higher, and breath-sound weaker.*

Died on the 16th.

Sectio 46 horis post mortem. Both lungs contain numerous miliary tubercles scattered through their texture; none hard, but some are grey, transparent, and offer some resistance. Others are red and soft, yet firmer than the tissue around. At the apex this distinction is most obvious, where are red bodies as big as a pea, sinking in water, while the intervening tissue is comparatively free, but the lower lobes are much congested, and the right partially hepatised posteriorly: even here the slightly firmer miliary tubercles can be felt scattered through it. A patch of recent lymph on posterior surface of right lung. Other organs healthy.

The remarkable points in this case are, the rapid production of miliary tubercles in twenty-four days, the suppression of the rash, and increase of the pulmonary oppression; and the soft plump character of the tubercles in their most recent state.

CASE 77.—*Acute Tuberculosis. Tuberculous Arachnitis.*

Miss K., aged 9, January 23, 1849.—Seen with Dr. Guillemard of Eltham. Delicate since inflammation of chest some years ago, but better than usual on her return from Dover in November. In December, had a cough with remittent fever, which much reduced flesh and strength. Four days ago came on pain in the head, and intolerance of light, with fœtid discharge from left ear; increase of cough and feverish heat, pain and tenderness of right hypochondrium; scanty urine. *No dulness, but general bronchial rhonchi through the chest masking all other sounds.* Pain was relieved by opium, but other symptoms increased, and death ensued in ten days.

Numerous miliary tubercles, yellow in parts, were found scattered through the lungs and spleen; and granulations on the peritoneum, the covering of the liver, and in the arachnoid and choroid plexus of the brain. The pulmonary tubercles were rather large, and could be crushed by firm pressure between the fingers (recent).

CHAPTER XXI.

CASES OF SCROFULOUS PHTHISIS FROM INFECTION THROUGH
LYMPHATICS, CONNECTED WITH GLANDULAR SCROFULA,
FISTULA, ABSCESS, &c.

*Twelve cases generally arrested for several years—Phthisis after Purulent
Otorrhœa—Fatal Dyspnœa from Caseous Bronchial Glands—Threatened
Phthisis after Empyema—Recovery.*

THE succeeding cases[1] are grouped together to exemplify
a connection between pulmonary consumption and several
local diseases which are commonly considered scrofulous;
for example, chronic glandular swellings, suppuration and
caseation—lumbar and other abscesses connected with
scrofula of the bones—fistula ani—and purulent otorrhœa.
In some instances the pulmonary disease and the local
one may be the result of one common or constitutional
defect, a decaying tendency of the whole bioplasm: but
in others the one has succeeded to the other so distinctly
as to warrant the inference that an infection has spread
from one part to another; and in all such cases the lymphatic system must be considered the conveying channel;
and if the result be not localised by an accidental inflammation, the disseminated phthinoplasms will begin in the
adenoid tissue in the form of miliary tubercles.

CASE 78.—*Scrofulous Glands and Abscesses. Phthisis.*

Mr. L., aged 35, first seen by Dr. Williams October 12, 1858. He had
had scrofulous abscess in the neck since childhood, and at a later date ab-

---

[1] These cases are not the best of the kind which could be produced, and
I regret that, after the long delay which has occurred in the publication of
this work, there is no time left for searching my large records for better.

.... hip and knee; but under the influence of cod-liver oil .... he gradually got well, the knee remaining stiff. Afterwards had several scrofulous abscesses, which all healed under the same treatment. In the last eighteen months the abdomen has become full of fluid, and tender to the touch; there has been occasional diarrhœa, and cough and slight hæmoptysis have come on. *Dulness and tubular sounds at and above right scapula. Superficial dulness and fluctuation in abdomen.* Oil was ordered in liquor potassæ and tincture of orange, and an iodide of potassium ointment for the abdomen.

March 7, 1861.—Abdominal swelling soon subsided, and he has generally improved, but still has infirm health, and has lately had ulcers in the foot and leg connected with diseased bone. Still has cough and occasional hæmorrhage from lungs and bowels. *Signs in the chest the same.*

May 1, 1866.—Continues infirm, but attends to business, generally at Brighton. Has lately had more cough with some hæmoptysis. Oil has been taken in above mixture. *Dulness and obstruction in whole right side. Tubular sounds in upper region.*—Oil ordered with sulphuric acid and ....

Not seen after. Heard of his death in 1870.

CASE 79.—*Phthisis arrested. Scrofulous Abscesses. Death Ten Years after from Subacute Pleurisy.*

Mr. G., aged 17. Fair complexion; family phthisical; mother afterwards died of scrofulous pneumonia.

First seen November 4, 1848. In May returned from Germany, and a fortnight after caught cold and spat a little blood. Cough continued after, and in August brought up large quantities of blood. Was starved, leeched, and cold vinegar kept constantly to the chest. Is very much reduced in flesh and strength, and breath is very short. Pulse 120, skin hot. Has been under the care of an eminent physician, who declares his case to be ...., and that he cannot live six weeks.

Dulness, defective motion, and crepitus superseding breath-sound throughout right lung. Moist cavernous sounds, and most dulness, in upper part. Some dulness and mixed crepitus at left apex also.

Cod-liver oil prescribed, with mixture of nitric and hydrocyanic acids tincture of hop and orange peel: morphia linctus for the cough, and a blistering liniment.

In a week considerable improvement. Pulse reduced to 100, appetite good, cough and expectoration less, strength increasing. *Cavernous sounds now drier, and extend from right clavicle to fourth rib.*

July 10, 1849.—Continued to improve in all respects, although shut up in London through the winter. Has gained much flesh and strength, but breath still short on exertion. Cough moderate, with opaque expectoration. .... oil regularly. *Collapse, dulness, and small dry cavernous .... below right clavicle to third rib. Obscure vesicular breath below* and in the back, with clearer stroke. Tubular sounds, but no crepitus at left apex. A few days ago, after walking in the heat, fainted, and has spit some blood since.

He afterwards gradually improved in flesh and strength, and the cough became little troublesome, with only morning expectoration. The next winter was spent in the neighbourhood of London, and the following year he went to Torquay, where he continued to improve, riding on horseback. Last year one of the knees became painful, and the joint swelled much. It proved to be a scrofulous abscess, which opened and has been discharging since; and another has since formed in the thigh, connected with diseased bone, and has discharged enormous quantities of matter. He was consequently so much reduced, that, when brought to London, Sir B. Brodie thought he would not live ten days. However, by resuming the oil with quinine, and taking liberally bitter ale and a very generous diet, gradual improvement followed in flesh and strength, and the discharge from the wounds diminished. The cough, which had entirely ceased, has lately returned, with some opaque expectoration.

Note of physical signs not kept.

May 31, 1854.—Abscess in thigh quite healed, the knee-joint anchylosed. His health is fair, with little or no cough. The last three years have been passed in London or at Fulham. He has continued the oil and a liberal diet. Lately, after the exertion of throwing a large dog into a river, he brought up an ounce of blood.

Right front still flattened and rather dull, but much less so than formerly, with some puerile vesicular breath-sound. Tubular sounds only close to sternum. More dulness and deficiency of breath in dorsal regions, and slight crepitus in parts.

[A sad but remarkable episode connected with this case deserves to be recorded. The patient's mother, who had most devotedly nursed him and dressed his wounds during his long and trying illness, was attacked with scrofulous pneumonia, which in a few weeks ended in excavation and death. Previously she had been quite healthy and strong.]

1858.—He continued in good health till the beginning of this year, when, travelling in Spain, he was attacked with ague at Madrid, and returned to England broken in health and very bloodless. On May 7, Dr. R. D. Harling found him suffering from pleurisy of the right side, with effusion, which resisted all treatment; and as the extensive effusion threatened suffocation, it was determined to attempt relief by paracentesis. This was performed by Mr. P. Hewett on May 17, with complete temporary relief, the fluid drawn off being clear serum, forming a fibrinous clot on standing. The dyspnœa, however, soon returned; and on the 20th the operation was repeated, a smaller quantity flowed, and was now somewhat turbid, but not purulent. In four days the breathing had again become as difficult as ever; but the patient refused to submit to another operation, and died on the 26th.

⬛⬛⬛, ⬛⬛⬛ examination was not permitted, and the ⬛⬛⬛ ⬛⬛⬛ of the chest at last remains doubtful; but, after the evi-⬛⬛⬛ of advanced consumption at first, and the wonderful recovery from this and from extensive scrofulous suppuration subsequently, the enjoyment of tolerable health for four years are all most remarkable; and no less so the fact, that the fatal attack brought on by adequate external causes did not ⬛⬛⬛ the purulent or consumptive character of his former diseases.

CASE 80.—*Phthisis (Scrofulous Pneumonia?) after Fistula. Long sea voyages. Recovery.*

Mr. —, aged 21. Towards the end of 1860 had an abscess near the rectum, which has left a small fistula. After much anxiety during that winter, in April, 1861, had left pleuropneumonia, which was treated by calomel and opium, salines, and repeated blisters. In June the fistula was still discharging. Much loss of flesh and strength. Still cough and purulent expectoration, and occasional recurrences of pain in the left side. *Dulness, deficient motion and breath in lower two-thirds of left chest. Loud bronchophony at and within left scapula; crepitus on deep breath.*—Ordered the oil, with nitric acid tonic. A saline with opiate at night. Cantharides liniment to the side.

November 9.—Rapidly improved and gained flesh. Had lost cough, but it has returned in last week. Fistula still open. *There are now coarse crepitation in left back, and cavernous sounds at scapula. General dulness rather less.*—To continue oil tonic and liniment.

May 28, 1862.—Wintered in Madeira, and pretty well; but after fast riding once spit three ounces of blood; and in April caught cold, with increase of cough and expectoration. Taken oil regularly, and not lost weight. *Still much dulness and obstruction in left chest. Obscure cavernous sounds in scapular region. Large tubular sounds above right scapula.*

June 6, 1863.—Passed winter in Natal and Capetown, returning by way of Brazil. Has taken oil and tonic regularly. Quite free from cough and expectoration; and is in good flesh and strength. Discharge from ⬛⬛⬛. *Signs of cavity more obscure, and some improvement in breath and percussion sounds.*

May 21, 1864.—In October went the voyage to Australia, and after a ⬛⬛⬛ has just returned. Quite well the whole time, except slight ⬛⬛⬛ at Capetown. Gained 7 lbs. *Loud tubular sounds at left ⬛⬛⬛; some breath-sound, weak in some parts and rough in others, on that*

⬛⬛⬛ 14, 1865.—To Australia this winter, and to the Cape and ⬛⬛⬛ last winter, taking the oil and tonic all the time; and quite well. ⬛⬛⬛ 5 lbs. in weight. *Left chest still rather duller than right, especially ⬛⬛⬛ part behind, which is contracted. Tubular sounds at scapula;*

peculiar dry vesicular breath-sound below, especially on full inspiration (flaccid emphysema).

May 12, 1868.—Last year took a voyage to the Cape, but this year has remained in London, quite well; stronger and stouter than ever. Takes oil only at times. Fistula still open, but discharges little, and gives no inconvenience.

This gentleman has been so well in the last three years, that his going away during the winter was a matter of inclination rather than of necessity; and the last winter was passed in London without inconvenience.

1871.—Heard of as quite well.

CASE 81. —*Phthisis after Scrofula in Glands.*

A dressmaker, aged 21, whose mother had died of consumption, saw Dr. Williams July 8, 1859. Seven years ago her cervical glands much swelled were lanced, and then healed; but every summer the swelling returns, and is painful. Had cough all the winter, with greenish expectoration, and has lost strength and breath. *Dulness and mucous rhonchus below left clavicle,* where there is pain.—Oil ordered, with iron quinine and phosphoric acid, and counter-irritation with acetum cantharidis.

July 15, 1860.—Took oil three months, and became much better, but cough still continues, with expectoration.—To resume remedies.

December 27, 1864.—Was quite well and active for four years, but lately, being much confined in business, has had pain in the left side and shoulder, and has lost flesh. *Still dulness and deficient breathing in upper left chest.*

October 15, 1868.—Continued better, but liable to occasional increase of cough, and often requiring the support of the oil and tonic, until the last three months, when, after a cold, the cough and expectoration, with feverishness, have much increased, and she has been obliged to lay by, and use various remedies, salines, blisters, &c. Is now better, but very weak and thin; and has not been able to continue the oil for any time. *More dulness and obstruction in left chest, with crepitus in parts.*

May 8, 1870.—Continued several weeks very ill, but at length the stomach bore the oil, and gradual improvement took place, regaining strength and some flesh, and almost losing the cough. In the last two months the cough has returned, with much opaque expectoration, sometimes offensive. Pain in left chest. *Dulness and tubular sounds in upper left and less in right bronchial rhonchi below.*

May, 1871.—This patient is reported to be living an invalid life, without much cough or suffering.

Case 82.—*Phthisis after Scrofula of Glands and Fistula.*

Mr. F., aged 37, consulted Dr. Williams, April 28, 1858. A brother died of phthisis. Had suffered during his youth from scrofulous glands of the neck, which had ulcerated. During the last three years had fistula, which had been operated on; but never healed. Cough came on a year ago, and had continued ever since with occasional hæmoptysis, and lately with opaque expectoration. Has lost much flesh, but regained under one year's course of the oil, and ten weeks spent at Torquay and Ventnor. *Dulness and loud tubular sounds in upper right chest, chiefly posteriorly.*

May 20, 1861.—Passed the first winter at Hyères, and left off oil, and became worse. The last two years have been spent in Guernsey, and oil has been steadily taken. He is much improved, but still has cough, with some yellow expectoration, and occasional hæmoptysis. *The physical signs are the same in the right lung, but some tubular sounds are audible also in the upper portion of the left.*

Case 83.—*Phthisis after Suppurating Bubo. Death Six Years after with Pneumo-Thorax.*

Mr. W. M., aged 19, was seen by Dr. Williams, in consultation with Sir James Clark, in December, 1843, for a suppurating bubo, accompanied by cough and expectoration. *Some dulness under left clavicle.*—Iodide of potassium, nitric acid, and sarsaparilla were ordered, and the patient apparently recovered, and remained well till July 1845, when he caught cold, and has had cough, expectoration, and occasional night-sweats ever since.

October 16, 1845.—*Dulness below left clavicle; more dulness and tubular sounds in right scapular region.* Was ordered a mixture of nitric acid and tincture of hop, and Iceland moss, and to winter in Madeira.

October 8, 1846.—Wintered comfortably in Madeira, and now well, except his breath is short. *Flattening and dulness, with click sound on deep breath, below left clavicle and above scapula.*

September 30, 1847.—Tolerably well, but still has cough and some expectoration. *Dulness; small tubular and click sounds upper left chest; obscure breathing in upper right.*—Was ordered cod-liver oil in nitric and hydrocyanic acids, and an acetum cantharidis liniment.

He wintered again in Madeira, taking oil, and returned home pretty well; but during the winter, which he passed in England, he caught severe cold; perforation of pleura took place, and he died of pneumo-thorax in 1849.

Case 84.—*Phthisis after Lumbar Abscess, and Empyema.*

Mr. S. was seen by Dr. Williams June 5, 1844. He stated that three years before, after rigors and pain, a swelling appeared in the right lumbar region, which opened in two points, and discharged a quantity of very offensive pus. Later on he coughed up much of the same matter, smelling like rotten eggs, for several months, and lost greatly in flesh and strength. He gradually improved, but the right side of his chest remaining dull and contracted, though less so.—Ordered a mixture of iodide of potassium and sarsaparilla ; counter-irritation, with an iodine liniment.

April, 1846.—Continued to improve till caught a fresh cold in March, and now has cough and soreness of chest. Physical signs not recorded. Died of phthisis in 1848.

Case 85.—*Phthisis after Syphilis, Mercurial Salivation, and Suppurating Glands. Cirrhosis of Liver and Ascites.*

Wm. M., æt. 28; admitted December 6, 1843.—French polisher. Lived irregularly. Four years ago had syphilis, chancre and bubo ; treated with medicines which made mouth sore, and two months after, whilst still weak, was laid up two months with pains and weakness of limbs; and under treatment his mouth and throat again became sore, and cervical glands swelled and suppurated, and remained open for several months, during which he continued weak, and has not been strong since ; but has not been confined. Two months ago had an abscess in groin (not syphilitic), which discharged, and healed in three weeks. At this time he began to cough and expectorate ; and the breath has become short, and he has lost much flesh. Sputa opaque, viscid, rather rusty. Tenderness and *dulness on percussion, and defective movement of left chest. Cavernous sounds below humeral end of left clavicle. Crepitus beyond and breath-sound obscure. Right side less dull than left, except above scapula.*—A blister was applied to left side, and a mixture containing tart. antimony and hydrocyanic acid given.

December 16.—Chest symptoms have been somewhat easier; but urine very scanty and high coloured, and there is some fluctuation in the abdomen. Liver dulness smaller than natural. Expectoration more opaque, less viscid. *Dulness and cavernous sounds as before in left lung, tubular in right.*

January 16.—Ascites increased rapidly, and cough for a time better. Diuretics and elaterium have been given, with only slight diminution of the swelling ; cough and breath again becoming troublesome, and appetite failing. Became delirious on the 22nd, and gradually sunk after. Died 22nd.

Moderate emaciation ; some œdema of legs. Abdomen contained many quarts of yellow fœtid serum and a few flakes of lymph. Right lung not adherent ; a few grey tubercles near apex, and much more in middle lobe, forming clusters, surrounded with black matter; some puckering of the pleura over it. Left lung closely adherent to chest ; the whole upper lobe consolidated, and of an iron-grey colour, with several cavities communicating, and some containing pus; lower lobe partially solid also, and containing a few cavities, but no tubercles ; lower portion healthy, and without tubercles.

... pericardial covering of heart. Liver very ... (.. lbs.), shrank up into a rounded mass in the ... nodulated on surface, of pale brick colour; right ... to diaphragm. Vessels on capsule fringed with opaque de... which could be seen also in the substance around the portal vessels. ... firmly adherent. Spleen very large (weight, 8 oz.) Patches of ... deposit on capsule.

Case 86.—*Phthisis after Purulent Otorrhœa.*

Mr. H. C., aged 17.—Maternal uncles and aunts have died of consumption.

March 28, 1860.—When a child he had an abscess under the jaw, and a purulent discharge from the right ear has gone on ever since. Has had ... every winter; increased during the present, and attended with pain in the chest, loss of flesh, and shortness of breath. Nevertheless he looks well, and is engaged in farming. *Deficient breath in front of both sides of ... Tubular sounds above right scapula.*—Ordered oil in phosphoric ... calumba, and tincture of orange, a cantharides liniment and an ... pill.

May 11th.—Has gained flesh and strength, but still has cough and expectoration. *Dulness and large tubular sounds, with croak on deep breath ... right clavicle.*

August 11, 1862.—Oil has been taken on and off ever since last visit, and the patient is much better, but he always has cough and yellow expectoration. *Tubular sounds in right scapular region and above it, but pretty good breath-sound.*

Case 87.—*Phthisis after Otorrhœa.*

An officer in the army, aged 24, consulted Dr. Williams, October 16, 1860. Has had otorrhœa, after scarlatina, from infancy. For last eight months ... slight and persistent cough. Six weeks ago, when in Canada, had ... to amount of three ounces after exertion, and has had some ... amount since. Had lost much flesh, which has been regained since. ... deficient breath in upper portion of right back, and some tubular ... upper left chest.—Oil was prescribed in a tonic of phosphoric ... calumba, and orange, and counter-irritation with acetum cantharidis ...

... 1861.—Wintered well, but complains of breath being rather ... During last few days, after hurrying himself, the expectoration was ... Physical signs same.

... 1862.—Well and stout, doing duty at Harwich, but has had slight ... occasionally, and has lately been suffering from cold and sore

CASE 88.—*Caseation of bronchial glands.* *Scrofulous* *Tubercles.*

Miss M., aged 3 years, was seen by Dr. Williams June 26, 18.. . had had severe cough for several months, and occasional attacks of .. lous inspiration, occurring especially at night. Did lose flesh, but .. gained. *Dulness and stridulous breath-sounds in right interscapular re..* —Ordered iodide of potassium, with sarsaparilla, and to use an iodine .. ment.

The little patient was removed to Clifton, where she improved du.. several months, then was suddenly attacked with bronchitis, and died .. two days. On post-mortem examination there were found consolidat.. with partial caseation of the lower lobe of right lung, with small tube.. nodules also, and a few miliary tubercles in middle lobe. There was co.. siderable caseous deposit in the bronchial glands, one of which was gre.. enlarged, and compressed the right bronchus.—*Reported by Dr. Symonds..*

CASE 89.—*Empyema threatening Phthisis.* *Paracentesis.* *Recovery.*

Miss B., aged 12, November 23, 1865.—Reported to have been qui.. well till ten days ago, when she was attacked with sharp pain of left si.. and shoulder, with shortness of breath and fever. Was treated by D.. Stokes, of Canonbury, for acute pleurisy, with salines, mercurials at nig.. and blister; but symptoms continue. Skin not hot. *Whole left side du.. without breath or voice. Heart to right of sternum. Abdomen large. Liv.. down to umbilicus.*

Pil. hydrarg. et scill., *bis die.* Haust. potass. iodidi et acetat., 4 horis.

November 25.—Dyspnœa increased. Pulse 130. Walls of chest œde.. matous; abdomen increasing; fluid in peritoneum; urine scanty; bow.. relaxed.

Further delay being judged unsafe, a trocar was plunged by Dr. Sto.. into the chest, above the fifth left rib at the side, and 10oz. pus flowed; th.. wound being covered with a poultice after the trocar was withdrawn, th.. discharge went on freely. No air was admitted into the chest during th.. operation; but soon after *there were signs of pneumo-thorax*; and about .. ten days the discharge became offensive. Much relief to the breathing an.. cough followed the operation; but the patient remained long very wea.. with quick pulse, night-sweats, and bad appetite. The abdominal enlarge.. ment, however, soon subsided.—Quinine, with mineral acids and cod-liv.. oil, was prescribed, and a generous diet with wine or malt liquor enjoin.. .

July 9, 1867.—Weakness and offensive discharge continued long, bu.. the first wound healed, and another opened spontaneously in front, and ha.. generally discharged from two drachms to two ounces daily. It has some.. times stopped for a few days, and then the cough has increased. The ..

pectoration as well as the discharge has the rotten-egg odour. In the last four months there has been considerable improvement in growth and strength, and she is able to walk two miles.—Half-an-ounce of oil twice daily has been regularly taken in wine.

The whole left side is still contracted and dull ; but less so in the upper half, where there is obscure breath-sound posteriorly, and loud tubular sound with slight crepitus in front. The heart beats under and to the right of the sternum.

The recommendation, made before, to go to the sea-side, and continue the tonics with the oil, was repeated., and was followed with great benefit.

May 1871.—The patient is reported to have completely recovered ; the discharge having stopped two years, all cough ceased, and the full development of growth having nearly restored symmetry of form.

I have notes of several more cases of empyema ending in complete recovery, although the compression of the lung and the long continuance of purulent formation around it, made the danger of infection imminent. Many other cases are less fortunate, empyema ending in phthisis. See Dr. Stokes on ' Diseases of the Chest,' p. 427.

CHAPTER XXII.

CASES OF CHRONIC PHTHISIS OR CHRONIC TUBERCULOSIS.

Anatomical difference between Acute and Chronic Tubercle—The latter more limited and local, and therefore more tractable—Cases of First Stage, Six Cases arrested and cured—Of Second Stage, Five Cases arrested and cured—In Third Stage, Twenty-five Cases retarded, arrested, or cured.

UNDER this head is arranged a large group which may be considered to present samples of the most common type of pulmonary consumption. If we except a few doubtful cases, we may add the designation 'Chronic Tuberculosis,' to express that the phthinoplasms occur in the form of tubercles, which are small miliary bodies, composed of indurated adenoid tissue. These cases of chronic tubercle differ from those of acute tuberculosis rather in extent than in kind. It may indeed be said correctly that the chronic miliary grey tubercle is much harder than the acute, which, as described in several of the cases, can be crushed by firm pressure (see p. 105), but this difference is only an affair of time, like that between acute hepatisation, which is soft, and chronic induration. The great difference is in extent. Acute tuberculosis is thickly scattered throughout both lungs. Chronic tubercles are comparatively few, limited chiefly to the upper parts of one or both lungs, and although they have a tendency to infect other parts both by contiguity, and through the lymphatics, yet there is much more chance of counteracting this than in the acute disease. Therefore, these chronic cases are generally not only more tractable than cases of acute tuberculosis, but, from their more limited extent, they may be arrested

~~or cured more completely than those~~ originating from ~~inflammation.~~

The short histories given are selected out of some hundreds of similar cases, not only to show what can be done by careful and continuous treatment, but also to exhibit various phases and changes in the disease under varying circumstances and remedies. It must be observed that, although all are classed as chronic cases, many have been acute, either at commencement or in some part of their course, and they altogether are fair samples of the most common form of pulmonary consumption as it occurs in this country.

The cases are arranged in some measure according to their stages and extent. First, those of the first stage, simple induration: second stage, induration with softening; third stage, induration with excavation—the last cases having cavities in both lungs.

CASE 90.—*Chronic Phthisis—first stage.—Recovery.*

Mrs. ——, æt. 33. December 14, 1852.—Sixteen years ago suffered much from a chest affection, with cough and expectoration, which continued four years. Took cod-liver oil, was frequently blistered, and long had an open issue. Eleven years ago she married, and has been much better since. Had six children.

In last three months cough has returned, with much pain in the right chest and back ; suffers from sickness, and cannot take oil.

Tubular voice and breath at and within right scapula. Loud long expiration above.

Oil to be taken in mixture with diluted nitric and hydrocyanic acids, tincture of hop, and infusion of orange peel; cantharides liniment to the chest.

December 30.—Takes oil well, and has been freely blistered. Much better in all respects ; much less cough and pain.

March 11, 1853.—Continued much better till a month ago ; became bilious and left off oil. Weaker since, and confined within doors.

Still tubular voice at right scapula. Breath-sound clearer. To resume oil, &c. &c.

November 4.—Continues in better health, but always with cough and expectoration, sometimes tinged. Worse in cold weather. *Signs as before.*

March 30, 1854.—Wintered at Notting Hill, pretty well ; but confined in cold weather. Taken oil pretty regularly.

· March 16, 1855.—In December had severe pain and an inflammatory attack of chest, and was much reduced, but has gradually improved. Still often pain in right chest. Appetite very bad; urine thick; bilious; cough and breath have not troubled much, and signs in chest as before. Anti-bilious pills and saline.

July 25, 1856.—Wintered well, suffering little in her chest; but lately weak and very bilious. Palpitation and occasional faintness. Heart-sounds loud and short.

February 6, 1860.—Chest continues better, but often suffers from palpitation and weakness, requiring iron, &c.

November 19, 1863.—Better, and become stout. Now fresh cold and cough.

1868.—Has had no return of lung symptoms, but always short breath, and palpitation on exertion. Was much benefited last year by several months in Switzerland.

1871.—Tolerably well.

CASE 91.—*Chronic Phthisis—first stage.—Cured by enforcing treatment.*

Mr. ——, æt. 23. June 19, 1863.—Quite well till twelve months ago, after close application in an office in Edinburgh, coughed up a dessert-spoonful of blood. Soon began to cough, which continued all the winter; worse in April, with expectoration, and rapid loss of flesh and strength. Is now returning from the south coast, weak, pale, emaciated, and in a most desponding state. Says that he cannot take cod-liver oil.

Much dulness, with loud ready bronchophony and deficient breath in upper half of right front and back. Tubular sounds within and above left scapula, and below left clavicle.

As the only chance of saving him, he was urged to take the oil in a mixture of phosphoric acid strychnia and orange. The chest to be blistered with acetum cantharidis, and a morphia linctus for the cough at night.

July 1.—Takes the oil very well, and is already better. Only occasional nausea. *More breath in right lung.* An occasional dose of blue pill and colocynth to be taken.

February 12, 1866.—Dr. W. heard that the patient had continued the oil and tonic ever since, and soon became wonderfully better. Has now hardly any cough, is regularly attending to business in Edinburgh, and is going to be married.

May 1871.—Heard from another patient that Mr. —— was quite well, and fully engaged in business.

The condition of this poor wasted young man, with his unhappy mother, was truly pitiable at the first visit. At the second, the unexpected discovery that he could take the oil had filled him with hope, and his amendment went on rapidly from that time to a happy issue.

CASE 92.—*Chronic Phthisis—first stage.—Arrested.*

A young gentleman, æt. 15. May 11, 1857.—Maternal aunt died of phthisis. In last Christmas holidays, after a chill, had pain in right side, and some cough ever since. Ten weeks ago had a severe chill after playing at football, and since has suffered much from cough and weakness, loss of appetite and breath. *Dulness, defective motion and breath-sound in whole right chest. Tubular sounds at and above scapula.*—To take oil, with nitric and hydrocyanic acids in orange infusion, and use acetum canthar.

June 16 —Much better. Cough nearly gone. Says breath is not short now. *Still dulness, and tubular sounds at and above right scapula.*

November 22, 1866.—Took oil at times for several years, and much improved in general health and strength, but always found himself rather short-winded on exertion, and sometimes rather wheezy. Still he has kept his terms regularly at Cambridge, and studied with such success that he came out Senior Wrangler last winter. Has continued well till six weeks ago, when he caught a cold, and has had slight cough since, with an occasional feeling of faintness. *Bronchophony above right scapula. Percussion and breath-sounds generally clear.*—To take oil, with iron tonic.

1868 —Continues well. Has now become Fellow of his college.

May 3, 1871.—Has continued well generally, but had cough several times last winter. None lately. Is pale and out of condition. *Chest-sounds good generally, but still tubular sounds in upper right.*—To resume oil and tonic.

CASE 93.—*Chronic Phthisis—first stage.—Recovery.*

A gentleman, aged 22, from Nova Scotia, visited Dr. Williams, November 5, 1856. He stated that August last year he had Asiatic cholera, for which he was given a great deal of mercury, and for two months after the attack he had a cough, which disappeared before May, when severe laryngitis came on, and cough had continued ever since. Oil had been taken for three months, with much benefit, and he improved more during the voyage from Nova Scotia. *Decided dulness and deficient motion at and above right scapula. Breath not tubular.*—Ordered oil, with tonic mixture, and cantharides liniment for the chest.

May 11, 1857.—Wintered at Hyères, and much improved in flesh and strength. *Still dulness and deficient motion and breathing at and above right scapula.*

June 16, 1858.—Returned to Nova Scotia, and wintered in Madeira, taking oil the whole time and gaining weight. At present he is apparently quite well. *Dulness hardly perceptible.*

June 24, 1859.—Returned from Italy and Switzerland quite healthy and active.

Three years later he appeared in perfect health.

CASE 94.— *Chronic Phthisis—first stage.—Arrested.*

Mr. ——, æt. 30. October 18, 1861.—A brother and a sister had died of consumption. Another brother had hæmoptysis and calcareous expectoration repeatedly. Has been twelve years in Syria, and three years ago, when on Mount Lebanon, was chilled, and since has had cough, sometimes spasmodic and sometimes hacking. Is now pale and thin. *Dulness; tubular sounds at and above right scapula. Bronchophony above left scapula.* —Oil ordered with phosphoric acid, and calumba, and a croton-oil liniment.

February 25, 1862.—Improved on treatment, but lately has been much bustled, and has now more cough and chest irritation. Has not used counter-irritation.—Ordered acetum cantharides liniment.

September 2, 1864.—Passed two years in Cyprus, but never free from cough, and several times had hæmoptysis, once to amount of half pint. Now resides at Tangiers, but has been home for the last three months. Has lost some flesh. *Dulness, large tubular sounds at and above right scapula. Small tubular sounds above left scapula.*

October 10, 1865.—Has been in better health during the last year at Tangiers, taking oil regularly. Within the last few days he has spit a little blood.—Oil to be taken with phosphoric acid and hypophosphite of soda.

September 17, 1866.—Pretty well, but always has some cough. Has twice expectorated calcareous matter. Sometimes has bronchitis, as at present, after voyage home.

July, 1868.—Has suffered more during the last two winters, from exposure at night at Tangiers. Last November had scarlatina, and expectoration has diminished since. Took oil and hypophosphite steadily, continuing them in the hottest weather, and has gained 10 lb. *Still dulness, tubular sounds at and above right scapula. Some tubular sounds in upper left chest.*

CASE 95.—*Phthisis—first stage.—Cured.*

Mr. ——, æt. 18. September 7, 1863.—Mother and sister died of phthisis. Pale and fast grown, but pretty well till a month ago; after a few days' cough, brought up several mouthfuls of blood. He was given perchloride of iron, and sent to Margate, where in the last week the cough has become much worse, with much wheezing, oppression, and feverishness. *Bronchial rhonchi all over the chest, but at right apex there is crepitation and dulness.* —To take oil and phosphoric acid and calumba twice daily, an effervescing draught at night, and use blistering liniment.

October 20.—Cough and fever continuing, it was necessary to give saline with antimony and opium, and continue the blistering for three weeks, when the fever abated, and he has since taken oil and an iron tonic. Bronchial rhonchi and crepitus have subsided. Still dulness, bronchophony, and whiffing breath-sound at and above right clavicle.

May 10, 1864.—Wintered at Torquay. Quite well, walking ten miles a day. Flesh and breath much improved. Has taken oil and tonic regularly. *Slight dulness, and tubular sounds above right scapula.*

October 7.—Generally well, but has had occasional returns of cough, *with crepitus at right apex.* A fortnight ago coughed up a little blood, and *cough continues. More dulness above scapula and below clavicle.*—Blistering to be repeated. Omit iron.

April 26, 1865.—At St. Leonard's. No cough, and quite well all winter.

May 8, 1866.—In town all winter, attending to business. *No remaining dulness. Only slight tubular in upper right.*

February 16, 1870.—Quite well, and recently married. A few months ago a slight tinge in expectoration, but no cough, and breath is good.

February 21, 1871.—At Christmas, and again in last fortnight, some cough and expectoration. Otherwise well, and has a fine little daughter. *Some tubular sounds and rhonchi in upper chest.*

This patient seemed threatened with acute phthisis at first illness. His sister was quickly carried off by a similar attack. Although in a measure cured for the last seven years, he must be considered predisposed to relapse, and will always need care.

CASE 96.—*Phthisis—second stage.—Cured.*

A clergyman, aged 32, of consumptive family, consulted Dr. W. July 13, 1853. For several months had cough and much expectoration, increased by heavy duty. Worse in last two months, and in last week much reduced by a feverish attack. Has lost much flesh and strength. Once brought up a teaspoonful of blood.

Moderate dulness and tubular sounds in upper left; obscure croak on deep breath.—Ordered oil in mixture of nitric acid, hop and orange-peel infusion; and cantharides liniment.

July 21.—Much better. Takes oil well. Still cough. *Tubular voice and thinness in upper left, especially near spine.*

January 3, 1854.—Taken oil, &c., ever since. Wintered at Torquay. Quite lost cough, and otherwise well, and has resumed regular duty.

May 11, 1854.—Continued pretty well, taking oil, &c., for three years. Last August, after unusual exertion, expectorated six ounces of blood; but was not worse after.

In January had cold and cough.

Still some dulness and tubular sounds within left scapula,

1868.—Heard that he is still alive and well, fifteen years after the first symptoms.

1871.—Continues well.

Case 97.—Phthisis—second stage.—Arrested.

Miss ——, æt. 24. June 2, 1852.—Father's mother died of [illegible]... a long time breath has been short on exertion, but cough first came in January, and has continued with more or less pain in left shoulder; weak and was losing flesh, but began oil three months ago and improved especially since she has been at Hastings three weeks. Dulness; deficient breath in whole left chest, with crepitus, coarse in upper parts. Tubular sounds above right scapula.—To continue oil, with nitric and hydrochloric acids, hop and orange tincture; and use cantharides liniment body of left chest.

August 12, 1853.—Wintered at Hastings. Much improved in flesh and strength, walking three or four miles daily. Cough moderate, but breath still short. Still dulness and deficient breath in left chest; tubular, with obscure creak in upper parts on deep breath. Large tubular sounds above right scapula.

October 20, 1854.—Continued to improve. Cough now only in [illegible]. Collapse and dulness below left scapula. Less tubular and no crackling sound in upper. Tubular above right scapula.

April 21, 1871.—In 1856 spent a year in Ross-shire, and became so strong as to be able to walk twenty miles in the day without inconvenience, and had no cough, except for a week or two from fresh cold. The breath was always short. Continued well, and passed several winters in Scotland. A year ago at Bournemouth over-exerted herself in reading and other ways, and became very weak and thin, and has not since regained flesh or strength. Occasional pain in left side. Little cough till the last week with slight expectoration. Pulse 90. Heat 100°.

Collapse and contraction of left front. Heart pulsation, and dulness to fourth rib. Obscure breath-sound and moderate dulness through left [lung]; only slight tubular above scapula; more so above right.

The oil, which had not been taken of late, to be resumed with a [illegible]. An effervescing saline at night, and iodine to be painted on left chest.

Case 98.—Phthisis—second stage.—Arrested.

Mr. ——, æt. 27. May 6, 1865.—Last February, when in a weak state of health, caught a severe cold, which ended with left pleurisy. Has ever since had cough, with little expectoration and frequent huskiness of voice. Not recovered his strength or breath. Bowels not free. No appetite.

Slight crepitus in upper third of left lung.

To take oil in mixture of nitric acid, tinctures of nux vomica and [illegible], and compound infusion of orange peel. A daily aloetic pill. Tincture of iodine to be applied to the chest.

October 6.—Cough continues, with viscid expectoration. Much [illegible] at night. Breath improved, but is still weak, and suffers from palpitation. *Mucous rhonchus and croak in upper left, front, and back. Tubular sounds at and within left scapula.*—To continue the oil with mixture of phosphoric acid, hypophosphite of soda, calumba, and orange infusion.

November 17.—Much improved in all respects. Gained 5 lb. Strength and appetite good. *Breath clearer, but still crepitus in upper half.*

May 29, 1866.—Wintered at Ventnor, pretty well; taking oil, &c., and out regularly till early spring, when he had congestion of left lung. Then the oil was discontinued; he has lost flesh; and expectoration, which had been free, has ceased, and cough and short breath have returned. Bowels costive. *Dulness, and neither breath nor vocal vibration through left lung. Tubular sounds above right scapula.*—Left side to be blistered with acet. cantharid. Effervescing saline, with iodid. potass to be taken every night. To resume oil and mixture and daily pill as before.

November 28.—Soon improved in breath and strength, and gained 4 lb. Cough slight, but still some expectoration. *Dulness gone in left chest. Breath-sound still mixed with crepitus in upper parts.*

May 2, 1867.—At Grimsby till February, then Bournemouth. Quite well, except slight cough. Has been out all through the winter, and gained 7 lb., but always continued oil, &c., and has occasionally blistered.

June 21, 1871.—Remained at Grimsby for last four years, quite well, except occasional cold and cough; and on active exertion a little wheezy. Flesh and strength better than ever.

Tubular sounds and subcrepitus in upper left. Emphysematous protrusion above left clavicle on cough.

Case 99.—*Chronic Phthisis—second stage.—Cured.*

Mr. ——, æt. 26. May 12, 1862.—Two sisters and one brother have died of phthisis. At the end of November, after two months' cold and cough, had hæmoptysis to amount of two pints in a week. Expectoration has since been yellow, and attended with loss of flesh and short breath. Wintered at Mentone and Cannes. *Dulness, tubular sounds, coarse crepitation in upper half of right chest. Less dulness, with weak breath-sound below.* Ol. c. acid. phosph. et calumb.: lin. acet. cantharid.: linct. morphiæ.

November 14, 1863.—Went to Madeira in October 1862, and gradually lost cough and expectoration; gained weight, increasing from 8 st. 9 lb. to 10 st. 2 lb.

July 9, 1865.—Has been at Madeira ever since, except a month absent in 1863. Has had no illness, except biliousness. In September last was attacked with vomiting, and lost 27 lb. in six weeks. Has since nearly regained weight (10 st. 1 lb.). Has occasional morning expectoration, but breath is pretty good. *Only slight dulness and weak breathing in upper right chest. No crepitation or tubular sounds.*

July 24, 1866.—At Torquay; gained 6 lb. Has had no return of cough, and only is occasionally bilious.

September ... 185...—Quite well, except occasional lumbago, and in last ... . Has oil for nine months. *Some dulness, obstruction, and ... in upper right.*

July 8, 1869.—Generally well, except occasional attacks of cold and cough, for which he blisters and takes oil, and is soon well, gaining 12 lb. or 15 lb. *Same dulness and tubular in upper right back.*

1869.—Heard continues well.

July 20, 1870.—Has been well, and attending actively to business as inn-keeper; weight, 11 st. In May got wet, and since has had cough, and lost flesh, but says his breath is good still. *Dulness and dry cavernous sounds in upper right and back. Breath heard below and in front.* Has taken oil only irregularly.

June 13, 1871.—Resumed oil and tonic steadily, and recovered flesh and lost cough; but it returned in winter, with expectoration. He was shut up, and lost appetite and strength. Not so regular with oil as formerly, and he again lost much flesh. *Collapse below right clavicle, and harsh vesicular breath below second rib. Above and to mid-scapula loud dry cavernous sound. Obscure breath, with subcrepitus below.*

August 7.—Gained 2 lb. Still cough and opaque expectoration, and ... sounds in right back.

This case records arrest of the disease for twenty years, with full enjoy-ment of life; then renewal of disease in the same parts, and again amelio-ration, twenty-five years after first attack.

Case 102.—*Chronic Phthisis—third stage.—Double Cavity— repeatedly arrested.*

Miss ——, æt. 21. April 27, 1849.—Always delicate, but with much pre-cocity and energy of character. Five years ago suffered for several months with cough and loss of voice. Well after till three months ago; cough and short breath, and a glandular swelling above left clavicle. Not lost flesh. Has never worn flannel. *Slight dulness and tubular expiration above left ...* Iodid. potass. et sarza.; flannel.

May 30.—Glandular swelling diminished; but still coughs, and has lost flesh and strength. *Signs continue.* Oil, with nitric and hydrocyanic acid mixture; capsicum liniment for the chest.

February 19, 1851.—Took the oil for six months, and lost cough, and was rather well till last November, when suffered long from sore throat, and in ... month the lump has reappeared above left clavicle, with much de-pression of strength and spirits. This swelling afterwards threatened to suppurate, but subsided without discharging, and its subsidence was fol-lowed by a fever, called 'bilious.'

In 1854 the throat again became troublesome; and then followed a cough, with opaque expectoration, which continued through a great part of the next ... Then were found *signs of disease in the left lung,* but the notes are not preserved. The oil and tonics were given as before, with the view of removing cough and other symptoms.

In 1857, after much vocal exertion and exposure to damp, had an inflammatory affection of the left lung, with dulness and crepitus in the upper lobe, which lasted several months, but was at length removed under the use of oil and free counter-irritation ; but tubular sounds remained above both scapulæ ; and, more or less, cough and chest irritation continued during that and the following year.

In 1861 was so much improved in health and strength that she undertook the superintendence of a charitable institution, involving a great amount of mental and bodily exertion.

In 1862, in the midst of this work, she left off all stimulants, and soon had a bad carbuncle on the leg, which for several months caused much discomfort and weakness.

In 1863 began to suffer again in throat and chest, *with return of crepitus in left apex, which in the course of that year showed signs of excavation.* Remedies were then more steadily persevered with ; and two winters were passed at Torquay, with very beneficial results as to general health : *but the left lung continued much obstructed, chiefly in its upper half, where there remained the large croaky sounds of a contracting cavity. The lower portion was imperfectly pervious, with emphysematous stroke-sound and crepitus; and tubular sounds were heard at and above the right scapula.*

In the summer of 1867, feeling so much better, this lady could not be restrained from her beneficent work, and with a view to its continuance, remained in London during the winter. At the commencement of this spell the trial of a coke-stove in her room brought on a severe attack of suffocative bronchitis, which very nearly proved fatal. Orthopnœa, with thrill, lips and nails, quick pulse and hot skin, a tight wheezy cough, and only scanty viscid expectoration. *Loud prolonged sonorous rhonchi in the chest, drowning all other sounds,* continued for several days ; yielding at length to ether, squill, and antimony, as expectorants, aided by blisters. The attack was of the nature of croupy bronchitis, and relief came with copious purulent and curdy expectoration ; and *then were heard moist crepitus in all parts of the lung, coarse and even cavernous in both scapular regions, chiefly the left; but the right now for the first time showed evidence of active disease.* Although the suffocative symptoms were relieved, the reduction of flesh and strength was fearful, and lapsing into rapid consumption seemed inevitable. Happily, however, the appetite returned, enabling the patient to take food, and to resume the oil with the cod-liver tonic which had served her so well during the previous years. Slowly and with interruptions during that winter, more decidedly and steadily during the following summer, improvement took place in flesh and strength, and imperfectly in breath, for only a portion of the upper and lower lobes of the right lung remained effective for respiration. About *the second and fourth ribs in front, and at the upper half of the scapula be-hind, was a loud cavernous rhonchus, assuming a stridulous or grating cha-racter at times, when the breathing was more oppressed. The left upper region also presented cavernous sounds, croaking or dry at different times: and in the lower portions the only sound was a short crackle on a deep breath. Yet the stroke-sound was clear, indicating the obstruction to be more from emphy-sema than from consolidation.*

This interesting patient had other ailments to distress her, although it is probable that, while adding to her sufferings, they may have contributed to avert the worst results. A succession of boils—some large and painful—broke out in various parts of the body, ending in pretty complete suppura-tion. These were eventually checked under the use of sulphite of soda (gr. x. or xv.) two or three times daily, which for convenience was combined with a morphia cough mixture. Another plague was an eruption of eczema, which appeared in the limbs and bends of joints, as the chest symptoms became mitigated. This was relieved by a carbolic acid liniment, and disappeared at length after several weeks' use of arsenic. The oil and strychnia tonics once a day have been steadily continued whenever possible.

After the improvement in the summer, several bad attacks took place during the winters 1868-9 and 1869-70, reproducing the croupy suffoca-tive symptoms of the former winter, and rendering recovery very uncertain. But she did recover, and during the summer 1870 made considerable ad-vances on her former improvement, enjoying a residence in the country of several months.

The last winter (1870-1) was a greatly improved one. Although shut up entirely for seven months, she gained flesh and strength, had no severe attack, and has been able to do much writing and other official work in connection with charitable institutions, of which she has long been a main-spring. And this lady, so limited in breath and strength, yet still so use-ful to humanity, has cavities in both lungs, with the greater part of one in an emphysematous, imperfectly pervious state : a condition balancing between consumption and asthma. Happily, the vigorous mind has not been over-come by the infirmity of the body; and by its resolute good sense, in strictly following the advice given through all trials and difficulties, it has been mainly instrumental in prolonging a valuable life.

CASE 103.—*Chronic Phthisis—third stage.— Arrested.*

Miss ——, æt. 26. June 22, 1863.—Often had cough, but one has been constant for the last twelve months, and in the last four months worse, with much opaque expectoration, and hoarseness, and losing flesh. *Dulness and crepitant obstruction through whole left chest. Bronchophony above right scapula.*—To take oil in phosphoric acid and calumba mixture, to paint chest with tinc. iodine, and use a linctus at night.

August 3.—Much better. Less hoarseness and expectoration. *Crepitus*

. . . . *While breath-sounds in lower part of left lung, and . . . . left scapula.*—To resume oil and tonic.

December 2, 1865.—Has remained in Norfolk during the last two years, comparatively well, and sometimes more active than was prudent. There is always some cough and expectoration. *Loud tubular sounds above both scapulæ, most on the right side, where they extend lower also, with dulness; but the breath is rough below left clavicle.*—The oil to be continued, with the addition of hypophosphite of soda to the tonic. Caution against exertion, &c.

May 16, 1867.—Improved very much, and had hardly any cough till last March, when one came on with catarrhal symptoms, and although then moved to Torquay, has continued to suffer with weakness and sickness. Being so much better, the oil and hypophosphite were not taken regularly through the winter. *Dulness and dry cavernous sounds in upper half of right back. Some vesicular breath in front. Tubular above left scapula.* —To take oil with simple strychnia mixture.

May 20, 1869.—After three months of suffering from sickness and renewed attacks of bronchial and pulmonary inflammation, was able to take the oil and tonic again, and rallied till end of winter, when the attacks recurred again, followed by improvement in summer. Has been generally in Norfolk, going for a month to Torquay in spring. *Physical signs little changed.* Flesh and strength not much diminished.

June 15, 1871.—Has been since to Norfolk, taking oil and tonic regularly, and has been generally free from attacks, but has always some cough and expectoration. Was out almost daily through the winter, but in the last three months has had inflammatory colds, and still suffers from their effects in pain on both sides of the chest, coupled with opaque expectoration, sometimes offensive, and some loss of flesh and strength. Catamenia regular. Lips and gums of good colour. *Moderate dulness with crepitus, and some breath in right front. The whole right dorsal region dull, with loud cavernous sounds in upper two-thirds, and coarse crepitus below. Tubular sounds with partial crepitus at left apex.*

July 7th.—Much better.

Case 105.—*Chronic Phthisis—third stage—Improved.*

Mr. ——, æt. 35, May 4, 1865.—Brother and two maternal uncles died of phthisis.

Two years ago, after a long bathe in the sea, became hoarse, with a cough and pain in the chest. Expectoration sometimes bloody. Passed winter of . . . . at a hydropathic establishment in Scotland, and lost much flesh. Next winter in Egypt, was better, and regained some flesh and strength.

Dulness and deficient breath in right chest, most upper front. Tubular sounds above right scapula.—Oil prescribed with nitric acid mixture. Tinct. iodine to chest.

Loud bronchophony below clavicle.

May 25, 1869.—Gained 7 lb. mo
tered again at Nice. Keeping well, a
and took cold, and has had much c
ness and moist cavernous sounds a
for more than a month.—To resum
phosph. soda.

May 26, 1870.—Again improved
December was yachting to Malta ar
creased, with more expectoration, i
found. Has lately been more caref
and is much better. *Dulness and l
at and above right scapula. Tubula*

1871.—This patient is still contin
making the care of his health the
risk, he is able to do this with much

CASE 106.—*Chronic Phth*

Miss ——, æt. 19. August 2, 18
had a slight cough ten months, and l
months the cough has increased, w
side, and loss of flesh. *Moderate dul
lung. Breath weak below.*—To take c

April 4, 1864.—Improved much in
passed the winter at St. Leonard's, a

.... regularly, and walking daily, sometimes .... had a cold, and the cough returned; but it is .... this, weighing only 7 st. *Cavernous sounds less* ....

.... 15, ...—Has been in Wales, walking well, and free from .... Now weighs 8 st. 10 lb. *No crepitus, but some dulness and collapse* *and dry tubular sounds to left of sternum.*

.......—This lady is reported as pretty well ever since, with only occa-......... ....

Case 107.—*First Acute, then Chronic Phthisis—third stage.* *Large Cavity. Retarded.*

Miss ——, æt. 25. September 21, 1867.—Mother and sister died of phthisis. Delicate before, but no cough till July, when she had a feverish attack, with ' congestion of the left lung.' Has continued extremely weak ....., with constant cough, and now copious, purulent, and clotted albumin-ous expectoration; hot skin; frequent pulse; profuse night sweats; no appetite; often vomits with the cough. Bowels relaxed. No catamenia .... *Dulness through whole left chest; liquid cavernous sounds in* *upper third; obstruction and crepitus below.*—To take sulphuric acid and .... mixture, with glycerine morning and noon. Evening and night ...., with morphia and hydrocyanic acid.

October 15.—Sickness began to abate in a week, and was then able to take more food, and cod-liver oil with the strychnia mixture; and there is considerable increase of strength, and reduction of fever and sweats, but the cough is still harassing at times. *Large cavernous sounds in whole left* *front. Some crepitus above right scapula.*—Continue oil and tonic, and blister side with acetum cantharid.

March 27, 1868.—Gradually regained flesh and strength, and cough ex-pectoration much moderated. Catamenia have returned twice, after five months' absence. Walks out a little, and appetite pretty good. Bowels have been costive and piles have been very troublesome; but after taking .... of senna and sulphate of potass, these are relieved. Has taken ...... tonic regularly, and frequently quinine has been added. *Large* *cavernous sounds still in front, but some breath in left back.*—Oil to be ...., with phosphoric acid and hypophosphite of soda mixture.

December 1868.—Has wonderfully improved in flesh, strength, and colour. Was frequently out during the summer, but now is shut up for the winter. Pulse 80. Skin cool. Catamenia regular. Feels pretty well, except for the short breath, cough and expectoration, which are, how-ever, much reduced. *Physical signs little improved; but there is more* *breath in left back, and now no crepitus at right apex—only tubular sounds.*

This reprieve continued till the winter of 1869, when the appetite began to fail, and it was necessary to discontinue the oil for a time. The heart also became troublesome, being compressed by the ribs collapsing over the

8

contracting cavity. This added to the ████████████; and
without any considerable increase of the ████████████, the ████
became albuminous, and the patient died dropsical in April, 1878.

CASE 108.—*Phthisis—third stage. General improvement, but
disease advancing.*

Mr. ——, æt. 30. April 6, 1864.—His sister and three or four
of her children died of phthisis. In the last month has had slight cough
and pains in his left side, and has lost flesh and colour. *Some tubular
breath and voice above both scapula.*—To take phosphoric acid and glycerin,
with tinctures of henbane and calumba; and to use acetum cantharidis
liniment.

June 28, 1866.—Regained his health, and, except a cough of six weeks at
Stockholm in December 1864, has been well till three weeks ago, when
began to cough and expectorate mucus, tinged with blood. Appetite bad,
and is losing flesh and strength. *Some dulness and tubular sounds at and
within right scapula. Less above left scapula. Mucous rhonchus in
several parts.*—To take oil in mixture of nitric acid, nux vomica and ██████.
Tinct. iodine to the chest.

September 25.—Cough continued troublesome several weeks, with yellow
expectoration and night sweats; but in last two months has improved
much and gained considerable flesh. *Tubular sounds chiefly confined to
right apex.*

November 22.—Continued better till lately out in the cold, which
brought on severe pain in right hip. This is removed, but in the last two days
has brought up 2 oz. of blood. Gallic acid first, and subsequently acetate
of lead, have been given. *Dulness below both clavicles. Coarse crepitus
upper left front and back.*—To take sulphuric acid and glycerine, with a
little opium. Blister with acet. cantharid.

June 12, 1867.—No more bleeding; and has since much improved, taking
oil and sulphuric acid; but still has cough, short breath, and night
sweats. *Whole left chest obstructed, with crepitus; coarse and tubular
upper part. Some crepitus at right base.*—To continue oil with phosphoric
acid and hypophosphite quinine, and to use cantharides liniment.

November 1, 1867.—Gained much flesh, and looks well, but breath very
short. Still much obstruction in left lung, and a cavity at apex.

September 22, 1868.—Wintered at home pretty well; but breath short.
In March brought up 6 oz. of blood, and less in April. Was much
weakened, especially in hot weather; but has recovered, taking oil with
hypophosphite of quinine. Feeds and sleeps well. *Extensive obstruction of
left lung. Excavation in upper lobe. Tenderness on percussion over it.
Crepitus at right apex.*

July 29, 1869.—Better through winter, regularly taking oil and ██████

██████ ████ ████████ ████ ███████ fail in hot weather, and lately blood
███████. Whole left side obstructed and crepitant. Cavernous sounds not
███████. Respiration puerile throughout right lung.

Case 109.—*Phthisis, third stage. Retarded Nine Years.*

A gentleman, aged 35, saw Dr. Williams July 6, 1861. Two years ago he
had cough lasting three months; was well afterwards, till in February he
brought up two pints of blood. Recovered, and had no cough till April,
when cough returned from fresh cold. Since then has taken oil and cream.
*Upper right chest tender. Some dulness, rough breathing in upper right.
Tubular sounds above left scapula.*—Ordered oil in phosphoric acid, calumba
and orange tincture; and counter-irritation with acetum cantharidis.

June 21, 1862.—Well till September, when suffered from heat. Passed
winter at Nice and Rome, with little cough. Taken oil irregularly. *Dulness
and tubular sounds upper right chest, with slight crepitus. Tubular expiration at left scapula.*

February, 1864.—Wintered at Pau; passed summer in Scotland; and at
Torquay since. No cough till last fortnight, but now one with feverish
symptoms. *Dulness and tubular sounds upper right chest. Slight subcrepitus at summits of both lungs.*

July 16, 1869.—Taken but little oil since last visit. Wintered at Pau
and Rome, where he had ague. Last summer was able to shoot; but at
Pau, after going out to parties, had congestion of right lung, and ever since
breath has been much shorter, and cough constant. *Extensive dulness in
right side, with crepitation; coarse in upper part. Tubular sounds and
crepitation in lower left chest.*—Warned to be more careful, and to persevere
with oil and tonic, and counter-irritation.

December 29.—Has taken oil, &c. regularly, and was much better till a
week ago, when he caught cold, with increased cough, and is now suffering
from biliousness and piles. *Small cavernous sounds at right apex; crumpling crepitus below. Tubular sounds above left scapula.*— To have blue
pill and confect. sennæ with sulphate of potass. Oil to be continued, with
strychnine mixture.

April 28, 1870.—Wintered at Torquay, pretty well, till a month ago,
had daily rigors, followed by heat every night, and is much weaker. Taken
quinine without relief. *Dulness and cavernous sounds in upper right; obstructed breath below.*—To continue the oil with a quinine mixture; effervescing opiate at night.

Case 110.—*Phthisis after Fever. Large Cavity. Great Improvement. Death from Pneumonia.*

Mr. M——, aged 46. First seen by Dr. Williams, with Dr. Pye Smith,
October 4, 1861. After twenty years in China, was long ill with fever, and
has been very weak ever since. Cough for more than a year. In low state

flesh, strength, and activity. Gained 6 lbs. and often walks twenty miles. Was out as usual last winter. Has still some cough and expectoration. Taken no oil for two years. *Tubular sounds at and above right scapula, left as much as right; but no crepitus or rhonchus.*

February 21, 1867.—In the last five years has taken little oil, as it made him bilious. Cough has increased; breath become shorter; and now can walk only two miles. Nails convex. *Dulness, collapse, and moist cavernous sounds below the right clavicle. Breath much obstructed all down the right back. Tubular sounds above the left scapula.*—To resume oil in mixture of nitric acid, strychnia, &c. Upwards of *nineteen years* have elapsed since this patient's first symptoms. His latter deterioration came on after long suspension of treatment.

CASE 112.—*Phthisis, third stage. Arrested.*

An officer in the army, aged 35, consulted Dr. Williams July 26, 1861. He had campaigned in the Crimea, and was afterwards ordered to West Indies, and then to India, where he distinguished himself in the Sepoy Mutiny; and was quite well till his return to England last summer, when camped at Shorncliffe, and found place extremely cold. In March caught severe cold, and had sore throat and cough, with hæmoptysis ʒi, and was much reduced. Improved since taking oil and iron; but is still thin, and has short breath. *Much dulness and tubular sounds upper half right chest; tubular sounds above left scapula.*—Oil ordered with phosphoric acid and quinine, the application of acetum cantharidis, and a morphia linctus.

June 19, 1862.—Improved much, and went to Madeira in November, where he took oil regularly, and rode on horseback. Lost cough, and gained much flesh and strength. *Dulness: dry cavernous sounds upper right third of chest, chiefly in back.*

February 6, 1865.—Recovered so much that he was on active duty in New Zealand during the war of 1864, endured all kinds of hardships, wet, cold, and starvation. In April had dysentery; in May spat blood, and was laid up with inflammation of the left lung three weeks, which much reduced him, but he recovered in all respects, except his breath being short. Improved much since his return, taking oil regularly. *Moderate dulness: tubular sounds high up in left lung: good breathing below. Tubular sounds above right scapula.*

May, 1866.—Wintered at Mentone, without cough; gained flesh and strength. *Physical signs improved.* The following winter left the army, and has since resided in Madeira; where he was well, and active in spring, 1871.

CASE 113.—*Phthisis, third stage.   Arrested.   Hæmoptysis and Death.*

A young gentleman, aged 14, whose family was consumptive, saw Dr. W. December 26, 1861. He had slight cough at Eton for two months, and three weeks ago he was sent home for a bilious attack. A week later had hæmoptysis to amount of ℥ss. Still had cough and pain in the shoulder. *Dulness: tubular sounds upper half left chest, most marked in the back.*—Oil ordered with phosphoric and gallic acids, and acetum cantharidis liniment.

April 22, 1862.—Passed winter well, but when taking iron in June, spat ℥ss. of blood, and also had epistaxis. *Still dulness; tubular sounds below left clavicle.*

July 17, 1866.—Heard that he died in September, 1864, having wintered for two years at Cannes and Hyères, where he improved very much, and appeared in restored health: but, after great exertion, large hæmoptysis came on: was treated with calomel daily for three weeks, and patient soon sank and died.

On post-mortem examination a large clean cavity was found in the upper part of the left lung, which was devoid of tubercles; but many were found scattered through the right.

CASE 114.—*Chronic Phthisis, third stage.   Much Improved.*

A barrister, residing in Canada, aged 42, who had lost a brother and sister from consumption, consulted Dr. Williams, June 25, 1859. Had lived in Canada, and enjoyed good health till a year ago, when he had a cold and cough, which had recurred several times since, accompanied by expectoration and oppressed breathing. Ten years ago he spat up about a dessert-spoonful of blood; has not lost much flesh or breath, but cough is still troublesome. Bowels costive. *Dulness and large tubular sounds in upper right chest, front and back. Tubular sounds above left scapula.* Formerly took oil, but lately iron.—Ordered oil in phosphoric acid and calumbo, with acetum cantharidis liniment.

July 15, 1863.—Oil has been taken regularly, and he has been generally better; especially during the cold weather. Has regularly officiated as Judge in Canada. Looks thin and pale, and yellow expectoration has increased. *Physical signs are about the same.*

June 29, 1865.—Still resides at Toronto, continuing his judicial office. Last winter took no oil, but cream. Has more cough and expectoration. *Collapse and more dulness in upper right chest. Cavernous rhonchus above scapula.*

July 16, 1868.—Has improved in general health and strength, and goes on circuit in Canada without interruption, but he is thin, and always has cough and expectoration. *Still loud tubular (cavernous) sounds in upper right chest. Tubular above left scapula.*

The patient was very sensible of the improvement in his health and strength under the oil, as compared with iron, cream, and other means which he had tried.

CASE 115.—*Chronic Phthisis. Cavity. Duration 18 years.*

Mr. M. F., aged 15, was seen by Dr. Williams, October 30, 1853. For three years he had been subject to occasional cough, which had become constant since June. Has been well and active till within the last few weeks, when cough has become worse. No expectoration at present, but a mucous rattle sound in the tubes. *Decidedly tubular sounds in both scapular regions.*—Ordered oil in nitric acid and calumba.

March 11, 1854.—Very much improved, but always has a loose cough. *Large tubular sounds above scapula, and within left scapula. Dulness at right scapula, and some mucous rhonchus.*

November 16, 1867.—Grew strong, and tolerably well; but breath was always short, and often had attacks of cough, which have been worse during the last few years. A year ago he had congestion of both lungs, relieved by blistering and other treatment. He took oil; and went to Nice and Italy; and there caught fresh cold; and since has had constant cough, with expectoration and short breath. Then tried several German baths, but received no benefit: and is now much reduced in flesh and strength. Nails convex. *Cavernous sounds in upper right chest; obstructed breath-sounds below. Whistling tubular sound at left scapula.*—Oil was ordered in phosphoric acid and strychnia mixture, and acetum cantharidis liniment for the chest. To winter at Cannes. Improved much under this treatment, gaining much flesh and strength for twelve months.

August, 1870.—Appears much broken in health, and is in great financial difficulties. Very feverish, and cough troublesome. Now quite an invalid, *with extensive cavernous sounds on right side and crepitation throughout left lung.*

Again improved on oil and tonics, and is living (May, 1871), eighteen years since his first visit.

CASE 116.—*Phthisis, with Cavity. First Acute, but Arrested.*
Recovery.

A delicate boy, aged 8, whose father had died of phthisis, was first seen June 28, 1853. Had cough, since influenza six weeks ago. Soon after was seen by Dr. West, who found *dulness and coarse crepitus in upper left.* Had lost flesh, and had profuse perspirations; but has taken oil for a fortnight, and much improved. *Dulness in upper half of left chest, with loud tracheal note on percussion at the top. Large tubular breath, and voice-sounds also, with coarse crackle in parts. Large tubular sounds above right scapula.*

The oil to be continued with acid tonic, and ██████ ████████ is to be applied from time to time on left chest.

1861.—For several years continued delicate, requiring constant ███, and always taking the oil with varied tonics; residing generally at Tunbridge Wells, or on the south coast. *The signs of cavity became very distinct, but in two or three years they diminished as the general health improved;* and now there are only *dulness, tubular sounds below the clavicle and above the scapula, and weak vesicular signs below.* Flesh and strength now pretty good for a lad of 16.

July 21, 1863.—Continued well and active till three months ago, when he had a severe cold, with signs of bronchitis affecting the right as well as the left lung; *and the large tubular sounds and coarse crepitus reappeared then.* After repeated blistering and continued use of the oil, he gradually recovered, and has had only moderate cough and rather short breath; but his strength is good, and he walks ten miles. *Still coarse crepitus in upper left front. Dry cavernous sounds above left scapula. Large tubular sound above right scapula, but breath quite good in other parts.*

1871.—Not seen since; but is reported to have recovered his health completely.

CASE 117.—*Phthisis, with Cavity, Cured.   Living and well Twenty-four Years after Attack.*

A gentleman, aged 22, first consulted Dr. Williams on October 4, 1847. Six months ago he had an eruption, followed by boils, and three months later cough and expectoration, which continued up to the present date. *Dulness and deficient breath in upper portion of the left side of the chest.*— Was ordered a mixture of nitric and hydrocyanic acids, tincture of hops, and henbane in decoction of Iceland moss; and counter-irritation with acetum cantharidis.

August 12, 1848.—Lost cough, and improved much in two months; but caught fresh cold a month later, and cough returned, with ████ and sickness, the latter having been caused by trying impure cod-liver oil. *Dulness and dry cavernous sounds in both mammary regions; large tubular in upper back.*

December 5th.—Has taken pure oil in a mixture of nitric and hydrocyanic acids, with tincture of orange-peel regularly at Ventnor, with ██████ of strength and appetite, and of weight amounting to 14 lbs.; cough ████ at Ventnor. *Physical signs the same, but croaky cavernous sound under left clavicle.*

May 5, 1849.—Generally better, and cough moderate. The oil occasionally sickens when exercise is not taken. *Dulness in left side; ██████ cavernous sounds below left clavicle; cavernous croak above scapula; tubular sounds above right scapula.*

... continued well till a week ago, when he had hæmoptysis, ...

May 4, 1850.—Had bilious fever some months ago, which much reduced him. Omitted oil for one month, but has since taken it regularly, and quite recovered flesh and strength; cough moderate: *physical signs the same.*

May 9, 1851.—Well since, and out all the winter at Ventnor, with only slight cough, and no expectoration. *No croaky or cavernous sounds in left lung; obscure bronchophony in scapular region, and breath weak above and hard below. In right lung, respiration tolerably vesicular; expiration long, but not tubular.*

October, 1852.—Embarked for New Zealand, but was wrecked in the Channel, and much exposed to cold and wet, without permanent injury. Wintered well at Torquay, and went to New Zealand in September, 1853.

October 28, 1863.—After arrival in Auckland, had more or less cough the first two or three years, but gradually lost it, and for the last six years has been quite well. Held a Government office in New Zealand till his return this year. Has been married several years. *Tubular breath in upper part of both sides of chest, most in the left, but good vesicular below.*

1867.—Has lived in England four years, wintering at Falmouth, and enjoys general good health.

1871.—Continues well.

In this case we may fairly conclude that cicatrisation of the cavities took place, and that no deposit of considerable amount remains. The patient has lived *twenty-four years* since his first symptoms, and for the last thirteen years has had no active disease.

CASE 118.—*Phthisis, Acute at first. Cavity. Arrested. Recovery. Living Twenty-seven Years after First Attack.*

An unmarried lady, aged 28, consulted Dr. Williams September 3, 1847. Had a cough for eighteen months, which commenced after taking cold baths, and had persisted ever since. Six months ago a remarkable purpura eruption came on her body, which had mostly disappeared, but was followed by increase of cough. Formerly had swellings under her jaws, but these had diminished. In the last two months, breath, flesh, and strength have been very much reduced. Had no appetite till she visited Margate, and on her return from that place she spat a few mouthfuls of blood, which relieved cough and tightness of chest. Patient at present very weak and much emaciated; has quick pulse and profuse night-sweats. *Marked dulness and cavernous sounds in more than upper half of left side of chest; stroke-sound clearer below, and moist crepitation; some moist crepitation in upper part of right side also.*—Ordered a combination of nitric and hydrocyanic acids, with tinctures of hop, calumba, and henbane, and a linctus containing morphia. A week later she was no better, and had loathing of food and increased emaciation. Cod-liver oil was then added to the above treatment, and two months later she had wonderfully improved in flesh, strength, and well-being, with little cough, no expectoration, and an excellent appetite.

January, 1848.—Continues to gain flesh and strength ; catamenia short ; *dulness and dry cavernous sounds in upper part of left lung.*—Ordered a nightly pill of aloes and iron, and the continuance of the oil, &c.

October, 1848.—Well and in good condition ; cough moderate ; able to walk several miles ; but breath still short, and lately has had diarrhœa ; catamenia now regular ; *dulness and dry cavernous sounds in upper left down to second rib ; obscure vesicular breath below.*

Was married in 1850 ; and Dr. Williams has not seen her since, but he heard that she was alive and well in 1871, twenty-four years after the first visit, and *twenty-five years and a half* after her first symptoms. When first seen the case presented all the aspects of galloping consumption.

CASE 119.—*Chronic Phthisis.   Cavity persistent 13 years.*

A lady aged 24, whose sister had died of consumption, was first seen by Dr. Williams July 14, 1858. Four years ago she coughed up about two ounces of blood, for which she was cupped, and remained pretty well afterwards, except a cough, which in the last four months had diminished, and she has gained flesh and strength by taking oil and good feeding. *Marked dulness, with loud cavernous sounds and crepitation in upper left chest ; most in front.*—Oil was ordered in a mixture of iron and phosphoric acid. The patient soon afterwards married.

January 12, 1859. Has been free from cough, and remarkably well till six weeks ago, when she was chilled during a long journey, and has got swelling of the ankle. This affection soon subsided under treatment.

1867.—Has become stout and healthy looking, and pretty well enjoys life ; but although little cough, there is slight opaque expectoration every morning, and the breath is always short on exertion. Twice or thrice in the winter has an attack of bronchitis, sometimes with moderate hæmoptysis, but soon recovers from them. *Limited dulness and cavernous sounds to upper left chest, which are generally dry, but now moist after a fresh cold.*

1868.—Well, except occasional attacks of bronchitis.

1871.—Continues stout and well looking. Has passed through much trouble, and had various ailments ; but of late little affecting the chest, which *presents the same signs of a cavity limited by consolidation at the apex of the left lung.*

CASE 120.—*Chronic Phthisis.   Persistent Cavity* 20 *years.*

A lady, aged 40, who had lost a sister from consumption, first consulted Dr. Williams June 20, 1849.   There had been slight cough and expectoration for a year and a-half, for which she had been long treated with steel without benefit. *Amphoric stroke and loud cavernous sounds above right clavicle and scapula; the same signs below clavicle, though less marked.* —Ordered cod-liver oil.

July 13.—Heard that she was suffering from increasing weakness, diarrhœa and hoarseness, and copious expectoration. *Oil had not been taken.* —Ordered a tonic of nitric and hydrocyanic acids, and tincture of orange, to be combined with oil at a later date.

November 20.—Has taken oil regularly, and much improved in last three months, having lost her cough for the first time in two years, and grown fat and strong.

Dulness, and loud cavernous sounds above right scapula, and to a less extent below right clavicle.

1856.—General health good, no cough, but *physical signs the same.*

1868.—Alive and well 20 *years after* first symptoms.   In this case the disease was limited to the very apex of the right lung, ending in a cavity which remained dry long after the patient's restoration to health.

CASE 121.—*Chronic Phthisis.   Third stage.   Arrested* 13 *years.*

A single lady, aged 46, consulted Dr. Williams December 2, 1858.   Three years ago she had severe cold and cough and became very thin.   She took oil and regained her flesh, but never lost her cough, and a year ago had hæmoptysis to the amount of ℥iii.   Her breath is always very short.   *Extreme dulness, deficiency of breath, and coarse moist crepitation throughout left lung.   Large tubular sounds above left scapula.*

Oil was ordered in a tonic of nitric acid and calumba and orange-peel.   A saline opiate at night, and counter-irritation with acetum cantharidis on the chest.

July 27, 1859.—Has been very ill in the winter, suffering from cough, frequent hæmoptysis, and much loss of flesh; but after much blistering and taking oil and tonic, gradually regained flesh and strength.   Now has fistula in ano.   *Same as at last visit, except dry cavernous or large tubular sounds in upper left chest.*

September 24, 1860.—Has wonderfully recovered, and is fat and pretty strong, but breath short, and has lately fulness above the right clavicle; from emphysematous protrusion.   *Crepitation still throughout left lung, but still more breath.*

October 11, 1862.—Is wonderfully well as regards flesh and strength, and free from cough. Fistula discharges only occasionally. *Physical signs much as before.*

May 17, 1864.—Now has only occasional cough, and is out walking all day long.

Dulness and cavernous croak in upper left chest, with obstruction much below. Tubular sounds above right scapula.

July 16, 1868.—Has continued well, taking oil in the winter. Has lately suffered from weak eyes. Now has an attack of severe nephralgia. Was relieved by effervescing saline with opium; (oxalate crystals in urine). Has no cough. *Collapse, with much dulness and croaky cavernous sounds in left front; croaky crepitation mixed with breath-sound in left back.*

January, 1871.—Heard of her continuing well. Walks out on fine days.

CASE 122.—*Chronic Phthisis, with Cavity, Arrested. Living and well 25 years after.*

A clergyman, aged 32, was seen by Dr. Williams in consultation with Dr. Hamilton Roe and Mr. Young, for the first time March 25th, 1846. He had lost four sisters by consumption. Three years ago, after great exertion of voice and close application to work, he became hoarse, and had remained so ever since. Cough came on five months ago, with expectoration and shortness of breath, but no wasting. Wintered at Ventnor. *Dulness and cavernous sounds in upper part of right side of chest. Breath rough below left clavicle. Sputa opaque and heavy.*—Was ordered a combination of nitric and hydrocyanic acids, iodide of potassium, and sarsaparilla, and to use iodine ointment. Lost cough at Ventnor, and went to Bridgewater, which did not agree with him.

August 21.—Has been at Minehead, taking cod-liver oil regularly, using salt friction three times a day, and keeping a blister wound open. Has improved, except in breath, and expectoration is still ramiform and opaque. *Slight and irregular dulness in upper part of right chest; tubular sounds above and below right clavicle and scapula.*

June 10, 1848.—Wintered first at Malta, which he found too irritating to his chest; next at Pisa, where he grew weaker, but was improved by the voyage. *Still slight dulness; loud bronchophony and irregular breath below right clavicle; but much good vesicular breath- and stroke-sound. Breath rather irregular below left clavicle.*—Ordered iron in combination with the oil, on which he gradually improved, wintering generally in Devonshire during the following years.

January, 1868.—Quite well and active; conducting a large school, which he has done for the last twelve years. Can walk, preach, and bear exposure to any extent; and has no cough. *Still dulness and tubular sounds in upper right chest, most above scapula. Marked tubular sounds above the scapula.* Although the physical signs have not entirely disappeared, they are greatly diminished since the first examination twenty-two years ago.

may be supposed to indicate contraction and obliteration of the cavity.   In fact, they may be considered signs of the vestiges of disease, rather than of actual disease, as the patient has enjoyed excellent health for the last twelve years. Alive and well in 1871. *Upwards of twenty-five years* have elapsed since the first symptoms appeared.

CASE 123.—*Chronic Phthisis. Cavities. Arrested. Living 13 Years.*

A solicitor, aged 32, first consulted Dr. Williams November 27, 1856. His brother died of phthisis. Was attacked with influenza two years ago, and ever since had cough and grey expectoration, increasing in winter and diminishing in summer. In last three months sputum has become pink, and patient has lost flesh, strength, and breath. *Some dulness and decided tubular breath at and above both scapulæ, mostly left.*—Ordered oil in a tonic of nitric and hydrocyanic acids with tincture of orange.

June, 1857.—Wintered at Pau, taking oil, &c., till April. Lost cough and expectoration, and gained flesh and strength. Then went to Eaux Bonnes, and left off the oil. Lost flesh, but otherwise remained well, walking three miles and riding twenty daily. Cough returned in last fortnight. *Physical signs the same.* To resume the oil.

May, 1858.—Wintered well in South of France and Italy, generally taking oil. Is stronger and stouter.

March 5, 1859.—Well till middle of January; since then cough and opaque expectoration. *Dulness and tubular sounds in upper part of both lungs, especially in left, where there is some moist rhonchus.*

June 24, 1861.—Well and taking oil till February, when he became bilious, and omitted oil for two months. After fresh cold, cough came on, accompanied lately by expectoration and pain in front of left chest. *Dulness, deficient motion and breath in upper part of left chest, front and back. Loud tubular sounds at and within scapula.* Urine scanty and high-coloured.—To continue oil in a tonic of strychnia and tincture of orange. Also to take an effervescing saline at night for a short period, and to use counter-irritation with tincture of iodine.

May 16, 1862.—Went to Scarborough, and gained three pounds. Physical signs also improved in autumn. Wintered at Pau, taking oil regularly, and out of doors a great deal. Cough slight, and strength good. *Dry tubular sounds at and above both scapulæ; mostly left, where there is dulness.*

October 15, 1862.—Well, and in London at his office the whole summer.

October 30, 1863.—Worked in London all the winter, and tolerably well till summer, when cough increased after exertion, and the expectoration became tinged with blood. Has taken the oil regularly. *Flattening and obscure breathing in left front; dry cavernous sounds above left scapula; loud tubular above right.*

May 16, 1865.—Continued well and in business, with only occasional cough till lately, when only took oil once a day (instead of twice). Patient at present weak and exhausted, with irregular pulse.—Ordered oil twice a day in tonic of hypophosphite of iron and strychnia. Soon improved, and has lost cough.

1867.—Has continued well, and at his business ever since. *Dry tubular sounds at and above both scapulæ.*

Thirteen years have elapsed since this patient's first symptoms.

CASE 124.—*Chronic Phthisis Arrested. Living 24 years after.*

A gentleman, aged 15. Several paternal aunts died of phthisis. September 24, 1847.—Nine years ago, after gastric fever, was very weak, and cervical glands enlarged, and discharged several times on both sides for a year and more. A year ago had measles, followed by whooping cough, and ever since has had cough and short breath, and been thin and weak.

Superficial dulness, tubular sounds, and moist crepitus below left clavicle. Loud tubular sounds and small spot of dulness within right scapula.

Prescribed cod-liver oil, and a vesicating liniment, occasionally.

May, 1848.—Wintered in Madeira, but did not continue the oil. Cough and breath better.

Less dulness and crepitation in left front. Still tubular at inter-scapular.

June, 1860.—Another winter was passed in Madeira, and two in Egypt and Italy. Taking oil irregularly. Cough generally better, but not much improvement in breath or strength. Dr. W. then recommended long sea voyages for two years. Accordingly he went to Australia and India, and returned much improved in flesh and strength, and quite lost cough and expectoration. Has since wintered chiefly in Egypt, which agrees well. *Chest and respiratory power increased. Stroke clear (emphysema) and breath-sound rather coarse and rough in left front. Tubular sounds at right scapula. Still loud tubular sounds within left scapula.*

1865.—Has enjoyed more uniform and vigorous health, and wintered three years in Scotland and England. Now in Parliament, and attends pretty regularly.

December, 1866.—After skating in Scotland, attacked with pain in chest, dyspnœa, and fever, with obstructed breathing and crepitus in both lungs, most left. This soon subsided under treatment, and chest returned to former state; but, after wintering in South Hants, stomach and bowels were disordered more or less, till the end of the summer, when he passed six weeks at Kissengen under the goat's-milk cure, and was much improved.

July 19, 1869.—Following winter at Cannes, which disagreed with him, causing much gastric and bronchial irritation. On return to England in spring improved, and regained flesh and strength. But stomach often out of order, and has occasional attacks of bronchitis, which now assume a wheezy character. Has lately had one; and also inflammation of the ear

.... in abscess. Still cough and opaque expectoration.
...... a day.—*Breath-sound superseded by crumpling crepitus in
...... and less in back. Large tubular sounds at and above left
...... at right scapula.*

September 26, 1870.—Last winter at Ventnor, with more care, and
... suffering from attacks. Flesh and strength fair. Still had recurrence of gathering in the ear and boils on the body. These have been
much better since, taking sulphurous acid mixture with the oil. When
free from bronchial attacks, there are always the *loud tubular sounds in
both scapular regions, and coarse breath-sound with a few large clicks in left
front. A fresh cold always blocks this up with crepitus, sometimes with bronchial wheezing at the roots and summit of the lung.*

June 1871.—Another winter at Ventnor, and with improved health and
more freedom from attacks. Flesh and strength fair. Attends to his
parliamentary duties.—*Less crepitus in the lung, but as before, the harsh
breathing and tubular sounds of old induration and emphysema in portions
of the lung.*—Continues oil and tonic.

CASE 125.—*Chronic Phthisis.   Double Cavity arrested 21 years.*

A gentleman, aged 26, first consulted Dr. W., June 15, 1848. He had
long been subject to occasional cough, which had become constant during
last two months, and was accompanied by expectoration, loss of strength
and breath, though not to any extent of flesh. Had improved on iodide of
iron and bark, and counter-irritation with tartarated antimony. *Dulness,
crepitation, and loud tubular sounds above and below left clavicle; loud
tubular expiration above right scapula.*—Ordered oil with nitric acid and
tincture of orange, and counter-irritation with acetum cantharidis.

August 23, 1848.—Has taken oil, and is much improved in flesh, strength
and breath. Cough stopped till last few days, when he caught fresh cold.
Physical signs same.

September 25, 1851. Continued well, taking 'gallons of oil,' but cough
has increased in last three months, otherwise strong and stout. *Dulness
and cavernous sounds above left scapula.*

September 21, 1857.—Well since, taking oil occasionally. Has had
hardly any cough till the last month. *Dulness and tubular sounds at
and above both scapula, most left.*

February 17, 1862.—Continued pretty well, but always short breathed
on exertion, and more so lately, with pain in left side. Has had no oil for
3 years, but has been living well and taken beer freely. *Dry cavernous
sounds in upper left chest; large tubular sounds above right scapula.
...... good in front.*—Ordered oil in above tonic, with tincture of calumba.

...... 1862.—Out all the winter, but lately distressed about his wife,
who is phthisical, and suffering from mental depression. Has now more

cough and expectoration. *Dulness, and dry cavernous sounds above both scapulæ.*

March 31, 1866.—Looks stout and well, but has always cough and expectoration, which have increased in last three months. Also has piles. Lost his wife a year ago. *Cavernous sounds at and above left scapula, obstruction and crepitus in front. Tubular and bronchial rhonchus above right scapula.*

October 27, 1866.—Has continued to take oil in various tonics, quinine and sulphuric acid, afterwards phosphoric acid, hypophosphite of soda, and quassia. When the urine was thick, occasionally an effervescing saline. Lately breath short, and occasionally blood in the expectoration.—Ordered oil in nitric acid and tincture of nux vomica. Living at Bognor.

October 23, 1867.—Has been tolerably well, except occasional slight hæmoptysis and piles. In last few days cough has increased. *Cavernous sounds in upper left chest, obstruction and subcrepitant sounds in lower part, puerile breath in right, except at and above scapula, where sounds are tubular.*

In this case cavities formed in both lungs, but in the right cicatrization probably took place. In the left the cavity has contracted, and other parts have become emphysematous. The puerile breathing in the sound part of the right lung testified to the extent to which its powers were taxed. This patient died suddenly of hæmoptysis, July 1869, on his way to the railway station; but up to that time presented a stout and ruddy appearance, and was able to enjoy life, but his breath was always short. He lived upwards of 21 years after the commencement of his illness.

CHAPTER XXIII.

MISCELLANEOUS CASES.

~~Slow Reduction in Phthisis—Arrest of Disease Twelve Years—Healthy Child born—Death Four Years after from Dropsy—Phthisis retarded Ten Years—With Baby and two dead Children born during the time—Phthisis during Pregnancy—Death after Childbirth—Phthisis arrested before Marriage—Relapse after second Childbirth—Arrested again, and Two more Children—Phthisis after Injury to Chest, Two Cases—Pneumo-thorax from Perforation of Pleura—Four Cases, all recovered—Phthisis with Heart Disease—Recovery—Caseous Pneumonia arrested—Calcareous Expectoration after, and Burns—Syphilis and Phthisis; Recovery—Senile Phthisis and Bronchial Glands enlarged—Phthisis arrested in Middle Age—Chronic Bronchitis for Thirty Years after—Death at Eighty-four from Hæmoptysis.

CASE 126.—*Phthisis, arrested Twelve Years. A Child born. Contraction of Chest. Emphysema and Dropsy.*

MR. T——, æt. 28, September 18, 1848. Two brothers and two sisters have died of phthisis. For the last six years has been suffering from cough, and copious opaque expectoration, occasionally bloody, short breath, and wasting. Has spent several winters abroad with temporary amendment. *Collapse and dulness in right front, with cavernous sounds in several spots, as from several small cavities. Dulness and larger cavernous sound above scapula. Partially obstructed breathing below. Tubular sound below left clavicle.*—To take oil in nitric acid and orange tincture, and use cantharides liniment.

Under this treatment, with generous diet, great improvement took place in flesh, strength, and general health. The breath was always short, but the cough and expectoration much diminished, except in occasional attacks, which subsequently assumed the form of asthmatic bronchitis, lasting two or three weeks, relieved by salines and small doses of stramonium. The oil was omitted only on these occasions. *The right side of the chest contracted much, and the size of the cavities diminished, with signs of emphysema below and in left lung.*

In 1856 she became pregnant, and in due time was happily confined, under chloroform, giving birth to a fine baby, who has lived to grow up in

T

health. She continued in invalid health, but enjoying life and highly use
ful in it, till the end of 1859; when, without decided attacks, the breathing
became so short and wheezy, that the least exertion became distressing.
This was from a gradual increase of the emphysema, *the resonance, crepit*
and wheeze of which almost superseded the dulness and cavernous sounds
the right lung. The veins and cellular tissue in the neck also became
swollen from the same cause. In this state, the oil did no good; some reli
was derived from iodide of potass. and digitalis, which acted on the kidney.
Orthopnœa and dropsy followed, and she died in 1860. No examination
allowed.

This is a remarkable instance of phthisis in its third stage being arrested
and, through the contraction of the scar-tissue, becoming converted int
habitual asthma. See Chapter XIX.

CASE 127.—*Phthisis retarded by Uterogestation.*

A married lady, aged 30, who had lost two brothers from consumption
first consulted Dr. Williams, September 20, 1861. Had always been del
cate, with small appetite. During the last two years had been living
bleak exposed situations; not wearing flannel. Cough came on six month
ago, and constant ever since, with loss of flesh and shortness of breath
Catamenia absent for two months: patient is probably pregnan
Loud tubular voice, with dulness at and above right scapula.—Oil w
ordered, with phosphoric acid and a bitter; and a South-coast residenc
recommended.

March 10, 1862.—Has wintered at Ventnor, going out of doors prett
regularly, and taking oil, and has gained flesh and strength. Expects co
finement in two months. *More dulness and tubular sounds at and abo
right scapula.*

March, 1868.—Has wintered three years at Torquay, one at Hyères, an
one at St. Leonards; generally taking oil once daily, with strychnia an
other tonics; sometimes with the addition of hypophosphite of soda. H
had three children, two living and one dead; and, though weak and o
pressed through confinements, has recovered pretty well, and her genera
health is not worse than it was seven years ago. Has had several attack
of bronchitis, and has never lost cough, which has been remarkably hars
and grating, but less so during the last four years, when there ha
been more or less opaque expectoration, sometimes tinged with bloo
In that time there have generally been *cavernous sounds, moist
dry, in right scapular and subclavian regions.* Now there are *dulness, co
traction, loud tubular or dry cavernulous sounds in upper right chest,
marked in the back, but blended with vesicular breath-sound. Long expira
in upper left lung.* Patient seems weaker, thinner, and her breath is shor

May 13, 1869. Was very languid all last summer, and her breath
tremely short, but gained strength in the winter at St. Leonards, fr
which she has just returned. Cough was not bad till March, when sh

.... affecting both lungs; but, although now better, still has, increased cough and occasional opaque expectoration. *Loud tubular or cavernous sounds in upper right chest, with occasional crepitation there and at left apex.* Stomach more fastidious than ever, and rarely takes oil, but pretty regularly glycerine with hypophosphite of soda and strychnia, or salicine once daily. In this feeble state she proved to be pregnant; and, after much oppression and weakness, gave birth to an imperfectly-formed fœtus about the seventh month.

Again there was a gradual recovery, so far as to permit of her being again removed to St. Leonards, where she remained till March, always suffering much from weakness, breathlessness, and cough; yet still in a limited manner enjoying the society of her family.

On her return to town, in the spring of 1870, there was increased feebleness of all functions; more frequent, but less violent cough, and more of the opaque kind of expectoration. *The dulness and cavernous sounds had hardly, if at all, spread in the right upper lobe; but there was crepitus mixed with harsh puerile breathing in the middle right lobe and in the upper lobe of the left lung.*

Even in this condition she again proved to be pregnant, and lived long enough to give birth to a dead child at the full term at the end of the year 1870, ten years from the commencement of the disease in the lung; having borne three living and two dead children within that time. The surviving children are well grown and hitherto healthy.

CASE 128—*Phthisis during Pregnancy. Death after Childbirth.*

Mrs. R., aged 33, first saw Dr. Williams, February 4, 1859. Several of her maternal cousins had died of consumption. Had delicate health from 16 to 25, was married at 24, and improved in health afterwards, especially during pregnancies, of which she had four. Now pregnant four months; and has been living since October in a damp cottage in Scotland, and has had a cough ever since accompanied by wasting.

Dulness, crepitation, and tubular sounds at and above both scapulæ, most marked on the left side.—Patient was ordered cod-liver oil in a tonic of phosphoric and hydrocyanic acids and tincture calumbo, to use a croton-oil liniment, and to winter at St. Leonards.

April 27.—Returned from St. Leonards, where she has taken oil regularly, and gained in flesh and strength, with decrease of cough, which has increased during the last fortnight. *Dulness and crackle in the upper part of both lungs, most marked on the left side.* This patient was prematurely confined at the end of May, and sank ten days later.

On post-mortem examination, in the lungs, tubercles with a great deal of emphysema were found at both apices, and a cicatrix and remains of a cavity at the right. Grey tubercles were also scattered through the lower lobes, the left one being in a state of pneumonic consolidation. The heart was large, both ventricles were dilated, and the walls easily lacerated.

Case 190.—Phthisis after Injury to the Chest. Cavities arrested. Living Twelve Years.

A gentleman, aged 25, of consumptive family, was first seen by Dr. Williams, October 6, 1857. A year ago, he was kicked by a horse in the left side of his chest, and since has experienced occasional pain there. A month ago, after a severe chill, coughed up an ounce and a half of blood; a less amount since, and has lost flesh and strength. At present there is a slight cough and yellow expectoration. *Dulness, large tubular sounds in both scapular regions, some deficient breathing in left lung.*

May 12, 1859.—After passing a winter at Pau, and taking oil for two months, he improved greatly in general health, the physical signs remaining about the same.

Last autumn he again brought up blood to the amount of 2 ounces. He spent last winter in Somersetshire. At present has pain in the left side, and is weak. No oil; a tonic has been taken. *More obstruction and crepitus in upper left chest. Large tubular sounds above the right scapula.*

October 20.—Had been taking iron tonic and oil for six weeks, and improved much during the summer; but still has morning expectoration and occasional hæmoptysis. *Extensive dulness and obstructive sounds in left front. Large tubular (or cavernous) sounds above right scapula.*

August 2, 1860.—Wintered at Pau, and remained pretty well, being able to ascend mountains. Considers that he has gained flesh and strength, but always has cough and expectoration. *Loud dry cavernous sounds in upper left. Coarse crepitation below in front. Large tubular sounds in upper right chest.*

June 20, 1861.—Passed the winter at Pau, doing well till the last four months, when he was bitten in the leg by a dog, erroneously supposed to be mad. Cauterization was largely used, which much weakened him. Since coming north has had some pain in right chest, but little cough; and lately coryza and sore throat. *Dulness, obstructive crepitation in left lung, with cavernous sounds in the upper portion, and some contraction of left chest. Tubular sounds above right scapula.*

April 29, 1864.—Has just finished his sixth winter at Pau. Cough and expectoration moderate, and breath improved. Two years ago a liver attack reduced him much, but he has regained his strength, and now walks some miles. *Physical signs much the same.*

December, 1869.—Has spent five winters in the south of England, and remained pretty well, being only short-breathed, and having little cough; but a year ago had pain in right front chest, which returned six weeks ago, and he brought up a teaspoonful of blood. *Dulness, cavernous sounds at and above left scapula. Considerable amount of crumpling crepitation and obstruction in left front. Tubular sounds and coarse crepitation above right scapula.*

The remarkable chronicity of this case, and the absence of general phthisical symptoms of late years, render it probable that the physical signs are partly due to dilated bronchi and air-cells, consequent on the original inflammatory lesion.

CASE 131.—*Phthisis after Injury to Chest. Arrested Eight Years. Death from Typhoid Fever.*

A young gentleman, aged 14, who had lost his mother and one sister in consumption, was first seen by Dr. Williams, June 12, 1860. Four years before, his chest had been crushed by a cart, since which time he had had more or less cough, and was thin, but was otherwise well, till the last four weeks, when it had increased, and was accompanied by expectoration. *Deficient breath and motion in upper part of both sides of chest, most marked on the right, where are large tubular and croaky sounds. Tubular sounds above the left scapula.*

Oil was ordered in a tonic of phosphoric acid and quinine; and counter irritation with cantharides liniment.

September 29.—Much improved. Cough slight. Gained 5lbs. in a month. *Dulness, large tubular sounds upper right chest, and some crepitation in parts.*

June 8, 1861.—Wintered well in Madeira, and out daily; but in April brought up three ounces of blood, in May one ounce, and on the voyage home, when a cold wind was blowing, five ounces. Nevertheless, has gained 14lbs., and physical signs are improved, *dulness being diminished in the right lung.*

June, 1862.—In the autumn gained 8lbs. more, and wintered again at Madeira, but was very sick on voyage to and from the island. Was out daily during winter, walking ten miles a day or riding twenty, but always had cough and expectoration, and once hæmoptysis to the amount of one ounce. Took oil only once a day, and lost 10lbs. in weight. *Dulness, dry cavernous sounds in upper right chest, with deficient breath below. Tubular sounds above left scapula.*

July 2, 1863.—Passed last autumn in South Devon and gained 14lbs.; afterwards spent the winter in Syria and Egypt, and remained pretty well, except at Cairo, where had diarrhœa, and brought up five ounces of blood in November. Then went up the Nile, and gained flesh, but lost it afterwards. Has taken no oil since March. *More breathing audible in right front. Tubular sounds still in upper portion, and some crepitation and obstruction in lower right back.*

Was seen again in October. Had brought up an ounce of blood in August, but had taken oil, gaining 9lbs., and was able to walk eighteen miles.

June 9, 1864.—Took a tour through Jamaica, Panama, Cuba, United States, and Canada. Was well and active all the time, but took no medicine, and has lost 3lbs. *Pectoriloquy in the right front, and tubular sounds above both scapulæ.*

September 28.—In Devon, and quite well, walking several miles a day at the rate of four an hour. Free from cough, short breath, and hæmoptysis. Physical signs improved.

June 1, 1865.—Wintered in Egypt well, except catching a slight cold, with tinged expectoration, at Beyrout, and since then has been taking oil. *Tubular sounds above both scapulæ, loudest above right, and some crepitant obstruction in the lower portion of the same lung.*

July 12, 1867.—Wintered during 1866 in Malta and Algeria, and last year in England, but caught cold when travelling, and had fever, and was much reduced. He nevertheless married in February, and went to Pau; but became very weak, and had slight hæmoptysis. In the spring visited Bagnères, and then Italy, where improved. *Dulness, dry cavernous sounds, upper right. Breath weak, with subcrepitus below.*

Died of fever in Devonshire, February 1868.

Pneumo-thorax from Perforation of the Pleura.

The occurrence of pneumo-thorax in the course of phthisis from perforation of the pleura commonly causes a serious aggravation of the malady, and accelerates its fatal termination. These cases are sufficiently familiar not to need exemplification; but I record four remarkable cases of recovery after this accident. To explain them, we need only bear in mind that the phthinoplasm which causes the rupture may be the only one, or nearly the only one, in the lungs, its accidental position near the surface leading to this peculiar result. In the same way, a large and fatal hæmoptysis may be caused by a small tubercle or patch of degeneration happening to involve a large blood-vessel and lead to its rupture.

CASE 132.—*Pneumo-thorax. Gradual Recovery. Lived Twenty-one Years.*

Mr. D. A., æt. 26, surgeon, March 17, 1846; seen with the late Dr. John Taylor. Sister died of phthisis. Declares that he was quite well till seventeen days ago, when, riding a very restive horse, he was suddenly seized with severe pains in the whole left front of the chest, catching the breath. This has continued more or less ever since, with short dry cough and quickened breath. Pulse 120, weak. No heat of skin, and other functions natural. *Left chest tympanic and tender on percussion. Loud amphoric breathing, metallic tinkling with voice, and sometimes with breath and heartbeat, which is a little to right of its proper place. Intercostal spaces not de-*

...and ...... vesisula. Dulness and little breath below; breathing ...... doth scapula.—To continue the oil in phosphoric acid tonic.

...... 12, 1862.—Quite well, and free from cough and expectoration, ... often exposed to wet and night-air in yacht. Is able to shout as ...... tree. Deficient motion and stroke-sound in whole left side, which is ...... contracted, but loud and vesicular breathing in front and at the side. With tubular sounds from the middle of scapula upwards. Tubular sounds above right scapula.

October, 1869.—Generally well, and has become stout, but more or less cough. Wintered at Caithness. *Still dulness and large tubular sounds at left scapula and above.*

The signs of pneumo-thorax were unequivocal in this case, and must have arisen from perforation of the pleura, by partial disease of the lung in the summer of 1861. Happily this disease was arrested, the air effused was absorbed, and the lung was gradually re-expanded.

Case 184.—*Pneumo-thorax. Complete Recovery. Well Four Years after.*

Mr. F., æt. 24, October 2, 1867.—Several half-brothers and sisters have died of consumption. Except a pain in the chest last November, from which he was well in a fortnight, has had no illness till the second week in August, when he again had pain in the front of the chest with a cough, which entirely ceased in two weeks; and in September was well enough to make a tour in Switzerland, and ascended the Eggischorn with no other inconvenience than short breath, and occasional pain in the left side. No cough. In the last three days he has noticed a splashing noise in his chest, but says he feels well. Seems nervous and anxious, and with quickened breathing. Pulse 90; heat natural. *Left chest distended, tympanic on percussion, and with no breath sound. Heart pulsation seen and felt to right of sternum and in epigastrium. Tubular breath and voice at left scapula; and below speaking or laughing is accompanied by a tinkling echo, which can be produced also by percussion. Dulness in lower third of left back.*—To take oil in tonic mixture. Left side to be painted with tincture iodine.

October 14.—Much the same. Complains only of short breath, and of the splashing noise on every quick turn of his body. Cough and expectoration slight, induced by change of posture. *Signs the same.*

October 22.—Continues pretty well, but breath short, and occasional pain in left chest, which is tender, especially in lower part. Hears noise less. *Left side smaller, with less tympanic distension. Tinkling and splashing sound higher in axilla and back. More breath sound above left scapula.*

November 18.—Weaker, and feverish at times, with pain in side. Sometimes ...... on exertion, and breath short. *Dulness, and absence of breath in lower half of left chest. Stroke clearer, with some breath sounds above. ...... above right scapula. Heart now in place, or a little higher and more to the left than natural. No tinkling, splashing, or other sign of cavity, nor flattening of walls.*

February 10, 1868.—Has continued steadily taking oil and tonic, and has much improved till the last week, when there has been much more pain in side, with feeling of weakness. No cough, but breath is shorter again; appetite bad. *Left chest more natural in shape, but lower third contracted; still dull, while in middle is less dulness, with obscure breath. Tubular sounds at and above scapula. Friction with deep breath in middle front (where has been pain). Heart to left of sternum, with its apex beating above fifth rib.* Nitromuriatic acid mixture, belladonna plaster to left chest.

June 9.—Quite well, except pain catching breath on exertion; felt since leaving off plasters. Strength good, and up to usual weight, 10 stone. *Same signs, except slight crepitus below left axilla.*—Continue nitromuriatic mixture, opium plasters to left side.

June 8, 1869.—Well all winter, without pain or cough, but breath oppressed by cold. Lately been a walking excursion, several miles daily, and uphill with a knapsack on back. Weight 10 stone 8 lbs. *Lower half of left chest rather duller, and moves a little left than right, but breath sound heard everywhere except at base, where is crepitus on deep breath.*

September 3, 1869.—Heard that he had been walking 30 miles a day, shooting, rowing, &c., without inconvenience.

In this case the discovery of the disease causing natural alarm, a late President of the College of Physicians was consulted, and expressed doubts as to the nature of the case. This led the patient to seek a third opinion, which was that of the present President of the same College, who fully confirmed the diagnosis first given.

CASE 135.—*Pneumo-thorax. Rapid and complete Recovery.*

Mr. M——— æt. 48; seen with Dr. Stutter, of Sydenham, May 16, 1868.— Lost a brother in phthisis. Has been quite well and gaining flesh lately. Has been in the habit of going quickly up and down a long flight of stairs twenty times a day, up to five days ago, and lately had found the exertion cause pain in the right side, and a feeling of oppression. On that day he consulted Dr. Stutter, who ordered a mustard poultice to the side. This relieved the pain, but the breath remained short, and then Dr. Stutter found signs of pneumo-thorax on the right side. Now complains of nothing but shortness of breath, and a feeling of fulness in the right side. Pulse quiet, urine scanty. Lower half of right chest tympanic on percussion down to lower margins of ribs, below which liver dulness reaches down four or five inches in abdomen. Breathing amphoric, with metallic tinkling on coughing in lower half of chest. Above breath sound obscure and stroke rather duller than on left side, particularly on the scapula.—An effervescing saline was given for a few days, and tincture of iodine to be painted on the right chest. Afterwards oil to be taken.

.... 18.... .... from Dr. Stutter that the signs of pneumo-
.... disappeared, and that the patient was quite well. ·

.... 5, 1871.—Mr. M. continues quite well, and continues to get
......

Case 136.—*Phthisis, with Cavity. Acute Rheumatism and Endo-cardial Murmur. Recovery.*

A married lady, aged 30, consulted Dr. Williams, October 13, 1860.
Lost her mother, two sisters, and one brother from consumption. During
the last four years she had had occasional cough and hæmoptysis, which on
one occasion amounted to three ounces. Did lose much flesh; but after
taking oil, and applying it externally also, became fat and still remains so.
Lately has been taking glycerine. Cough has increased in last two months,
and now she has a bad cold. *Extensive dulness, cavernous sounds and surrounding crepitus in upper right chest. Tubular sounds above left scapula.*
—Oil ordered with phosphoric acid calumbo and orange; a morphia linctus
at night; cantharides liniment.

December 24.—At the end of October, severe rheumatic pains came on
with tenderness of wrists and ankles, was soon relieved by opiate salines;
but she has been confined for two months. Looks well, but still has a
cough. *In addition to former signs there is a loud diastolic murmur at
mid-sternum.*

February 5, 1861.—Much better in every respect. Little cough. *Physical
signs same, only a trace of crepitation above scapula.*

September 18, 1861.—Looks quite well, and has only slight cough and
short breath, with occasional pain in right chest. Catamenia irregular
and in extremes. *Less dulness and more breath in upper right; no cavernous, but tubular sounds.*

November 10, 1862.—Weathered last winter fairly in Ireland, being free
from cough. From May to September took a cold sponge bath every morning. A scaly eruption appeared on arms and legs, which Dr. Noligan cured
by arsenic. During last fortnight she has had a cold and cough. *Still dulness
and tubular sounds in upper right chest, with slight crepitation. Cardiac
murmur not audible.*—Effervescing saline with opiate at night, and continued oil and tonic.

May 30, 1865.—Living at Woolwich, and wonderfully well. ˙ Only occasionally suffers from cough and rheumatic pains. Has taken a great deal
of oil, but is less stout, though in good condition. *Still dulness and tubular
sounds through upper third of right lung.* Loud diastolic murmur audible
to right and along upper portion of sternum.

November 2.—Had hæmoptysis to the amount of 1oz. a month ago, and
since then has had violent cough, with mucous expectoration. Now she is
taking oil with sulphuric acid. *Dulness, tubular sounds, and coarse crepitation in upper half of right lung.* The patient was seen again in the summer
of 1867; she was then stout, but her breath was short with some cough.

March 13, 1868.—Has lost cough, is ruddy and stout, but occasionally has palpitation, and has lately had a vesicular eruption on the hands, which was soon cured by lotion. No catamenia for twelve months. *Physical signs of heart and lungs much improved. Only slight dulness and loud tubular sounds above the right scapula. The second sound of the heart is dangerous, but without murmur.*

1871.—Has been heard of as in good health, fifteen years after first attack.

CASE 137.—*Acute Phthisis arrested. Afterwards Calcareous Expectoration. Lithic Acid. Nephralgia. Eczema.*

Mrs. V——, aged 34, who had lost a sister in consumption, was seen by Dr. Williams, September 28, 1858. She stated that in July she had scarlatina and quinsy, followed by cough, diarrhœa, night-sweats, and great loss of flesh and strength.

Much dulness, and large tubular sounds at and above right scapula. Oil was ordered in a tonic of strychnia nitric acid and orange peel, and a morphia linctus.

June 28, 1859.—Heard that she quite lost her cough in four months; and increased in weight from 9st. to 10st. 10lbs. She also is able to sing as formerly, but her breath is still short. After this she suffered two nephralgia, and passed some red gravel.

July 26, 1860.—Has become stout, and is free from cough. Has had occasional diarrhœa, and passed some red gravel. Physical signs same as at first visit.

July 24, 1865.—Was shut up during the last winter, but had only occasional attacks of cough and expectoration. Breath always short, and there is constant morning expectoration.

June 26, 1866.—Was well till two months ago, when, after a cold severe cough came on with green expectoration, and several times she spit up calcareous matter. Was ordered to resume the oil and tonic and linctus as before. Physical signs same.

October 18, 1866.—Heard that she had had some more calcareous expectoration and wheezy cough, and that she had been suffering from eczema over various.parts of the body, accompanied by very acid urine.—Before cing citrate of potass with iodide potassium and quassia. Good habits.

In this case the first disease was probably inflammation, caused the beginning to caseate and infect the system. This was arrested by the treatment, the caseous matter remained quiescent, and, becoming petrified, was expectorated in a subsequent bronchial attack.

CASE 138.—*Syphilis. Phthisis. Cavity. Recovery.*

Mr. ——, aged 30, who had lost a brother from consumption, consulted Dr. Williams, June 30, 1843. Three years ago he had ulcerated sore

...of it occasionally since, affecting the voice, which is at ... and ... voice during last six weeks by cold; copious ... Has lost flesh. Formerly had red and coppery patches on ... and now has them on abdomen. *Dulness in upper right chest, with ... sounds below clavicle.* Cicatrices are visible on fauces.—Ordered full doses of iodide of potassium, with sarsaparilla, and to use an iodine and ammonia liniment.

August 25, 1846.—Wintered in Italy, and quite recovered.

CASE 159.—*Senile Phthisis. Bronchitis. Enlarged Bronchial Glands.*

T. C., aged 74, admitted into University College Hospital, December 12, 1845.—A shrivelled, deaf old man, many years subject to cough and short-ness of breath, which have much increased in the last few weeks, with ... expectoration, and much tightness across chest. Bowels cos-tive; pulse 84, weak; urine turbid, specific gravity 1010, contains a little albumen.

Loud wheezy breathing on both sides. Expiration loudest in upper parts, especially on left side. Some dulness in upper left front and back. Inspi-ration louder in lower parts. On right side expiration loud and sibilant. ...mixed with submucous rhonchus in lower right, which sounds dull ... percussion.—Blisters between scapulæ. Calomel and henbane at night, ... draught in morning. Squill, ipecacuana, and stramonium three times a day.

18th.—Cough and breathing have been rather easier. Urine free; no albumen. Is very weak, and the expectoration very purulent. *Loud wheez-ing in all parts, with crepitus in lower half of both lungs.* Carbonate am-monia was given, but he died on the night of 19th.

Post mortem 18 horis. Emaciation moderate.

Extensive adhesions of both pleuræ. Those on right side most general, those on the left confined to apex and base of the lung, but very tough; several patches of dense membrane on the pleura; cartilages of bronchi much ossified, especially near the root of the lungs, which were compressed ... mass of enlarged bronchial glands, quite black. Bronchial membrane ... and covered with bloody mucus, but many of the bronchi were full of pus.

...ture of lungs generally much congested, but on scraping away the ... appeared dark grey, very tough and resisting, with numerous hard-... granulations scattered through it. In posterior part of left lung, the ... passed into partial hepatisation at the lower part, but not ... in water. In front this lung was not congested, but very dark grey, ... at the apex were tough consolidations, extending half an inch into the ... with a patch of dense membrane on the pleura. Some similar ... of dark induration near anterior margin. No yellow or recent grey tubercles were found. Lower lobe emphysematous, with large projecting air cells, quite flaccid and transparent. Right lung presented similar appearances, but with less recent hepatisation. Numerous, very dark, tough consolidations, and one contained an encysted calcareous body. The lower lobe of this lung also was emphysematous.

Heart large, weight 15 ounces. Right ventricle thick. Kidneys slightly mottled, and granular on removing capsule. A few cysts.

In this case the tubercles were all dwindled and obsolete. Dyspnœa and death caused by bronchitis passing into pneumonia in a subject previously suffering from emphysema and pressure on large bronchi by enlarged glands.

CASE 140.—*Inflammatory Phthisis in Middle Age. Arrest; and Asthmatic Twenty-nine Years. Death from Hæmoptysis at 84.*

Dr. G., æt. 55, April 14, 1848.—Seven years ago had inflammation of the left chest, which was said by one doctor to be pleural abscess, and by another condensation of the lung. Was sent to Cadiz, and gradually improved in health; became a wine merchant; able to attend to business, but always short breathed, and often suffering from gout and neuralgia. Has been in England eight months, and has generally had some cough and wheezing. Has lost flesh lately. Now has fresh cold, with cough, hoarseness, and wheezing, and gout in his feet. *Collapse, dulness, and defective breath in left front. Bronchophony below clavicle. Tubular sounds and wheeze at and above scapula. Crepitus at right apex. Clear stroke and emphysematous crackle at both bases.*—Iodide and carbon. potass., with colchicum. Croton liniment (which he is in the habit of using).

1870.—Was soon relieved from attack, but had recurrences of bronchitis, with violent cough and wheezy dyspnœa two or three times every year, generally in winter. He continually suffered in his digestion, which was often tried by free living; and he was occasionally visited with gout. In the last ten years cataracts formed in both eyes, and very much impaired his vision, but he continued to get about and enjoy society when not confined with severe bronchial attacks, which generally ended with opaque expectoration. *The signs latterly were only those of bronchitis and emphysema, and the former contraction, and dulness having diminished.* After an attack, however, in 1870, he began to cough up blood in large quantities, and so died. No post-mortem.

We can only conjecture that a rupture took place in some degenerated vessel in the old phthinoplasm after an arrest of 29 years.

CHAPTER XXIV.

THE DURATION OF PULMONARY CONSUMPTION.[1]

By Dr. C. Theodore Williams.

Estimates of Portal, Laennec, Andral, Louis, and Bayle compared with those of the Brompton Hospital, Fuller, and Pollock—Differences explained by Class of Patients and Mode of Treatment—Author's Thousand Cases selected from wealthy Classes—Ground of Selection explained—Method of Tabulation of Cases—Sex—Age of Attack—Family Predisposition—Origin and first Symptoms—Cases of Inflammatory Origin; their Proportion and Course of Symptoms—Hæmoptysis—State of Lungs at first Visit as evidenced by Physical Signs—Classification of Stages adopted with Restrictions—Majority of Patients in First Stage, and consequent favourable Prognosis—Mortality in each Stage—State of Lungs at last Visit—Classification of 'Healthy,' 'Improved,' 'About the same,' and 'Worse;' and Percentage of each—Relative Liability of Lungs to Attack, Excavation, and Extension of Disease—Number of Deaths—Causes—Long Duration—Living Patients more numerous and with higher average Duration—Present State described as 'Well,' 'Tolerably well,' and 'Invalid'—Large Proportion of First Two Classes—Hopeful Prognosis—Causes of long Duration—Influence of Age and Sex on Duration—Among Females Duration shorter, Age of Attack earlier, and Age at Death less advanced than among Males—Great Age reached by some Patients—Relation of Age of Attack to Duration—Prolonging Effect of Inflammatory Origin—Pneumonic, Pleuro-pneumonic and Bronchitic—Duration of Pathological Varieties of Consumption difficult to determine—Diagnosis of Tuberculous and Caseous Phthisis obscure.

We need not dwell on the importance of the subject which we propose to treat of in this chapter. In a country where, according to the Registrar-General, one death in every eight is caused by phthisis, it is obvious that a true knowledge of the duration of the disease and

[1] This chapter is an abstract of a paper on 'The Duration of Phthisis Pulmonalis, and on certain Conditions which Influence it,' contained in the LIV. volume of the *Medico-Chirurgical Transactions*.

the conditions which modify it, is of the greatest consequence to the community. Many estimates have been formed of the duration of phthisis in this and other countries, and these estimates will be found to vary to such a degree that a reader may well despair in attempting to harmonize them. A due consideration, however, of the conditions under which each estimate was made—i.e. of the number and of the social class of the patients, of the form of disease, of the mode of life and of the treatment pursued, will serve to explain many of the variations. Portal's saying that phthisis may last from 10 days to 40 years is undoubtedly true, but far too indefinite for our present state of knowledge. Laennec gives 34 months as the mean duration; Andral the same; Louis and Bayle 23 months, founded on the examination of 314 cases.

The first Brompton Hospital Report, in 215 fatal cases, found that 40·8 per cent. died less than 1 year after attack, 45·3 per cent. between 1 and 4 years after, and 6·5 per cent. had a duration of more than 4 years.

Dr. Fuller, in 118 cases investigated by himself at St. George's Hospital, found that by far the greater number died from 3 to 18 months after first attack, whereas in 46 cases in his private practice he found the usual duration varied from 1½ to 7 years, and he remarks that this discrepancy cannot be wholly explained by the social position of the sufferers and the advantages the latter enjoyed with respect to medical treatment, change of air, and proper regimen. He accounts for it by the greater jealousy with which the upper and more educated classes are wont to watch their health, and note the earlier inroads of disease. Dr. Pollock, in his valuable work, which has contributed more than any other to our knowledge of the prognostics of consumption, gives from 2¾ to 3 years as the average duration of 129 cases ending in death. These occurred among 3,566 hospital out-patients, the rest of whom, at the end of 2½ years, were living and in a state of health favourable to the expectation of life for a considerable term.

Louis' and Laennec's cases seem to have been chiefly of a rapid kind, treated with depletion, antimony, starvation, &c., or else on the expectant method, with little or no medicine. It has been urged in connexion with this that a more acute form of consumption prevails in France, but no facts have been hitherto adduced in proof of this; and, on the other hand, if anyone compares English hospital cases of forty years ago with those graphically described in the pages of Louis, he will find the greatest possible similarity in symptoms and duration, and in what, to my mind, affords some explanation, in their treatment.

In the days of bleeding, antimony, &c., the great majority of cases of phthisis were distressing tragedies, as those who can look back on a very long experience of consumption strongly testify, and at that time the prognosis of English physicians was as unfavourable as that of French, as far as the disease was concerned, though the different constitutions of the two races may have exercised some slight modifying influence on it. Moreover, from what I saw of French consumptive patients, when residing in the South of France in 1863, there appeared to be no material difference in the nature of the cases, but a very great one in the hygienic and medicinal treatment. Climate was almost entirely relied on; cod-liver oil and tonics, though recommended, were seldom persevered with.

The estimate of the first Brompton Hospital Report refers to deaths occurring among the in-patients; and those, owing to various causes, and chiefly to their having to wait so long before admission, are exceptionally bad cases. Some died within a week after admission.

U

Dr. Pollock's statistics are taken from the broader and very extensive set of cases which the out-patient department at Brompton furnishes. These may be said to embrace all classes below the wealthy one, and what is more to the purpose, all varieties and degrees of the disease; the fortnightly visit to Brompton, not as a rule, interfering with the necessities of occupations or home cares, and thus securing the attendance of a large number who could not afford to become in-patients; while, at the same time, information as to the state of those not able to attend, is given through a form of note supplied to the patients at the hospital, or else by a letter from the relatives. Dr. Pollock's statistics, when viewed in relation to the few deaths and the expectation of life for the survivors, give the most favourable results for the lower classes ever published.

The cases on which our estimate of the duration of phthisis is founded amount to 1,000, and have been selected from private practice, the patients, for the most part, belonging to the upper and middle classes of society, and consequently enjoying many advantages over hospital patients in the avoidance of those ills which arise from poverty, exposure to cold, unhealthy atmospheres and occupations, and in the opportunities of rest, change of climate, better living, and exercise. As statistical information of disease among the upper classes is rare, we hope that these statistics may prove acceptable, as affording some facts capable of comparison with results of hospital experience, which have been well set forth by some of the abovementioned authorities.

The broad definition of pulmonary consumption, as stated at the beginning of the book, includes all the cases we have now to deal with, and also includes the most acute forms of the disease, as acute tuberculosis and scrofulous pneumonia; but some of the worst forms of these are excluded owing to the ground of selection, which will be shortly explained.

The 1,000 cases have been selected from the records of patients who first consulted Dr. Williams between the years 1842 and 1864, a period of twenty-two years. The chief ground of this selection has been the time during which the patients have been under observation. Considering phthisis to be, in most instances, a chronic disease, and that observations of its course and how it can be modified by treatment can hardly be satisfactory, unless carried on for some length of time, we have judged it advisable to select, out of a mass of records, those cases which have been under treatment twelve months and upwards.

A large majority of the patients who consult physicians are seen once only, or two or three times within a short period, and there may be no opportunity of learning their subsequent history. Such cases, although supplying useful information as to the origin and varieties of the disease, are of no value in relation to its treatment, results, or duration.

Yet because these cease to attend is no proof that they derive no benefit. Many come only to ascertain the physician's opinion, and are unable, through scanty resources, or through distance from town, to repeat their visits. We must not conclude, however, that because they do not continue to attend, they are unfavourable cases, and likely to terminate within the year. On the contrary, all the evidence at our command points to a different conclusion. Patients frequently appear on the scene years later, having, after one or two visits, been lost sight of, who had been prevented, by various causes, from visiting the physician, but had been carrying out treatment steadily.

Were we, however, to include all the cases, our numbers

would be enormously swollen, but the addition could only
be a large quantity of indefinite and useless material,
more likely to obscure the statistics than to render them
lucid.

Still we must not lose sight of the fact that certain
cases of phthisis prove fatal within twelve months; for instance, the forms known as acute tuberculosis and scrofulous pneumonia, though the latter does not always terminate rapidly, but is sometimes brought by treatment into
a comparatively chronic state, and in this condition may
last on some years. These early fatal cases, which have
been excluded, form, among the mass of consumptive
patients, a very small percentage; estimated variously at
three or five per cent.

Against these we would balance the much larger number of patients reported as having much improved after a
few months' treatment, and as affording promise of permanent recovery. As our limitation shuts out these, the
few deaths may also be fairly excluded.[1]

[1] In order to form some estimate of the proportions which the cases fatal
within the year bear to those more or less improved within the same period.
I have carefully examined the records of every case of phthisis occurring
during one year, the year being selected at hazard, as a sample, from the
period of 22 years. Of 433 consumptive patients who consulted Dr. Williams for the first time in 1863, 245 were seen only once, and no more was
heard of them; 84 were one year and upwards under observation, and were
among those, therefore, selected for our tables. Of 104 patients whose subsequent history was known for periods under one year, 8 died, 13 were at
the last visit rather worse, 3 were about the same, 75 were more or less
improved, and 5 were quite restored to health. Thus those improved
and cured were ten times more numerous than the deaths. It can hardly
be said, then, that in taking the fact of the patient being at least one year
under observation as the basis of our selection, we increase the balance of
favourable results, but we thereby deal with facts more carefully observed,
and more conclusive in relation to the real efficacy of treatment.

Note by Dr. C. J. B. WILLIAMS:—In determining in the first instance
to select for analysis only those cases which had been under my care
for a year and upwards, I was guided by the desire to obtain more
sure and reliable results than could accrue from cases during shorter

As the duration of phthisis is such an important subject, we must crave the indulgence of our readers, if we give a considerable amount of preliminary information about the 1,000 patients, before stating the results of the statistics.

The cases were extracted from the note-books of Dr. Williams, and arranged in tables containing twenty-five each, under the headings of

> Age.
> Sex.
> Family Predisposition.
> Date of first Symptoms.
> Origin of Disease.
> Occurrence of Hæmoptysis.
> Date of first Visit.
> State of Lungs, as evidenced by Physical Signs.
> Treatment by Medicine, Climate, &c.
> Result.
> Duration.

The obituary of the newspapers has been closely watched, and where the patients had been lost sight of for several years without having been announced as dead, a correspondence was opened, either with themselves or their

periods of observation. I wished to ascertain the power of nature, aided by art, to control or arrest the course of pulmonary consumption ; and knowing the deep-seated and enduring nature of the disease, I distrusted all results not confirmed by time, and I rejected reports of temporary amendment or even cure, as unsatisfactory and inconclusive. Deaths were indeed conclusive, although not satisfactory ; but the few deaths which did occur within that period were the issue of that degree and form of the disease, over which treatment never had, or is likely to have, any control. I already knew such cases to be hopeless—too rapid and overwhelming to be stayed by human power—therefore I put them out of calculation. I am quite content if our accounts are debited with the three or five per cent. which such deaths may be supposed to amount to ; for although, as my son argues, the ten times more numerous ' improved and cured' cases may be ' set off ' against them, yet this is balancing a certain against an uncertain quantity, which brings no definite result. But it cannot be fairly said, that our selection gives nothing but chronic cases, for many of the cases are acute at commencement, or in some part of their course, and are reduced to a chronic state by treatment.

friends, to ascertain whether they were alive and in what
state of health—a correspondence which, when addressed,
as it often had to be, to the individual whose life was sus-
pected, sometimes evoked ludicrous answers.   Reference
to the various lists, the ' Army and Navy,' ' University,'
' Clergy,' and ' Law,' to the ' Court Guide,' and to the
' Peerage,' has often afforded valuable information ; and
on this point private practice has great advantages over
hospital practice, for in respect of the former, by some
means or other, patients can be traced through a number
of years, whereas in the latter they are generally lost
sight of when they quit the hospital.

Nevertheless, a certain number of the tabulated cases
could not be traced up to the present time ; and of these
the date when last heard of, with notice of their state, is
registered.

SEX.—Of the 1,000 cases, 625 were males and 375
females, or 62·5 per cent. of the former, and 37·5 per
cent. of the latter.   This preponderance of males cannot
be regarded merely as accidental, for it is closely in accordance with the evidence of the first report of the
Brompton Hospital, where the percentage of males was
61, and that of females 39.   Among Dr. Pollock's out-
patients, 60·75 per cent. were males, and 39·25 females.

AGE.—The ages of the patients have been arranged in
the following table.   This table differs in one point from

Age at Time of Attack of 1,000 Cases of Phthisis.

Age at Time of Attack	Males	Percentage	Females	Percentage	Total	Percentage
Under 10 years .	10	1·60	3	·80	13	1·3
10 to 20 . .	86	13·79	96	25·60	182	18·2
20 to 30 . .	245	39·20	173	46·13	418	41·8
30 to 40 . .	183	29·28	66	17·60	249	24·9
40 to 50 . .	70	11·20	24	6·40	94	9·4
50 to 60 . .	22	3·52	8	2·33	30	3·0
60 and upwards .	9	1·44	5	1·33	14	1·4
	625		375		1,000	

Average age at time of attack, Males . . 29·47 years.
" " " Females . . 26·06 years.

many similar records. Instead of the age at first visit, the
age at first attack is tabulated; and this is arrived at by
subtracting the history from the age at first visit. The
date thus obtained is of far more consequence in esti-
mating the duration of disease, and the conditions which
modify it, than the age at first visit, which depends upon
shifting circumstances; as, for instance, the feelings and
opportunities of the patients, who may come under the
observation of the physician either at the commencement
of their disease, or many years after, near its termination.
The record of their age at the time of the first visit would
therefore afford us but slight information as to the time
of attack or its duration. It may be objected, that it is
difficult to arrive at accuracy as to the date of first symptoms. And undoubtedly this is true in the case of hospital
patients, with whom it is necessary to pursue a system of
close cross-questioning, in order to evoke the necessary
information. Dr. Fuller[1] truly says on this point: ' The
average duration of the complaint is ordinarily, I believe,
very much understated, from the fact that the inferences
respecting its duration are drawn from the statements of
hospital patients, who pay little heed to the earlier, and,
as they imagine, unimportant symptoms of the disease,
and pertinaciously date their malady from the occasion on
which they first experienced pain in the chest, or were
frightened by the occurrence of hæmoptysis, or found
themselves unequal to their daily work.' Private patients, with whom we have now to deal, hardly err on
this side, for the upper classes generally remember and
narrate, almost too fully for the physician, every symptom,
early or late, of their illness.

The results of this table accord with the commonly
received opinion as to the period of attack. Taking the
sexes collectively, 41 per cent. were attacked between

[1] *Op. cit.* p. 413.

20 and 30 ; about 25 per cent. between 30 and 40 ; 19·5
per cent. under 20 ; and 13 per cent. above 50.   When
we examine the relative liability of the two sexes in the
various decades, we find some important differences to
exist.   Between 20 and 30—the most common period of
attack for both sexes—about 7 per cent. more females
were attacked than males ; and again, between 10 and
20, 11·8 per cent. more.   On the other hand, after 30
the reverse was the case.   Between 30 and 40 the males
attacked exceeded the females by 11·68 per cent., and
above 40 by 6 per cent.   These results may be said
nearly to agree with those of the first Brompton Report.

The average age of attack was—for the males 29·47,
and for the females 26·06.

Family Predisposition.—The results under this head
have already been given in Chapter XV., to which the
reader is referred.   This feature was traced in 48·4 per
cent. of the 1,000 cases.

Origin and First Symptoms.—In 385 cases the disease
came on without any antecedent illness, and was characterised by the usual group of symptoms, more strongly
marked in some cases than others, and it pursued its
course free from complications, besides the ordinary ones
of phthisis.   In 315 cases it either originated in, or
followed closely after, other diseases, as the subjoined
table will show :—

Phthisis was preceded by Pleurisy and Pleuro-pneumonia in 149 Cases.

,,	,,	,,	Bronchitis	.	.	118	,,
,,	,,	,,	Asthma (spasmodic)	.	.	7	,,
,,	,,	,,	Scrofulous Abscesses	.	.	12	,,
,,	,,	,,	Fistula .	.	.	5	,,
,,	,,	,,	Hooping Cough	.	.	6	,,
,,	,,	,,	Croup .	.	.	1	,,
,,	,,	,,	Scarlatina	.	.	4	,,

302

Brought forward 302 Cases.

Phthisis	was	preceded by	Measles	2	,,
,,	,,	,,	Continued Fevers . .	3	,,
,,	,,	,,	Peritonitis . . .	1	,,
,,	,,	,,	Malformation of the Chest .	2	,,
,.	,,	,,	Injuries to the Chest and other Organs . . .	5	,,

315

The number arising from pleuro-pneumonia and bronchitis is very large, reaching a total of 267, or more than one quarter of the whole, and deserves attention as showing statistically the influence of these diseases as direct sources of consumption. It is well known to physicians connected with hospitals for diseases of the chest, how often a neglected case of pneumonia or bronchitis becomes, under depressing causes, one of consumption; but statistics proving this frequency are rare, if not wanting. This number, 267, or 26·7 per cent., is high, considering that it is taken in a class which has opportunities of protecting itself from many depressing conditions; but high as it is, it is probably much below a correct estimate for hospital patients, among whom the prevention or rapid cure of these diseases is much more difficult, and therefore less common than among their wealthier brethren.

In the cases of phthisis arising from pleuro-pneumonia (pneumonic phthisis), the course of events was generally what was painted in the examples given in Chapters VIII. and X. After the attack, some portions of the lungs remained consolidated or compressed by dense pleuritic adhesions, or both these lesions existed, and tended to cripple the lungs for their respiratory work. The breath remained short; the patient seldom or never lost the cough, which a fresh cold or some disordering influence caused to increase, muco-purulent expectoration and sometimes hæmoptysis accompanying it. Signs of softening were detected in one or both lungs, followed by those of excavation, and the case assumed a consumptive aspect.

Of the cases of phthisis following bronchitis, which may be termed catarrhal phthisis, some arose from acute attacks, others from chronic. These last patients generally lost their cough and other symptoms in the summer, or in warm weather, but were subject to a return of them every winter, or during inclement weather. A longer, or more severe attack than usual, greatly prostrated them, and the cough now remained persistent, and was also accompanied by permanent feverishness, heat of skin, and wasting. On examination of the chest, in addition to the ordinary bronchitic sounds, patches of consolidation were detected; these did not clear up, and in some cases softening and excavation eventually took place, and the patient lapsed into phthisis. Examples of this transition of bronchitis into phthisis have already been given.

Of the 149 cases originating in pleuro-pneumonia, in 85 no family predisposition could be traced; and this was also the case in 57 out of 118 instances arising from bronchitis.

We see, therefore, that 142 phthisical patients or 14·2 per cent. owed their attacks entirely, as far as could be ascertained, to inflammatory attacks of the lungs, thus endorsing the views of Alison, Broussais, and Addison, as to the origin of the disease from inflammatory attacks.

Hæmoptysis.—This symptom was recorded to have been present in various degrees, at some period of the patient's history, in 569 cases out of the 1,000; i. e. 57 per cent.—a percentage lower than that of the First Medical Report of the Hospital, which was 63 per cent., but nearly agreeing with that of Dr. Cotton's[1] 1,000 hospital cases, which was 53·6 per cent., and that of Dr. Pollock's[2] 1,200 hospital cases, which was 58·4.

State of the Lungs as evidenced by Physical Signs.— We shall now endeavour to describe, as briefly and

[1] *Op. cit.*   [2] *Op. cit.*

succinctly as possible, the state of the lungs of these patients when they came first under observation, and afterwards to give some report of the changes which had taken place at the date of their last examination; and the reason we do so is to give our readers some account of the local changes, whether for the worse or better, which took place in these patients, and thus enable them to form an opinion as to how far the improvement in the general health was accompanied by improvement in the state of the lungs. The relation, or in many cases the want of relation, between these two, must strike all physicians. How often does a patient gain flesh and strength and colour, and improve in breathing in a few months, and yet the physical signs show no perceptible improvement, but remain stubbornly at about the same! The converse is more rare, though we have known instances of cavities contracting and the general health making no great progress.

The record of the physical signs has been perhaps more carefully carried out than any other point in these cases: and in perusing it, a fair idea can be easily obtained of the amount of disease present in each case, with its subsequent progress; but the selection of similar cases for the purposes of statistics, and their arrangement into as few classes as possible has been attended with great difficulty. The classification of the conditions of the lung, consolidation, softening, and excavation, into first, second, and third stages, is open to objections, because such stages are not always well defined, it being sometimes difficult to distinguish between the end of the second and the beginning of the third, and again various parts of the same lung may be in different stages. What different amounts of consolidation, too, may not the first stage include! Sometimes only a small portion of the lung, like that underlying the supra-scapular or the interscapular, or the infra-clavicular region, is consolidated; in other cases two-thirds or more are involved. However, it has been found difficult to avoid some such classification for the purposes of statistics, and therefore that of stages has been adopted, with the understanding that the first stage embraces various amounts of consolidation, and that the second and third are sometimes only different degrees of the state of softening and excavation. In none of the present cases is the evidence of physical signs alone accepted; in all it has been amply confirmed by the clinical symptoms and the course of the disease. The results have been embodied in a table, divided into two parts, showing the 'state at first visit,' 'state at last.' From this it will be seen that 660 patients or two-thirds were in the first stage at the first visit; 181, or 18 per cent., in the second; 145 or 14·5 per cent. in the third; and 14 patients presented the physical signs of other lung diseases, namely, bronchitis, pneumonia, pleurisy, and asthma, on which shortly afterwards supervened signs of consumption. Those in the second and third stages hardly constituted a third of the total, which shows how large a proportion came in the stage of consolidation, of which the prognosis was likely to be more favourable. As regards the relative liability of either lung to disease, of those in the first stage both lungs were affected in 205; the right alone in 287, and the left alone in 168. Of those in the second stage, 55 had the right alone affected, 69 the left alone; 55 had both lungs involved, and in many instances both in the second stage. Of the 145 in the third stage, 43 had the right lung alone affected; 53 the left, and 49 both; but in only 4 cavities were detected in both lungs. This indicates a greater liability of the right[1] lung to consolidation, but of the

---

[1] This agrees with Laennec's conclusions; but it is at variance with Louis' and Cotton's, both of whom found the left lung more frequently affected.

TABLE.—Showing State of Lungs at First and Last Report in 1,000 Cases.

Stage	No.	Percentage	State at First Visit	State at Last Visit						
				Dead	Healthy	Improved	About the same	Worse	Unknown	
1st	660	66·0	287 had the right lung alone affected . . .	39	15	75	19	110	29	= 248
			168 had the left lung alone affected . . .	25	9	48	16	64	6	= 143
			205 had both lungs affected .	40	6	61	25	59	14	= 165
			660		30	184	60	233	49	= 556
2nd	181	18·1	55 had the right lung alone affected . . .	15	1	13	5	20	1	= 40
			11 had the right in the 2nd stage and the left in the 1st	5	—	4	1	1	—	= 6
			69 had the left lung alone affected . .	20	1	18	4	23	3	= 49
			35 had the left lung in the 2nd stage and the right in the 1st . .	5	—	16	3	9	2	= 30
			11 had both lungs in the 2nd stage . .	3	—	2	—	3	3	= 8
			181		2	53	13	56	9	= 133
3rd	145	14·5	43 had the right lung alone affected . .	11	—	16	9	3	4	= 32
			5 had the right lung in the 3rd stage and the left in the 2nd .	2	—	2	—	—	1	= 3
			23 had the right lung in the 3rd and the left in the 1st	9	—	6	3	4	1	= 14
			53 had the left lung alone affected . .	14	1	13	10	14	1	= 39
			1 had the left lung in the 3rd and the right in the 2nd	—	—	1	—	—	—	= 1
			16 had the left lung in the 3rd and the right in the 1st	8	—	3	2	3	—	= 8
			4 had both lungs in the 3rd stage . . .	—	1	2	1	—	—	= 4
			145		2	43	25	24	7	= 101
	14	1·4	presented physical signs of other diseases, but the signs of phthisis supervened after first visit.							
			4 had signs of bronchitis ⎫ 4 „ pleurisy ⎪ 3 „ pleuropneumonia ⎬ 1 had signs of asthma ⎪ 2 had doubtful physical signs ⎭	2	—	—	4	8	—	= 14
			14 Totals . .	198	34	280	102	321	65	= 802

left [1] to softening and excavation: a conclusion confirmed by the evidence of the second report of the Brompton Hospital, and by other authorities. Having briefly considered the state of the patients at first visits let us turn our attention to their state at last report. Of the 1,000 patients, 198, or nearly one-fifth, died; the deaths being distributed as follows:—

Of those who came in the first stage, 104, or 15·75 per cent. were ascertained to have died.

Of those who came in the second, 48, or 36·51 per cent.

Of those who came in the third, 44, or 30·34 per cent.

Thus we see that the percentage of mortality of the second and third stages was very much higher than that of the first; the third showing actually a double proportion of deaths: and the fact must not be overlooked as demonstrating that, although cavities may be tolerated for years, yet the danger from blood infection, after their formation, is considerably increased. In 80 out of the 150 in the first and second stages, cavities were ascertained to have formed before death.

The state at last visit of the *living* patients is arranged under five headings: (1) *Healthy*; where the physical signs of disease had entirely cleared up, and could no longer be detected. (2) *Improved.* (3) *About the same.* This last term is used to include, not only the cases in which no change has taken place, but also those which, after various fluctuations towards better or worse, presented at the last about the same amount of disease as at the first. (4) *Worse.* This heading is intended to signify extension of the disease, either in the same lung or in the opposite one, as well as progress in the way of softening and excavation. (5) *Unknown.* The table shows that among 802 living patients, the last recorded state of the lungs was 'healthy' in 34; 'improved' in 280; 'stationary' in

---

[1] Cotton, Walshe, and Pollock confirm this.

102; 'worse' in 321; and 'unknown in 65. Excluding the unknown ones, the relative percentages are :—
Healthy, 4·5 per cent.; improved, 38· per cent.; worse,
43·53 per cent.; and stationary, 13·39 per cent. If we
take the cases in stages, and compare the numbers under
'Healthy' and 'Improved' with those under 'Worse,' we
find that, whereas in the first stage the 'Worse' somewhat
outnumber the 'Improved;' in the second they are nearly
equal; and in the third the ratio is entirely changed,
the number of the 'Healthy' and 'Improved' being
nearly double that of the 'Worse.'

Some further particulars about the changes that took
place in the lungs may not be unacceptable. Where
registered as 'healthy' or 'improved,' the improvement in
the physical signs of patients in the first stage consisted
of dulness diminishing, either in extent, or degree, or in
both; of the breath- and voice-sounds becoming less
tubular, and more vesicular; and, in some few instances,
of the signs disappearing altogether, the percussion- and
breath-sounds being normal. In those of the second
stage the crepitation diminished, and was replaced by
breathing generally having some roughness or tubular
character, which, in some instances, eventually gave way
to healthy sounds. The favourable change in the physical
signs of the third stage was shown by the dulness decreas-
ing, the moist cavernous sounds becoming croaking and
drier, and pectoriloquy being less marked and audible
over a smaller portion of the lungs, sometimes being
replaced by the dry whiffing or crackling sounds of
emphysema, but generally by tubular breathing and
bronchophony. These last signs have, in some instances,
disappeared, except above and within the scapula, where,
with some remaining dulness, they generally could be
detected after they had vanished from other parts of the
chest.

The cases of restoration to complete health number 34, and include 30 recoveries from the first stage, 2 from the second, in each of which only one lung was involved, and 2 from the third stage, in one of which, wonderful to relate, were cavities in both lungs—but they were small, and the long duration of the case, viz. 22 years, afforded time for their contraction and obliteration. In 16 cases out of the 1000, calcareous expectoration is noted; in 20, contraction of cavities; in 2, contraction of the lung without the formation of a cavity; and in 16, emphysema of the lungs were recorded. So much for the ' Improved ' and ' Healthy ' classes.

Under the heading of ' Worse ' we find that, in cases of the first stage, in 77 or 15·18 per cent., cavities formed in one lung; in 10 in both lungs; and that softening took place in 24 others. Of those in the second stage at first visit, cavities are reported to have formed in 32 or 28·8 per cent.

In order to arrive at satisfactory data as regards extension of the disease from one lung to the other, the results of the deaths are included, and thus the whole number of cases is brought into use. We find that, exclusive of 325 patients who had disease of both lungs, and 80 of whom the results at last visit are unknown, 585 had one lung only attacked at first visit; of these the disease spread to the other lung in 131 instances, or in 32 per cent. Of those in the first stage, the disease extended to the other lung in 85 cases; of those in the second in 24; and of those in the third in 18. These numbers indicate that, after a certain period, the disease has less tendency to spread, but rather is apt to remain limited to one lung. As regards the relative tendency of the two lungs, the right seems rather more liable to extension than the left, and this greater liability exists in whatever stage of disease the left lung may be.

The results of the changes in the lungs may be summed up as follows :—

A cure was effected in 4·5 per cent. of the cases; great improvement in 38 per cent.; the disease was stationary in 13·4 per cent.; but in 43·5 per cent. there was more or less increase.

The right lung was attacked more frequently than the left; but the left, when attacked, was more prone to softening and excavation.

Where the disease extended from one lung to the other, the right lung was more liable than the left to such extension.

In former times it was hardly admitted that phthisical disease of the lung was ever cured; though it might be sometimes arrested. The 34 cases, however, mentioned as cured, were undoubted instances, as far as the disappearance of all physical signs can attest the fact. Yet how few were they, contrasted with the whole number of phthisical cases, and especially with the 'Improved' class, in which the various steps towards arrest of the disease were to be found.

We have now laid before our readers sufficient information to show the nature of these cases; and we think that we are not far out in stating that they include and fairly represent all forms of Phthisis, except the very acute cases, which are rare. The main questions of this chapter can now be considered. How long did these patients live? What did they die of?

Of the 1,000 patients, 198 are ascertained to have died; and the greater part of these succumbed to the gradual waste and decay of phthisis; 15 died of phthisical complications as seen below:—

4 died of haemoptysis.
1 „ haemoptysis and diarrhœa.
2 „ diarrhœa.
1 „ diarrhœa and dropsy.
2 „ dropsy (from contraction of lung).
3 „ pneumothorax.
1 „ emphysema.
1· „ ulceration of the intestine.

How long did these patients live ?—

```
 8 lived 1 year and under 2
22   „    2   „     „      3
18   „    3   „     „      4
23   „    4   „     „      5
75   „    5    to          9 inclusive.
31   „   10   „           14   „
12   „   15   „           19   „
 9   „   20   „           30   „
───
198
```

Of 21 patients who survived their first attack from 15 to 28 years,—

```
2 lived 15 years.          1 lived 22 years.
2   „    16   „            2   „   24   „
6   „    17   „            1   „   26   „
1   „    18   „            2   „   28   „
1   „    19   „                 ──
3   „    21   „                 21
```

The average duration of the disease in these 198 patients was 7 years 8·72 months: *the highest average among deaths from phthisis yet published.*

The chronicity of these cases is very remarkable; and it may be noted that 64 per cent. lived five years and upwards, while only 36 per cent. lived less than that period. In the above list the greatest number is included under '5 to 10 years;' the next under '10 to 15,' and the smallest number 'under 1 to 2 years.' Taking the duration of life by stages,—

In 106 of the first stage, the average duration was 7 years, 11·8 months (nearly 8 years).

In 49 of the second stage the average duration was 8 years, ·04 months.

In 43 of the third stage the average duration was 6 years, 8·3 months.

What results do we obtain from the 802 patients who were alive when last heard of? The average duration of life in these has been 8 years 2·19 months: a somewhat higher duration than among the deaths (which were probably the worst cases), and one, which considering the still favourable state of many of the patients, bids fair to increase further.

The average was thus composed :

71	have lived	1 year and less than		2
97	,,	2 years	,,	3
96	,,	3 ,,	,,	4
68	,,	4 ,,	,,	5
224	from	5	to	10
124	,,	10	,,	15
54	,,	15	,,	20
65	,,	20	,,	30

3 have lived 30 years and upwards.

This table shows that 332 or 41·4 per cent. have lived from 1 to 5 years, and that 470 or 58·6 per cent., have already lived 5 years and upwards. The class of 10 to 30 years' duration is a large one, forming 30 per cent. of the whole, and affords remarkable evidence of the chronicity of the disease. Still more remarkable is the fact, of as many as 68 patients having lived 20 years and upwards, and the distribution of these it is worth our while to note further.—

11	have lived	20 years.		3	have lived	28	years.
7	,,	21	,,	1	has lived	29	,,
13	,,	22	,,	1	,,	33	,,
12	,,	23	,,	1	,,	36	,,
10	,,	24	,,	1	,,	47	,,
3	,,	25	,,				
2	,,	26	,,	68			
3	,,	27	,,				

The question naturally arises as to the state of the 802 living patients at last report? Were they complete invalids, lingering out a miserable existence? or was their health sufficiently good to permit of their returning to the duties, if not to the pleasures of life? Observation on this point leads us to divide the patients into three classes :—

Firstly, those who have apparently quite recovered their general health, and are able to follow their occupations without any recurrence of their former symptoms. Those we describe as *well*.

Secondly, those who are able to follow their occupations more or less actively, but owing to their being subject to a return of their symptoms, are obliged to use precautions and to limit their exertions. These we designate *tolerably well*.

Thirdly, those who are obliged to devote themselves entirely to the care of their health, are described as *invalid*.

The 'well' class numbered 285 or $35\frac{1}{2}$ per cent; the 'tolerably well' 293 or $36\frac{1}{2}$, and the 'worse' 224 or 28 per cent. The two first classes, therefore, comprise 72 per cent. of the whole, and show a great preponderance over the 'invalid' class, which is only 28 per cent. This is remarkable, and proves what reparative power nature puts forth, if only the time is allowed for her to do so. In considering the patients, we must remember, that though their social status exempted them from absolute want, it by no means exempted them from exposure to other injurious influences. Among these patients were men of every profession, members of parliament, officers in the army and navy, clergymen, practitioners of law and medicine, men of business, etc., and were therefore liable to the trials consequent on each calling : as exposure to great varieties of temperature, from which military and naval men suffer; or close confinement in hot rooms and occasional pressure of work, the lot of many professional and business men; or again, the strain on the lungs which public speaking entails on members of Parliament, clergymen, barristers, public lecturers, and the like. When we remember these facts, it must be considered highly satisfactory that so large a majority are found in the 'well' and 'tolerably well' classes. The greater part of the 'well' class could not be distinguished in ordinary life from healthy persons, and many are sufficiently strong to undertake exertion of an arduous kind, whether physical, like long walks and mountain ascents, or mental, like close application to study or business.

Numerous illustrations of the arrest and retardation of the disease will be found among the 'Abstracts of Cases.'

If we compare our results with those of the authorities given at the beginning of the chapter, we find Dr. Fuller's 46 private cases to be the only ones which resemble in duration to our own ; which might be expected, as they are taken from the same class of society. As regards the French authorities, the contrast is most striking; the average duration of our 1,000 cases is four times greater than Louis's or Laennec's, and far exceeds any estimate yet formed. We must not forget that the restrictions which we have adopted exclude the very acute cases; this very limitation, however, indicates a decidedly favourable inference, viz., that if the average duration of life, in consumptive patients who survive their first symptoms one year, is 7 or 8 years, and the possibility of longer life, extending to 10, 15, 20, 30, 40 years, and even to the natural term, is often realised ; then surely the time is come when we can hold out a fairly hopeful future to the consumptive patient. We can tell him that if he is prepared to make certain sacrifices of time, of money, and of liberty for some years ; to rigidly carry out certain common sense rules which long experience of the disease inculcates, he may, under favourable circumstances, live on for a long period, even to the ordinary span of life ; and, as he lives on, may gain sufficient strength to resume his former occupations and duties.

The long duration of these cases may be attributed—

Firstly, to the early detection of the disease, two-thirds

of the patients being in the first stage when they came
under observation.

Secondly, to the perseverance with which they carried
out the various healing measures at their disposal, whether
medicinal, hygienic, or climatic.

The average duration of pulmonary consumption having
been ascertained, let us see how far it may be modified by
certain varying conditions, as those of age, sex, origin,
hæmoptysis, and family predisposition.

The influence of the last two elements on duration
having been fully discussed in their respective chapters,
need not be entered into here, but we will direct our
attention to the other points.

Sex exercises an important influence on duration.
Among females the disease lasts a shorter time than
among males, as the following abstract from our tables
demonstrates :—

Average duration of disease in 119 males (dead), 8 years, 4·72 months.
   „   „   „   „   79 females „   6 „ 8·67 „

This shows a difference of 1½ years in favour of the
former. When we call to mind that the age of attack
with females was earlier than with males by an average
of 3½ years, we see clearly that women succumbed much
more quickly to the fatal disease. This is borne out by
an examination of the average age reached by the sexes
before death. The females died, on an average, at 34½ ;
the males, on an average, at 40—showing a difference of
5½ years between the expectation of life in the two sexes.

Age has always been held to exercise considerable
influence on the duration ; and, according to our researches, the age of the patient at time of attack exhibits
this most strongly.

Our annexed table shows that this feature is more
marked in the males than in the females :—

TABLE.—Showing Influence of Age of Attack on Duration in 198 Deaths.

Age when Attacked	Males	Duration yrs.—mo.	Females	Duration yrs.—mo.	Total	Duration yrs.—mo.
Under 10 yrs	2	16—11	1	7—0	3	*13— 7
10 to 20	15	6— 6	19	6— 6·47	34	6— 6·23
20 to 30	40	8— 9·12	35	6— 6 97	75	7— 4·28
30 to 40	36	8—11·13	15	6—10·06	51	8— 3·76
40 to 50	15	8— 2 20	3	6—10	18	*7—11·5
50 to 60	8	8— 0·12	2	6— 4	10	*7— 8·1
60 and upwds	3	2—11·66	4	8— 5·25	7	*6— 1·14
	119		79		198	

* Numbers too small to yield a fair average.

Of those attacked in the decade 10 to 20, the duration is the same for both sexes; but of those attacked between 20 and 30, the duration for the males is 8 years 9 months, for the females 6 years 7 months—a difference of more than 2 years; and the result was much the same in the decade from 30 to 40.

TABLE.—Showing Age at Death of 198 Patients.

Age at Death	Males	Females	Total
Under 10 yrs	0	0	0
10 to 20	6	7	13
20 to 30	19	32	51
30 to 40	38	17	55
40 to 50	28	14	42
50 to 60	19	4	23
60 to 70	8	1	9
70 to 80	1	4	5
	119	79	198

The ages that some of our patients reached were remarkable: about 50 per cent. of the males, and 29 per cent. of the females, survived 40; 9 males and 15 females lived over 60; and of these 1 male and 4 females lived beyond 70. The majority of the males died between 30 and 40, and of the females between 20 and 30. These are the results which our 198 deaths give; but we may

1stly.—The duration is l
age of attack is later, the ret
more conspicuous among ma

2ndly.—Among the femal
an average, earlier than amc

3rdly.—The duration of t.
4thly.—The age reached
less.

These conclusions natura
tions as to the different ope
or predisposing, of phthisis c

Although phthisis is more
females, yet we see that t
subjected to the action of a
offers less resistance to its
because the causes which par
are more powerful and less
because females attain full c
earlier age than males?

If the former suppositio
menstruation, pregnancy, ar
causes than any which aff
disease would be more fre
not being the case, it seem:
to the latter hypothesis, anc
between the period of cessa
ment in each sex and the

duration of the malady in females may be explained by the stronger frame and better power of resistance possessed by the male, which enable him to battle with the disease for a longer time, and allow more chance for treatment, etc., to have effect.

Origin.—Does the mode in which a case of phthisis commences affect its duration? or is it immaterial, when the disease has once attacked the constitution, what the mode of origin may have been—as, when the heavens are thickly covered with clouds, and no blue sky is visible, it is then too late to look towards the quarter from which the storm commenced?

There is little doubt that this is not the case with phthisis, for the mode of origin has great influence over the form and character of the disease and its duration. Compare a case of phthisis originating in bronchitis, which is gradual and local in its development, and the general eruption of miliary tubercle following an attack of typhoid fever! Our statistics do not at present include a sufficiently large number of instances of the different modes of origin to estimate the effect of each on the duration, but we are able to do so in the case of inflammatory origin. It will be remembered that 149 of the cases originated in attacks of pleuro-pneumonia, from which the patients recovered, with lungs more or less crippled by adhesions, by consolidations, or by both. Did these patients live a longer or a shorter time than the average? Among 29 who have died, the mean duration was 9 years 6¾ months, and the 120 who still survive have on an average also lived 9½ years, thus exhibiting an extension of life beyond the ordinary, of nearly 2 years for cases having an inflammatory origin. In 64 of these cases hereditary taint was traced; but it is not worth while to consider the duration of these separately, as the number of deaths is small, and it has been already demonstrated that family predisposition ~~exercises no cur~~ tailing influence over the duration of the disease.

To further investigate the influence of the inflammatory origin on the duration of consumption, at Dr. Burdon Sanderson's suggestion, I selected a small number of cases which exhibited the inflammatory origin most strongly, and were entirely free from family predisposition. Not only was the disease directly traceable to the pneumonic or pleuro-pneumonic attack, but in every case lesions more or less extensive, the result of such attack, remained behind, and were easily detected by the physical signs. The duration of these cases confirms still more strongly the conclusion, that inflammatory origin has a prolonging influence over the duration of phthisis. Among 10 patients who have died the average duration was 12 years 10 months: among 20 who still survive it is 11 years 8¼ months.

Bronchitis was the origin of the disease in 118 patients —19 dead and 99 living. Here a different conclusion presents itself, though we hesitate in accepting it on account of the small number of deaths. The average among these was less than 6 years; among the living 99 it was slightly over 8¼ years: a great contrast to the deaths, and one which rather invalidates any conclusion arising from them. We may assume, however, that if the origin from bronchitis has any prolonging influence on the duration of phthisis, it is not equal to that of pleuro-pneumonia.

We should have been glad to arrive at some conclusion as to the duration of such varieties of phthisis as have been demonstrated by *post-mortem* examination; for instance, of caseous phthisis free from miliary tubercle, and of the same in which it is present, of the contractile form of phthisis, of acute and chronic tuberculosis, but for this purpose a vast number of *post-mortems* are neces-

██████████ have not at present available. A perusal,
however, of the clinical examples already given will give
the reader some idea of the good or bad prognosis of a
certain group of cases.

Looking at the forms of phthisis from a clinical point of
view, we have been led, from careful observation among
the in-patients and the still more numerous out-patients
of the Brompton Hospital, as also among private patients,
to believe that the varieties of consumption merge im-
perceptibly one into another, and that while duly recognising them, it would be unadvisable to draw a hard and
fast line between them.

How can we lay down a strict rule as to what cases
are tubercular, and what are not ? Or again, as to the
time when a case of chronic catarrhal pneumonia becomes
tubercular ? Niemeyer[1] admits that ' the development of
tuberculosis in lungs which are already consumptive, as a
result of inflammatory action, sometimes takes place in a
manner so latent as to make it extremely difficult, if not
impossible, to recognise the fact with certainty.' And
Wunderlich[2] says ' that even by the behaviour of the
temperature it is not possible to distinguish acute tuberculous from acute non-tuberculous phthisis.' We quite
agree with these opinions; and though we have been often
able to detect the supervention of acute tuberculosis during life, and to prove our diagnosis by *post-mortem*
examination, yet when grey tubercle is formed in the
lungs more gradually, and the process has a very chronic
course, we admit that it has sometimes escaped our observation, as it has that of others.

[1] *Op. Cit.*   [2] *Medical Thermometry*, p. 409.

CHAPTER XXV.

SUMMARY VIEW OF TREATMENT IN PULMONARY CONSUMPTION.

By Dr. C. J. B. WILLIAMS.

Author's Retrospect of Forty Years—Discovers a Great Improvement in the Results of Treatment, chiefly due to the use of Cod-liver Oil and the Tonic plan—Duration of Life in Phthisis Quadrupled—Modern Treatment chiefly sustaining and Tonic, but not excluding moderate Antiphlogistic Measures where required: soon returning to Tonics and Oil—Mode of Action of Oil—Plan of Exhibiting it—Cautions—Necessity of Enforcing its Continued Use—Adjuvant Remedies—Iodine—Hypophosphites—Sulphurous Acid—Inhalations—Mineral Waters in Consumption—Mountain Cure—Air and Climate.

On taking a retrospect of an experience of forty years in the treatment of Pulmonary Consumption, I can trace a remarkable improvement in its success, as judged by the results. During the first ten years of that period the beneficial effects of the treatment were very limited, being chiefly confined to incipient cases, and to those patients who were able at an early stage and for long continuance to resort to more favourable climates, such as can be obtained by voyages to Australia or India. My general recollection of the histories of the developed disease at that time is that of distressing tragedies, in which no means used seemed to have any power to arrest the malady; the tardative and palliative treatment employed was little satisfactory; and life was rarely prolonged beyond the duration of two years, assigned by Laennec and Louis as the ordinary limit of the life of the consumptive.

In the next period of ten years (from 1840 to 1850) a marked improvement took place in the results of treatment, apparently in connexion with the allowance of a more liberal diet, and the habitual use of mild alterative tonics, as they might be termed, particularly iodide of potassium with sarsaparilla or other vegetable tonic. These were first given in conjunction with liquor potassæ or an alkaline carbonate; but the lowering effect of the alkali led to the substitution of a mineral acid, generally the nitric; and a combination of this description (iodide of potassium, two grains; dilute nitric acid, fifteen drops; tincture of hops and compound fluid extract of sarsaparilla, of each one drachm; with an ounce of water or infusion of orange-peel) became the favourite prescription, until it was superseded by something which was much more efficacious. Several of the earlier of the cases recorded were treated in this way, and with improved results, in respect of the general health of the patients and diminution of the cough and expectoration.

It was in the latter half of this period that chemists began to produce cod-liver oil of sufficient purity and freshness to be fit for the human stomach; and I have no hesitation in stating my conviction that this agent has done more for the consumptive than all other means put together. And so far is this remedy from having 'had its day and gone out of fashion,' that in my experience its usefulness and efficacy have gone on increasing in proportion to the greater facilities for obtaining it in a pure state, and to the improvements in the manner of administering it, in combination with various tonics, and in connexion with certain rules of diet and regimen. Many of the cases narrated in the preceding pages are striking proofs of the efficacy of this remedy, not only in the general results of cure or prolongation of life, but also in detached passages of the abridged histories, in which improvement or deterioration in the symptoms corresponded respectively with the regular use of the oil, or its discontinuance.

The cases selected to exemplify the present volume have been taken chiefly from the records of my experience during twenty-two years. They are a very small sample compared with the whole number under my care during that period; but they are selected, not as being more favourable, but simply because they remained under observation for a year and upwards, and therefore gave the opportunity of more correctly judging of the results of treatment than those seen for a shorter time; and although this very ground of selection implies that the cases eventually became chronic, yet many were acute in the first instance, and their surviving into the chronic state may fairly be ascribed to the treatment. When I state that the average duration of life in Phthisis has during my experience of forty years been at least quadrupled, or raised from two to eight years, I say what is below the actual results, as calculated by my son; for of the 1,000 cases, 802 were still living at the last report, and many of these are likely to live for years to come.

Before entering into the details of the treatment of Consumption in all its varieties, I will give a brief general view of my usual plan of treatment. As we have been led to conclude that consumption is essentially a disease of degeneration and decay, so it may be inferred that the treatment for the most part should be of a sustaining and invigorating character. Not only the most nutritious food, aided by a judicious use of stimulants and of medicinal tonics, but pure dry air, with such varied and moderate exercise in it as the strength will bear, and the enlivening influence of bright sunshine and agreeable scenery, and cheerful society and occupation, are among the means best suited to restore the defective functions and structures of frames prone to decay.

This is the most comprehensive view that can be taken
of the means found to be most effective in the prevention
and cure of consumptive diseases ; but when we come to
examine the details of cases, we find that the treatment is
by no means so simple a problem, and that varied and
even opposite remedies are required to control the different
morbid actions concerned in developing or in aggravating
the malady. Inflammation is by no means an essential
part of pulmonary consumption, and yet, as we have seen,
many cases originate in inflammation, and in many more
this process is mainly instrumental in aggravating and
spreading the destructive ravages of the disease ; therefore
remedies that may be called antiphlogistic frequently
have to be used in its treatment.

I apprehend that most practitioners in this country are
agreed in considering that consumption should be generally treated on a tonic and sustaining plan ; and that the
nourishment and strength of the system should be supported by varied tonics and cod-liver oil, as well as by
the most nutritive articles of diet. But when the disease
is ushered in with symptoms of acute bronchitis or pneumonia, with its attendant fever and scanty disordered
secretions, it is obvious that such treatment is wholly un-
suited for the occasion ; and that remedies of the mild
antiphlogistic kind, such as salines with or without antimony, blisters, and cataplasms, and sometimes even moderate leeching or cupping, will give most relief, and will
prepare the patient for the safe administration of the sustaining class of remedies. In former years in this country (as still in many places abroad), the antiphlogistic and
starving plan was carried on too long and too far : I fear
that some of my early hospital cases are open to this imputation : but it appears to me that there is now a tendency
too much to the opposite extreme, so that consumption is
treated too exclusively with tonics, stimulants, and full diet.
I quite admit that this is the better extreme of the two ;

and it may fairly be stated that the sooner, and the more
constantly, patients can be treated on this plan, the better.
But in case of active inflammation, continued heat of
skin, hard racking cough (dry, or with viscid and tinged
expectoration), much pain or soreness of the chest or side,
it answers well to withhold or withdraw the stronger stimulants and tonics, and for a time—it may be a few days
only—to substitute cooling and soothing remedies, with
moist epithems or counter-irritants on the chest, and,
more rarely, local depletion.   But this discipline, which
is exceptional, should as soon as possible be replaced by
what may be called the *antiphthisical* treatment, by cod-
liver oil and tonics, and a more generous diet.   The
transition need not be abrupt.   So far as regards cod-
liver oil, and the mild acid tonics, with which I generally
combine it, the change may be made long before the
inflammatory complication has subsided.   A dose of these
may be given after the morning, and perhaps after the
midday meal, whilst still the saline is taken in the evening
and night, and whilst blisters or other counter-irritants
are in full operation.

So soon as the diurnal heat of skin subsides and the
cough becomes less urgent, and the urine more free, the
salines may be replaced by a mere cough linctus, if that
be needed; the counter-irritation moderated, and the
tonic, given with the oil, gradually strengthened by the
addition of small doses of salicine, quinine, or iron.
These two last tonics are of great use where they are
well borne, as their influence in strengthening the muscular system and in improving the condition of the blood
is greater than that of any other drug; but their use re-

bowels. It therefore often happens, where the patient cannot be seen frequently, that it is safer to be content with a milder tonic—such as calumbo, cascarilla, or chiretta,—which may be continued for weeks and months together in conjunction with the oil, than to give those that are more powerful, but which by occasional disturbances may prevent the continuance of the remedy.

But the great remedy, more essential and more effectual than any other, is the cod-liver oil ; and we may well bestow a little consideration on the mode of using it to the best advantage.

It is now pretty generally admitted by the profession that the pure, pale oil, simply extracted from the fresh, healthy livers of the fish, is that most suitable for the majority of patients, as being less unpalatable and at least as efficacious as the impure kinds. Since I first recommended this pure oil (*London Journal of Medicine*, January, 1849) it has been so extensively prepared and used that it is now one of the most important articles in the materia medica ; and the universality of its introduction is a strong proof of its claim to public favour.

On the mode of operation of the oil, and on the best methods of administering it, I have little to add to what I published fifteen years ago ('Principles of Medicine,' 3rd edit., p. 487). The subject will again be under consideration in the details of Treatment ; but I may here give a brief summary of my opinions and experience on the subject.

Cod-liver oil, when taken into the system in sufficient quantities, and for a sufficient length of time, acts as a nutrient, not only adding to the fat of the body, but also promoting the healthy growth of the protoplasm and of the tissue-cells, and in some way, as an alterative, counteracting the morbid tendency to the proliferation of the

Y

decaying cells of pus, tubercle, and kindred cacoplastic
and aplastic matters.

That its efficacy depends much on its being absorbed
freely into the blood, and through the circulation pervading all parts of the body, and thus reaching to the
very seat of morbid deposits and formations.

That the more fluid part of cod-liver oil surpasses all
other oils and fats in the facility with which it forms
emulsions, which are tolerated by the stomach and readily
absorbed into the blood, without causing the nausea and
bilious derangement that commonly result from an excess
of fat food. This peculiarity may depend on the biliary
and other matters contained in the oil, and which in other
instances of disease are found to act beneficially on the
liver and other secreting organs.

That the best time for the administration of the oil is
immediately after, or, to those who prefer it, at or before,
a solid meal, with the constituents of which the oil
becomes so intimately blended that it forms a part of the
chymous mass, and is less likely to rise by eructation than
when the oil is taken into an empty stomach. From this
chymous mass, the oil, being absorbed through the lacteals
with the chyle, is less apt to disorder the liver, than if
absorbed through the veins of an empty stomach.

That as the use of the oil should be continued for a
long time—perhaps for months, or even years—it is of
great importance to conciliate both the palate and the
stomach by giving it in a vehicle which may agreeably
disguise its flavour and strengthen the stomach to bear
it. For this purpose an aromatic bitter, such as the
compound infusion of orange-peel, acidulated with a
mineral acid, both to help to cover the taste of the oil,
and also to suit the stomach, which should be duly supplied with acid during digestion, generally answers well.
Syrup may be added according to the taste of the patient ;

or, still better, some bitter tincture, such as calumbo, cascarilla, or quinine, in every case in which it is desirable to improve appetite and tone. In cases of peculiar weakness of stomach, with tendency to retching or nausea, strychnia, in a dose of from $\frac{1}{12}$ to $\frac{1}{4}$ of a grain, proves a most valuable adjunct to the vehicle. By its means I frequently overcome the fastidiousness of stomach arising from debility, hysteria, or indulgence in alcoholic liquors. Salicine is another efficacious alternative of the same kind. Either of these, although a powerful tonic, has none of the heating properties of quinine or iron. When the strong bitter taste is objected to, a pill, containing extract of hop or chamomile, or salicine, or quinine, may be taken after, or before, the oil and its vehicle.

The bulk of the whole dose of oil and vehicle should be small, so that it may be swallowed at a single draught; therefore the vehicle should not exceed a tablespoonful, with, at first, a teaspoonful of oil, to be gradually increased to a tablespoonful. The dose of oil should rarely exceed a tablespoonful twice or thrice daily: when a larger amount is taken at a time, generally either it deranges the stomach or liver, or some of it passes unabsorbed by the bowels.

The acid may be varied according to circumstances. The nitric generally suits best in inflammatory cases, and those attended with much lithic deposit in the urine: but its tendency to injure the teeth is an objection to its long continuance. The sulphuric is more eligible where there is liability to hæmoptysis, profuse sweats, or diarrhœa.[1] But in most cases, and for long continuance, I have found reason to prefer the diluted phosphoric acid, which may be termed the most physiological of the acids,

[1] The sulphurous proves useful in cases of purulent or offensive expectoration; and when a suppurative tendency is manifest in the system.

tending to derange the chemistry of the body less than the others.

With some individuals the oil agrees so well, and so much improves their digestive powers, that they require few or no restrictions in diet; but this is not the case with the majority. The richness of the oil does prove more or less a trial, sooner or later, to most persons; and to diminish this trial as much as possible, it obviously becomes proper to omit or reduce all other rich and greasy articles of food. All pastry, fat meat, rich stuffing, and the like, should be avoided; and great moderation observed in the use of butter, cream, and very sweet things. Even new milk in any quantity is not generally borne well during a course of oil; and many find malt liquor too heavy, increasing the tendency to bilious attacks. A plain nutritious diet of bread, fresh meat, poultry, game, with a fair proportion of vegetables, and a little fruit, and only a moderate quantity of liquid at the earlier meals, commonly agrees best, and facilitates the continued exhibition of the oil in doses sufficient to produce its salutary influence in the system.

In case of a bilious attack coming on, indicated by nausea, headache, furred tongue, offensive eructations, high-coloured urine, and sometimes pain and tenderness of the right hypochondrium, it is necessary to suspend the oil, lighten the diet of the patient, and give blue pill or calomel with an aperient on alternate nights, and an effervescent saline two or three times during the day. A few days of this treatment will generally set the stomach and liver to rights, and the oil may be resumed, beginning with small doses as at first. In all cases during the use of the oil the bowels should be kept regular in action; and if this cannot be done by regularity of habit and diet, it should be effected by the use of a mild daily pill of rhubarb or aloes.

Such are the directions which have proved most effectual in the administration of a remedy which may truly be said to have so much altered the prospects of the consumptive as to give hope of cure in not a few, and of· much prolonging life in by far the greater number. But. to induce patients to follow these directions, and to overcome their aversion to a remedy which the prejudice of some represents as disgusting, and the experience of many may find trying to continue for so long,—the practitioner will often find it necessary to use all his powers of argument and persuasion. The great plurality of patients are. amenable to reason, and are willing to follow any advice that is given with *confidence* and *clearness*. To those who demur or rebel, it is generally expedient to tell the plain truth—that they have a serious disease, pretty sure to increase, and sooner or later to destroy life, if left to itself; but *here is the remedy*—the only one worthy of the name, which, if carefully and faithfully used, may arrest and cure the disease, and is pretty sure to retard it and prolong life more than any other known means. If the physician believes this himself, he will rarely fail to carry his patients with him. I believe it firmly, and I rarely fail to make the patient take the oil, and to persevere with it, in the experience and conviction that it is, essential to his well-being and improvement. The proportion of recusants, either from waywardness of temper, fastidiousness of taste, or from intolerance of stomach,. altogether does not exceed five per cent.

Although my long experience assigns to cod-liver oil a place far above all other remedies in the treatment of pulmonary consumption and its allied maladies, it has taught me to believe also in the limited efficacy of certain other agents, and it would not be fair to pass these over in this brief summary of Treatment.

I have already mentioned a combination of iodide of

potassium and nitric acid with a vegetable tonic, as having distinctly wrought some good in consumptive cases before the pure oil was introduced. I still sometimes use this medicine in the rare cases in which cod-liver oil disagrees or cannot be taken, and I think that it is improved by the addition of a drachm or two of pure glycerine to each dose. Glycerine by itself is of little use, but it is valuable as a lubricant, and to sheathe the acrimony of mineral acids and other pungent medicines.

The hypophosphites of soda and lime, so strongly recommended by Dr. Churchill, of Paris, have in my hands proved decidedly beneficial in certain cases. They have been tried by Drs. Quain and Cotton, at the Brompton Hospital, with only negative results; but having met with several patients who distinctly ascribed their improvement to Dr. Churchill's treatment, I have thought it right to try them myself, both as a substitute for the oil and in addition to it. In the former way the results have not been generally satisfactory: the hypophosphite does not disagree, but there is no marked improvement as under the oil; and when they have been doing well under the oil, the patients generally lose flesh and strength when the hypophosphite is substituted for it. On the other hand, it has happened to me in several cases that a patient has long been taking the oil, and, after having derived great benefit from it, halts in his improvement, or even loses ground, and then the addition of the hypophosphite has been followed by a marked change for the better; flesh and strength have been gained, and the chest symptoms have been more or less improved. In these cases I have merely added four or five grains of the hypophosphite to each dose of the vehicle in which the oil is given, always selecting the phosphoric as the acid, and generally substituting glycerine for the usual syrup. Such precautions are necessary, because the hypophosphites are very unstable in composition; the addition of nitric acid, or mere exposure of the solution to the air (if not guarded with glycerine or a good deal of syrup), being sufficient to convert them into inert phosphates. In my mixture of the hypophosphite with phosphoric acid, I presume the hypophosphorous acid is set free, and is the active agent in the compound. How it acts is quite uncertain. I cannot say that I agree with Dr. Churchill's views on the subject, even if I understand them. The hypophosphites seem to increase the failing powers of respiration and circulation. Can this be by increasing the affinity of the blood for oxygen, so that it can attract it and maintain the blood-changes even under the increased difficulties and obstructions produced by disease?

Perhaps the efficacy of the sulphurous acid—Dr. Dewar's remedy for consumption—may depend on an influence not altogether unlike that of the hypophosphites. My experience of the use of the spray of sulphurous acid is limited in phthisis, and as far as it has gone has not been conclusive. But I have found the spray a most useful and agreeable remedy in various affections of the throat, whether diphtheritic or aphthous; and it has proved cleansing and soothing in some cases of foul ulceration of the throat, affecting both larynx and fauces, generally syphilitic in origin, and sometimes ending in pulmonary consumption. If the blighting effect of damp and impure air on the bioplasm or living sarcophytes is dependent on parasitic germs or spores, as some have conjectured, the utility of sulphurous and carbolic acids as potent parasiticides would be intelligible; but the whole subject requires further investigation before we can confide in it as a basis for practice.

In connexion with this subject, I must notice remedies administered by inhalation, which are really useful in certain cases, especially those in which the larynx and trachea are much affected, and in those attended with convulsive cough or offensive expectoration. I have generally found the use of inhaling instruments fatiguing and unnecessary. A quart jug of hot water, with a napkin thrown over the nose down to and around the jug to confine the steam, is all that is needed. To the hot water is added the drug to be inhaled; and creasote or carbolic acid, iodine, chloroform, oil of turpentine, and juice or extract of hemlock, are the articles which I have found most beneficial. A few drops of one, or of several of these combined, being put into the hot water, the inhalation is practised through both mouth and nostrils without restraint or difficulty, and may be continued for five or ten minutes every night, and, if need be, repeated once or twice in the day. Although the chief operation of this medicated vapour is on the guttural and bronchial surface, yet a portion penetrates into the lungs, and is absorbed into the system; for iodine and oil of turpentine can be detected in the urine within a few minutes of the inhalation being made. Still, although proving very serviceable in certain cases, I cannot rank inhalation higher than as a subordinate remedy in the treatment of consumption. I may add, that the practice of painting the chest with tincture of iodine every night, as a gentle counter-irritant, is not without a certain influence in the way of inhalation; for a portion of the iodine evaporates, and slightly impregnates the air around the patient, and this atmosphere of iodine may not be without its influence for good. In the advanced stages of phthisis, when much purulent and often decaying matter is continually thrown off, it is very important to keep the surrounding air as pure as possible; this may be done not only by a free supply of fresh air, not fast enough or cool enough to cause a draught, but also by the purifying influence of antiseptic agents. Condy's fluid, freshly prepared, char-

lime, kept in the room in open vessels, or the vapour of carbolic acid or creasote diffused through the air, would answer this purpose.

It is hardly possible to compress into a summary the principles to guide us in the recommendation of baths and watering places for the benefit of consumptive invalids. As a matter of experience, we cannot report very favourably of the results of sending consumptive patients to the sulphur springs of the Pyrenees, or to the alkaline and saline waters of Ems and other German spas. The temporary ease to the cough and other symptoms of irritation, which they sometimes afford, is outbalanced by the increase of weakness caused by the discontinuance of the oil and tonics, which these places of water-cure generally require.

There is much better evidence in favour of those establishments in which consumptive patients can breathe the pure air of lofty mountains without being exposed to extremes of weather and temperature common at those heights. The strong claims of the 'mountain cure' have been already favourably noticed (see p. 106), and will be again considered. It may suffice here to state that experience has already justified the sending pulmonary invalids during the summer to any Alpine abode between 3,000 and 6,000 feet in height in South Europe, where good accommodation can be had, and there is shelter from the coldest winds and security from damp. The advantage, or even safety, of such patients remaining at these heights during the winter, although strenuously asserted by several respectable authorities, is more questionable, and cannot be affirmed without larger experience. Probably it will be suitable only for certain cases.

This has brought us to the subject of change of air and climate, which is of the highest importance in the treatment of pulmonary consumption. It is of the greatest

SUMMARY OF TREATMENT.

consequence to the phthisical invalid that he should
breathe as pure an air as possible, and that the influence
of this pure air on the blood and on the body should be
increased by such gentle and varied exercise in it as ·his
strength and the condition of his organs will permit.
This is the great object in sending him to a warm
and sheltered climate in winter, and to a high and dry
locality in summer.   It is a great but common mistake to
suppose that a hot climate has any power to cure consumption.   On the contrary, it is more likely to hasten
its course; and we have already noticed that the most
rapid forms of consumption are more common in hot
climates than in cold. (See p. 106.) We send patients
south in the winter, not to extreme heat, but to avoid
extreme cold and damp and changes, which, by causing
inflammatory attacks, develope the disease, and hasten its
course :—to avoid, therefore, the inflammatory causes of
the malady ;—whilst we also counteract the decaying or
phthisical tendency by the invigorating influence of OPEN
AIR, with its exhilarating and vivifying qualities of purity
and freshness, and the attendant accessories of sunshine
and beautiful scenery.   •

CHAPTER XXVI.

TREATMENT OF VARIETIES AND FORMS OF PULMONARY
CONSUMPTION.—ANTIPHLOGISTIC TREATMENT.

Acute and Chronic, not synonymous with Inflammatory and Non-inflammatory—May be acute from rapidity of decay, as well as from Inflammation—Sthenic Inflammation only requires decided Antiphlogistic Measures—Otherwise limited—Blisters very useful—Their management—Croton Oil—Opium and other Sedatives—Treatment of Asthenic Inflammation by Stimulants and Tonics—Cautions—Treatment of Sub-acute and Chronic Inflammations—Chronic Pneumonia—Rest and Quiet—Conservation of Strength.

CASES of consumption may be divided into acute and chronic, according to the rapidity or slowness of their progress; and the distinction between the well-marked cases of the two classes, as regards both symptoms and treatment, is commonly well marked. Again, there is an equally appropriate division into the inflammatory and non-inflammatory forms, which we have traced in their pathological varieties. And so far are these (acute and chronic, inflammatory and non-inflammatory) from being convertible terms, they mean really quite different things; and both inflammatory and non-inflammatory consumption may be either acute or chronic. If we bear in mind, that the course of consumption may be accelerated either by an abundance of the phthinoplasms, or by their low vitality and tendency to decay, we can understand that either element in excess—inflammation, which produces them, or their dying nature, which decays them—may render the disease acute; and that the most galloping

consumption of all must be that in which both the producing and the decaying elements go together—as in
scrofulous pneumonia and acute tuberculosis.   On the
contrary, disease will be both slow and partial where the
consumptive or decaying tendency is moderate, and where
inflammation can be either averted or kept to a high
standard.

It is necessary, therefore, in the treatment of every
form of consumption, to keep in view its consuming and
decaying character, and yet to look out for inflammation,
which, in some form or other, is in many cases concerned
in developing or aggravating it.   As before stated, the
rule or leading principle of our practice should be to
sustain the vital powers by all suitable and available
means; the use of depressing or debilitating measures
will be only exceptional and occasional, and limited to
the short periods when acute inflammation supervenes,
and calls for such restraint.   For it is not every kind of
inflammation that requires what used to be called antiphlogistic treatment.   In these days we successfully treat
patients under asthenic and erysipelatous inflammations
with nutritious soups, various stimulants, quinine, and
iron; and the low forms of pneumonia and bronchitis
which usher in or complicate phthisis are best managed
by a moderate application of the same plan.   Iron and
quinine, indeed, are apt to aggravate the cough and
dyspnœa, and other stimulants have the same effect; but
diluted stimulants, infusion of bark and senega, or serpentaria, with ammonia and chlorate or nitrate of potass,
are generally well borne in asthenic pneumonia or bronchitis in phthisical subjects.

It is only in the sthenic inflammatory attacks in consumption that antiphlogistic measures are called for.   In
case of hard as well as frequent pulse, hot dry skin,
scanty high-coloured urine, together with tight hard

cough, viscid or sanguinolent expectoration, pain in the
chest and side, quickened or distressed breathing,—the
abstraction of a little blood from the chest, followed by a
large, warm, thin linseed poultice, covered with oiled
silk; an effervescing saline draught every four or six
hours, with fifteen or twenty drops of antimonial wine,
and three or four of solution of morphia,—will be about
as much as can safely be done in the antiphlogistic way
in a phthisical subject; and the antimony may be withdrawn when the skin becomes moist; when also the time
for blistering is come, if the breathing and cough
require it.

Of the utility of blistering in inflammations of lungs
or bronchi, after the skin has become moist, I have not the
slightest doubt; and many thousands of facts, and the
testimony of countless relieved patients, have made it to
me a matter of certainty, in spite of all the modern de-
nunciations against it. Neither is the practice so irra-
tional as it has been represented; but I cannot afford
space here to discuss its principle. And so far from their
doing good by causing pain which disguises that of the
disease, I find that they do most good when they cause
least pain. I therefore recommend a good-sized blister,
oiled on the surface, and kept on only a short time—
from six to eight hours—and followed immediately by a
linseed poultice, as the first dressing. If the blister have
not fully risen before, it will rise under the poultice, and
discharge with little pain or irritation; soon healing,
and leaving the part ready for a renewal of the remedy,
if needed. This, for acute and subacute attacks, is preferable to the practice of keeping the blister open by irritating applications, which sometimes prove painful and
unmanageable, and often fail in the desired result. In
more chronic inflammations other modes of counter-
irritation may be preferable.

In acute bronchitis in a phthisical subject, attended
with violent hard cough, with scanty or very viscid expectoration, croton oil liniment or ointment rubbed over
the whole front of the chest, is sometimes more effectual
than a blister.   In the proportion of one part of croton
oil to four of lard or soap liniment, it quickly produces a
vivid erythema, which in a few hours breaks out in a crop
of fine pustules : this eruption will sometimes altogether
carry off the bronchial inflammation, and it generally
considerably mitigates it.[1]

Of other aids useful in subduing inflammation, the
most important is opium or morphia.   Small doses are
frequently required as palliatives to mitigate the cough,
but from a quarter of a grain to a grain of opium or its
equivalent in Dover's powder, or from one-sixth to one-
third of a grain of acetate or hydrochlorate of morphia
once or twice during the night, have considerable effect
in subduing inflammation attended with much pain or
other nervous disturbance.   It is generally expedient to
combine a grain or two of calomel to prevent the astringent effect of the opium on the biliary and other secretions.   I have never found any evil effect from this limited
use of mercury in phthisical subjects, and the combination also is less apt to check the expectoration than opium
alone.   It is of the greatest importance to do all we can
to aid those secretions which have a natural tendency to
relieve the inflammation—these are, the expectoration,
the urine, and the perspiration.   The free flow of these
may not remove the inflammation, but it rarely fails to

---

[1] Patients or their attendants must be cautioned to wash their hands after
rubbing in croton oil, otherwise its effects are apt to appear in other parts
touched by the hands, where they are not wanted.   When croton oil is
combined in a liniment with turpentine or camphor, or other volatile matters, it rises in the vapour, and may cause an unpleasant eruption of the
face.   On this account the ointment is best.

mitigate the acute forms; and if, at the same time, the attendant pain, cough, and other irritations are assuaged by the opiate, the best steps are taken towards a natural resolution or cure before the mischievous increase of phthinoplasms can take place.

Some other sedatives deserve mention as useful in helping to subdue inflammation and fever. Aconite, in tincture or extract of the root, has considerable power in lowering the pulse and diminishing inflammatory pains; but its use requires caution and watchfulness, as it may weaken the heart too much and cause dangerous syncope. The same may be said of hydrocyanic acid, which is, however, in small doses, a useful adjunct to a saline. The veratrum viride has a steadier influence in reducing both pulse and heat in inflammation: its chief inconvenience is in its inducing nausea. The same objection applies to digitalis, which, without any power over active inflammation, is sometimes very useful in steadying the pulse, and relieving the breath after the acute stage.

This brings us to the subject of the asthenic stage and form of inflammation, which is common in phthisical subjects; and, because it is so, they neither require nor bear any continuance of lowering measures. Whether the inflammation be pneumonic or bronchial, it throws out bioplasms or sarcophytes: which, if they languish and concrete, block up the tissues and interfere with respiration and circulation; but, if kept alive and active, may migrate and clear out of the affected tissues and membranes in the form of pus and mucus-cells and other excretable matter. Now we may in some measure promote this result by the judicious use of stimulants and nutriment, in such forms and quantities as the patient will bear them. Often the stomach is weak and cannot digest much or solid food, and then beef tea and other soups and broths, in small

quantities and at short intervals, together with the diluted
wine or spirit most agreeable to the patient. Some
medicinal stimulants called diffusible, such as carbonate
and other salts of ammonia, spirits of chloroform and
ether, are also often beneficial in promoting the same end;
tending to improve the flagging circulation and secretions,
and aiding the processes of respiration and expectoration.
Some medicines are supposed to have a special power in
this way: squill, senega, and serpentaria, for instance;
but as they sometimes disorder the stomach, I do not rely
much on them. And at this time it becomes an indication to improve the tone of the stomach by the milder
tonics, such as the dilute mineral acids and light bitters;
for by their help more substantial kinds of nourishment
may be borne, and, together with them, that greatest of all
aids to nutrition—cod-liver oil. After such attacks of
inflammation as have required the use of antimony and
salines, or even after those lower forms benefited by carbonate of ammonia, the operation of dilute mineral acids
—especially the nitric—is often very grateful to the
palate and stomach, cleansing the tongue and restoring the
appetite and the power to take and digest solid food; and
the sooner this can be effected the better. It may sometimes be commenced during a remission of the febrile
symptoms in the morning, even when salines are still
necessary in the evening and night; and if the remission
increases to intermission of the fever, quinine, salicine, or
calumbo may be added to the morning dose. This should
be our aim: to attempt as early as possible to change the
treatment from the antiphlogistic to the tonic and sustaining, still retaining the aid of nocturnal soothing salines
and moderate counter-irritation, to keep in check any remains of the inflammatory irritation. I feel quite sure that
this is a much safer and more successful practice than that
which has been much recommended of late, that of giving

strong tonics, such as iron and quinine, boldly throughout
an inflammatory attack without regard to their immediate
effects of increasing pain, cough, tightness of breath, and
heat of skin.   I am equally opposed to the practice of
keeping patients in pneumonia and bronchitis in a state
of constant semi-intoxication with brandy in quantities
much greater than are necessary merely to sustain the
failing powers.   No doubt patients do sometimes recover
under this treatment, but their recovery is more tardy
than that from a more moderate and rational plan ; and
convalescence and subsequent health are often impaired
by the craving for, and indulgence in, stimulants which
this practice produces.   I have known several, and have
heard of, more, cases of dipsomania which dated their
origin from this spirituous medication.

The subacute and chronic forms of inflammation occurring at the commencement or in the course of phthisis,
require only the mildest antiphlogistic remedies.   When
the urine is scanty, high-coloured, or loaded with
lithates, an effervescing saline once or twice in the evening and night, an occasional mercurial aperient if the
liver be tender and full, and counter-irritation over the
affected parts by acetum. cantharidis, or croton oil liniment, or the nightly application of poultices of linseed-
meal and mustard,—are usually all the measures of this
kind necessary ; and in most instances the usual sustaining treatment for phthisis, with cod-liver oil and tonics,
may be continued in the morning and noon; with a
generous diet, and a moderate allowance of stimulants.

In the more persistent forms of chronic pneumonia,
with extensive induration of the lung of the fibroid or
contractile kind, iodide of potassium in doses of three
or four grains, with fifteen of bicarbonate of potass,
every evening and night, together with daily painting
the chest with tincture of iodine, so long as the skin

z

will bear it, has proved beneficial in many instances; but always combined with the usual treatment with the oil and acid tonic once or twice in the earlier part of the day. Whatever may be its mode of operation, iodine certainly has some resolvent effect on lymphatic swellings and inflammatory effusions; but it is a wasting and depressing agent if its histolytic action be not counteracted, and this is most effectually done by cod-liver oil and generous living. The influence of iodine seems to be restricted to the living sarcophytes, the proliferation of which forms the bulk of soft lymphomata, bronchocele, and inflammatory swellings; it has less power over them in the purulent form, or when indurated, and none at all in a state of caseation. The action of mercury on inflammatory products seems to be still more limited to the early stages; and its destructive or histolytic operation on the gums and salivary glands rather favours the notion, which has been commonly entertained, that it tends to hasten the decay and softening of tubercle.[1]

---

[1] The effect of mercury on the gums reminds me that these boundaries of our flesh claim close attention in all diseases affecting the nutrition of the body. The late Dr. Theophilus Thompson particularly directed the attention of the profession to the state of the gums as a symptom of phthisis. I have long observed this, that not only in phthisis, but in other diseases of malnutrition, the gums recede, and often become inflamed and spongy, independently of any cause in the teeth, before loss of flesh or strength attracts attention. The mere advance of age causes the receding of this flesh border, and this may be accelerated by anæmia or bad living; but in many phthisical cases, in addition to the recession, there is a redness and turgidity, and sometimes a partial ulceration of the margin, indicating an unhealthy congestion or inflammation. It is not usually attended with soreness, in fact, often patients are not aware of its presence. It is commonly diminished under tonic treatment, and generous diet; but the gums rarely become quite natural again. Mouth-washes or tooth powder containing tannic and carbolic acid, or other antiseptic astringents, are of some use, and correct the fœtor often present in the breath.

Not the least important part of the antiphlogistic treatment of inflammatory varieties of consumption is rest of body and mind, and confinement to a uniform temperature.   In all acute and febrile attacks, the repose and warmth of bed are required for some days at least; and it is remarkable how this simple nursing, with time, will sometimes soothe away acute symptoms without any active measures; and in all cases they make these measures more effectual, especially in cold seasons.   The exercise of the voice must in like manner be limited. In a phthisical subject, to save the strength by avoiding its expenditure, is a wiser and safer course than to allow it to be wasted, and then to rely on regaining it through strengthening agents.

CHAPTER XXVII.

ANTIPHTHISICAL TREATMENT.

Its Objects to sustain Vitality of Bioplasm and counteract Decay—Remedies, Medicinal, Dietetic, and Hygienic—Of Medicinal, Cod-liver Oil the chief—Its beneficial Effects—Mode of Action as an Oil, on the Bioplasm and on concrete Sarcophytes, promotes resolution and ripening of Exudates—To be effectual must be given largely and constantly, to act on Phthinoplasms and counteract Decline, which may exist without Phthinoplasm—Cod-oil proper for Decline also—Notice of other Oils and Fats—Pancreatic Emulsion—Reasons for preferring pure Cod-liver Oil—Mode of preparing it—Sources—Modes and Times of Exhibition—Cautions—Tonic Medicines—Best combined with the Oil—Mineral Acids—Nitric—Sulphuric—Phosphoric—Sulphurous—Hypophosphites—Bitters and Tonics—Prescriptions of various Forms—Doses to be few—Antiseptics—Inhalations—Arsenic.

MORE or less of the preceding measures may properly be brought into operation to remove or counteract various forms and degrees of inflammation which may usher in or accompany the course of Pulmonary Consumption; and they are more often required in cold and changeable seasons and climates, which derange the circulation and cause colds and inflammatory congestions. But the paramount and most constantly required treatment is not antiphlogistic, but ANTIPHTHISICAL—that directed against the consumptive element; that which may improve and sustain the vital activity of the bioplasm, and remove or counteract all blighting or hurtful agencies, which tend to pervert it from its proper fitness for the quickening and reparation of the body, into a dying and decaying matter, carrying with it waste and destruction.

It is pretty obvious that to do all this—to renovate the

life and material of the bioplasm and to remove or correct that which is already degraded, is not to be accomplished by any one remedy or any one class of remedies. Tonics, stimulants, antiseptics, cod-liver oil, the best kinds of nourishment, pure dry air, regulated temperature, judiciously adapted clothing and exercise, are all needed to complete the antiphthisical measures; and their success will depend on their being so used, proportioned, and directed, as to restore and sustain the healthy functions of the body in their proper activity, and thereby to keep the protoplasm of the blood, lymphatics, and tissues in full life and vigour, and to promote the removal or quiescence of any that may have already degenerated into phthinoplasm. It is obvious, then, that no routine plan, or fixed course of treatment, can succeed in working out this complex problem. The leading indications are, to nourish the textures, and to sustain the several functions of the body; and experience has proved that certain agents have such power in this way that their use may be considered almost indispensable: but in the use of these and of all other means, much intelligent discrimination is constantly required, and success will depend in great measure on the care and skill with which this is carried on.

In the following sketch of the principal antiphthisical remedies, our time and limits require brevity; and we shall most concisely attain our end by considering them in succession, under the heads of Medicinal, Dietetic, and Hygienic measures.

Medicinal remedies include cod-liver oil and other fats, tonics, stimulants, eliminants, and antiseptics.

Dietetics include food and stimulants.

Hygienic means refer to air, temperature, climate, habitation, exercise, and clothing.

Medicinal Remedies.

Of all means hitherto tried for the relief of the consumptive, unquestionably cod-liver oil has been found the most successful.   This I stated in 1849, after three years' trial of its use; and so I repeat, after a quarter of a century's experience, that it is the only agent in any degree deserving the title of a remedy in this disease.   Its mode of action is still a matter of uncertainty; but we can at least offer some reasonable conjectures, in addition to those already proposed in the Summary of Treatment.   That it is in itself a nutriment cannot be doubted; and that its nutritious properties go farther than to augment the fat in the body is proved by the well-ascertained fact, that the muscles and strength also increase under its use.   In fact, it has been proved to increase the proteinaceous constituents of the blood, except the fibrin, which is diminished.[1] In truth, the beneficial operation of cod-liver oil extends to every function and structure of the body.   In cases most suitable for its use, there is a progressive improvement in digestion, appetite, strength, and complexion; and various morbid conditions perceptibly diminish. Thus, purulent discharges are lessened, ulcers assume a healthier aspect, colliquative diarrhœa and sweats cease, the natural secretions become more copious, the pulse less frequent.   It is difficult to comprehend how it can produce such marvellous and manifold salutary effects; but the extent to which it has been, and still is, administered, pretty well prove that it has properties which render it congenial to the animal economy.

Cod-liver oil forms an emulsion more readily than other oils, and leaves no greasy feeling in the mouth, and this corresponds with its easy digestibility and absorption

[1] *Simon's Animal Chemistry*, by Day, vol. i. p. 280.

from the alimentary canal. This may depend on its containing some biliary principles; it often has a marked
effect in increasing the secretion of the liver, and if this
is sufficiently carried off by the several processes of com-
bustion and elimination, no tendency to sickness results
from its use. It is, therefore, not surprising that cod-
liver oil can be administered in larger quantities and for a
longer time in cold seasons than in hot; to persons who
take exercise than to the sedentary; and especially to those
whose bowels act regularly and sufficiently. With many
weakly persons it assists the digestive process by promoting the biliary secretion: and, in not a few instances,
I have found it effectual in improving and rendering more
fluid this secretion in persons liable to gall-stones, or ob-
.structions from inspissated bile. On the other hand, it is
apt to disagree in cases of inflammatory dyspepsia, especially that affecting the duodenum; in those of hepatic
congestion, with fulness and tenderness of the hypo-
chondria; and in all states of high fever or inflammation.
All such affections should be relieved by saline effervescing
draughts, mild mercurial aperients, and such means,
before the oil is given; and, in case of persons prone to
these disorders, they may be required occasionally during
its use.

Thus we have an oily matter, well'borne by the stomach,
easily diffused by emulsion through the alimentary mass,
readily absorbed by the lacteals, where it contributes to
form a rich 'molecular base' in the chyle; apt to saponify
with the basic salts of the blood; and, when diffused in
this fluid throughout the capillaries of the body, capable
of penetrating to all the textures, and of exercising its
solvent and softening action on the solid fats of old
deposits, whilst it affords a rich pabulum for the living
sarcophytes and bioplasm of the blood, tissue-cells, and
lymphatics.

Its superior penetrative and suppling properties render cod-liver oil valuable in the process of currying
leather, and previously to its introduction into medicine,
this was its chief commercial use.   Its fluidity and divisibility enable it to pervade all tissues of the body, and to
penetrate even into caseous and imperfectly organised
deposits, and so to dissolve their solid fats and soften their
concrete sarcophytes, as to render permeable and supple
their whole mass, and open them to the immigration of
new and active bioplasm, by the operation of which their
vitality and nutrition may be improved and maintained,
or if incapable of such improvement, their substance may
be gradually dissolved and carried off.

If we call to mind also the large share which fatty
transformation seems to have in the processes of resolution and suppuration which terminate inflammation and
clear away its products (as explained in Chap. vii.) we can
see why the administration of cod-liver oil proves so emi-
nently beneficient in promoting these salutary results.
For that very process of fatty transformation which is so
injurious and fatal when it affects vital organs, as the
heart, or when it spreads destruction in the caseation of a
lung, is salutary and conservative when it helps to soften
and carry off the obstructing and irritating products of
inflammation.   We can thus understand why under the
use of the oil the cough becomes softened, and the expectoration easy, being thereby fattened and ripened (*sputa
concocta, crachats gras, cuits*).

Much more might be said respecting the action and
valuable qualities of this wonder working agent ; but we
cannot afford space here, and must refer to the ' Principles
of Medicine,' (3rd Ed. p. 484 *et seq.*) for further particulars,
and for its history and the best mode of taking it. I would
only add here that longer experience has further convinced
me of its value as a remedy, and has proved that there

need be less limitation to its use than formerly was thought necessary. For instance, it was, and often still is, said that it ought not to be given in warm weather, or in hot climates, or during the existence of any fever, inflammation, or hæmorrhage. We now have abundant evidence that it may be taken throughout the summer, in the East and West Indies, in Madeira, and in other tropical climates. Under these circumstances, it is generally expedient to reduce the dose or the frequency of its exhibition: and the same moderation may be required in continuing it during feverish or inflammatory attacks; but, as before stated, it may commonly be given after a morning meal, long before the attack has subsided, and it may contribute not a little to their removal. So soon as a patient is able to take and digest solid food, he may take a little oil after it. With respect to hæmoptysis, so long as the discharges of blood are so large or frequent as to require the constant exhibition of styptics, there is no time for the oil; neither ought solid food to be taken which fits the stomach for it; but I have found no reason to suppose that the oil has any tendency to increase the hæmorrhage; whereas it certainly promotes the healing the phthinoplastic ruptures which produced it. But in such a case the oil may be given in conjunction with a styptic, and a mixture containing sulphuric, tannic, or gallic acids, separate or combined, or tincture of perchloride of iron, or liquid extract of ergot, with judicious flavouring, may be made an agreeable vehicle for the oil.

A most important point to be observed in order to obtain the greatest benefit from the oil, is that its use should be persevered in regularly, and for a sufficient length of time. Neither the public, nor the profession, is sufficiently aware of this, and it is the more necessary to insist strongly on it. To prove truly remedial, it must

be taken in quantities sufficient so to diffuse it through the
system that it may affect the nutrition of every part. This
cannot be effected by giving unlimited doses, as these
would be either not retained or not absorbed. The doses
must be moderate, and therefore they must be steadily
continued for an indefinite length of time; not only until
there is an amelioration in the symptoms—even although
such an amelioration may amount to the patient thinking
himself quite well, which is a common case,—but until
all signs or symptoms of the existence of phthinoplasma
are removed, and the nutritive functions are restored to a
healthy state. Doubtless, it will be objected, in that case,
many persons once seriously affected must continue to take
the oil all their lives. So they must, I reply. It is the
staff of life to them, and it is a great boon thus to have
a life, otherwise despaired of, prolonged and made enjoy-
able at the trifling inconvenience of taking daily a dose
of oil with one or two of their meals. The cases requiring this perpetual oil-preserving are chiefly those in
which phthinoplastic matter has already formed to such
an extent, chiefly in the lungs or lymphatic glands, that
although it may have become quiescent for the time,
trifling causes may bring it into activity, and spread its
infecting influence through the frame. This phthino-
plastic influence may be exerted, not only locally—producing crepitus, cough, expectoration, &c.—but also con-
stitutionally, by impairing the nutrition of the body, and
causing a *general decline* of its powers. So, even without
cough, a person in whom consumption has been arrested,
may go into a *decline*, wasting and dwindling, without any
obvious increase of local disease. This decline may commonly be counteracted by the oil, aided by suitable
tonics and generous living and healthy air: but all these
latter are of little avail without the oil.

A similar declining state of general health sometimes

precedes the development of pulmonary consumption, which may supervene at any time on the application of an exciting cause. If we endeavour to examine more closely in what this general decline consists, we find loss of flesh a prominent feature. The nutrition of the body is at fault; and in the absence of any cause in the supplies, or in the digestive or assimilating organs, we are led to suspect the bioplasm itself to be wanting in quantity or quality, or both : it lacks some of those wonderful vital properties of action, motion, growth, and multiplication, by virtue of which it normally renovates and sustains the tissues of the body in the wear and tear of life.   Here is what may be called predisposition to consumption, whether hereditary or acquired ; whether the result of conformation, or arising from the operation of some depressing or deteriorating agency.   As yet there may be no local development of disease.   There is a general phthisis, but no phthinoplasm to begin the decay of an organ.   But this soon follows.   The first cold taken excites an inflammation, with its proliferating sarcophytes, and these partaking of the declining vitality of the general bioplasm, form concrete and decaying products, beginning with obstruction, and ending in destruction, of the part. Or it may be some blighting influence conveyed by damp or impure air, which palsies the sarcophytes of the lymphatics in the glands or in the lungs, and thus localises the work of consumption.

Now it is manifestly most desirable to prevent this destructive work before it attacks an important organ; and, in reference to our present subject, the use of cod-liver oil, here is a case for its most appropriate application in conjunction with other invigorating measures.   A general wasting or falling away of flesh may be sufficient to mark the decline in question ; but we may be confirmed by the appearance of swellings of the submaxillary or cervical glands, or any other symptoms connected with the lymphatic system. In children especially the state of these glands should be observed, and wherever they are enlarged, whatever may be the cause—teething, sore throat, otitis, or skin eruptions—such cases are sure to derive benefit from the cod-oil. The same remark applies strongly to enlargement of the bronchial glands, several times before mentioned as having for its sign a tubular sound within or above a scapula. This bronchial lymphoma may be a sign of disorder, not merely of the bioplasm in general, but specially of that in the pulmonary apparatus, from which the bronchial glands receive their lymph stream; and the concreting of sluggish sarcophytes in them, besides possibly causing bronchial asthma, may be preliminary to their accumulating in the adenoid tissue of the lungs also. (See Case 88.)

Now all these are appropriate cases for the use of the oil, together with other antiphthisical remedies, and their beneficial operation is generally soon manifest in the improved aspect and condition of the patient. But to work a durable and effectual change, the remedies must be continued regularly for months, and even for years, and assisted by all available dietetic and hygienic means.

Considering it to be most consonant with fact to conclude that cod-liver oil acts rather as oil, than by virtue of the iodine, bromine, phosphorus, or any other peculiar element which it may contain, it is hardly necessary to discuss the possible share which these may have in its remedial powers. Not only is the proportion of these elements too minute to have much influence in determining results so prompt and so considerable as those often obtained from cod-oil, but these elements have been used in various other combinations without an approach to such satisfactory effects. On the other hand, certain other oily matters have been exhibited with a success more resembling that commonly attending the use of the cod-oil. Thus cream, bacon, mutton suet in milk, cocoa-nut oil, and neats'-foot oil, have been found by several practitioners to answer like the cod-oil; and although the testimony in favour of all these falls far short of that in favour of the latter agent, yet it approximates them to it more nearly than any evidence which can be brought in favour of iodine, bromine, or any other chemical element or combination.

But it is quite possible that, in addition to its remarkable fluidity and penetrative power, cod-liver oil may owe its congeniality with the animal economy to one or other of these elements, which are wanting in common fats, or it may be to its biliary constituent. I have tried various other oils and fats, and have heard the results of their being tried by others, and although it is certain that if persevered with, they fatten the body and so counteract the waste of consumption, they fail to produce the general salutary effects which result from cod-oil, and, in most instances, sooner or later disagree, and cannot be continued for months and years like the latter.

Of Dr. Dobell's remedy, the 'Pancreatic Emulsion,' I have little personal experience. Not admitting either his leading idea, that failure of the function of the pancreas is the starting-point of consumptive disease, or his mode of supplying the supposed want by giving mutton fat beaten up with the pancreatic secretion of an animal, I have not been forward in making trial of the new remedy; and I confess that my hesitation has not been diminished by the manner in which 'Pancreatic Emulsion' has been advertised and paraded before the public, as exclusively prepared by one particular chemical firm. I have heard various accounts from patients who had taken this emulsion. Some declare that they have derived benefit from it; others do not admit this. Many declare that it is quite as bad to take as cod-liver oil; and I have never found that enthusiasm with respect to its good effects which is so common among those who have been benefitted by the oil.

As some difference of opinion seems to exist as to the kind of oil that is best for exhibition, it may be well to say a few words on this point. The dark-brown cod-liver oil of commerce, which is used by curriers, was that employed by Dr. Bardsley of Manchester in this country seventy years ago; and was recommended by the late Dr. Darling of London, who prescribed it with great success in scrofulous affections during fifty years. A brown oil of more or less impurity has also been in use as a remedy, first by the people, and subsequently by the profession, in Holland, Germany, Norway, and other parts of the Continent, for a century past. In 1841 Dr. Hughes Bennet published his first book on the oil, recommending its use on the authority of several Continental practitioners, and giving preference to a light-brown oil. At this date I began to prescribe this oil; but I found so much objection on the part of patients, and sometimes such real disorder produced by all attempts to take it, that I came to the conclusion that, however Dutch and German stomachs might bear it, English ones could not, at least among the upper classes. It was not until the pure pale oil was brought under my notice, that the difficulties in administering it gave way; and during the last twenty-five years I have prescribed it for between twenty and thirty thousand patients, and with such success that it was taken without material difficulty by about 95 per cent. of the whole number; and of those who thus took it, fully 90 per cent. derived more or less benefit from its use. This experience, which is in accordance with that of many of my professional friends, is at least quite as strong as any that can be adduced in favour of the brown or impure kind of oil; and it does seem absurd to recommend the exhibition of the remedy in its offensive form, when the pure fresh oil has been proved to be at least equally efficacious.

The dark coloured and strong smelling oils owe their offensive properties to the partial decomposition and putrefaction which the livers undergo before and during the process of separating the oil from them. They thus acquire a strong fishy smell and taste, like that of lamp-oil, which, although highly disgusting to most persons, are not disliked by a few who resemble Russians and Laplanders in their tastes. Dr. De Jongh, who has given the sanction of his name to an article widely advertised in this country for many years, strenuously advocates the superiority of the light-brown oil; but, as Dr. Garrod has well shown ('Brit. and For. Med.-Chir. Rev.,' January 1856), the facts which he adduces by no means bear out his assertions; and the general results of chemical analysis, as well as of clinical experience, are altogether in favour of the pure pale oil as carefully prepared in this country and in Newfoundland. The process is thus described by Dr. Garrod :—' The livers are collected daily, so that no trace of decomposition may have occurred; carefully examined, in order to remove all traces of blood and impurity, and to separate any inferior livers; they are then sliced, and exposed to a temperature not exceeding 180° Fahr. till all the oil has drained from them. This is filtered, afterwards exposed to a temperature of about 50° Fahr. in order to congeal the bulk of the margarine, and again filtered,¹ and put into bottles well

---

¹ I have always recommended the oil without the solid margarine and stearine, both from the experience that it agrees better with the stomach, and from the views which I entertain as to its mode of action. Dr. Garrod has tried the solid residuum of the oil, and found that the few patients who were able to take it, derived no advantage from its use.

secured from the action of the air' ('Brit. and For. Med.
Chir. Rev.' January 1856). In fact, the great object to
be kept in view in the preparation of the oil, is to separate
its more liquid part in the simplest and speediest manner
from all contaminating matters, so that it may be administered in the pure state in which it exists in the cells
of the liver of the living or recently dead fish. Much
meddling or tedious elaboration will injure it as much as
carelessness or roughness of preparation; for exposure to
the air soon turns it rancid, and spoils its freshness as
much as if it remained in the livers until they became
stale. The sweetest cod-oil, if rubbed on the skin, ac-
quires a very offensive smell in a few minutes; hence the
stench produced by the practice of rubbing the oil on the
surface of the body is so sickening as to render this mode
of exhibition intolerable with many individuals. For the
purposes of inunction, recommended by the late Sir James
Simpson, it would be much better to use almond- or olive-
oil rather than cod-oil; for I feel sure that, among the
upper classes at least, it would soon bring the latter into
disgrace to attempt to administer it in a mode which
renders it truly disgusting.

The wonderful penetrative power of cod-liver oil on
animal tissues has long caused it to be used in the leather
trade, and proofs of this action in the living body occur
in the smell of the oil being occasionally detected when
scrofulous abscesses are opened, after the patients have
been taking it for some time previously.

When we consider the amount and variety of beneficial
effects which result from the use of cod-liver oil, and that
its exhibition ought to be continued not for days and
weeks only, but for months and years, we shall perceive
the vital importance of obviating as much as possible all
objections of taste, smell, nauseousness, and other causes
of offensiveness to the senses, stomach, or system, which

may impede its continued administration. I will, therefore, add a few directions as to the particulars of its exhibition.

(1). *The Oil.*—It should be as fresh, and as free from taste and smell, as it can be procured. Several of the leading chemists in London prepare during the winter season an oil, which, for sweetness and freshness, surpasses any obtained from abroad; and from December to the end of June I have found the London-made oil generally prove the best. Soon after midsummer, a supply is imported from Newfoundland, and is generally excellent, being at this season quite equal to the home-made oil, with the recommendation of being considerably cheaper. The fine oil which is now largely imported from Norway is remarkably free from unpleasant flavour, and has the advantage of keeping better than the Newfoundland, its price being about the same. The oil should be kept in a cool place, in moderate sized bottles, well corked, and not opened or exposed to the air more than is necessary.

(2). *Mode of Exhibition.*—Many persons, especially children, take the oil alone without any difficulty; and in such a case it seems needless to recommend any adjunct. Yet even with these, if the remedy is to be continued for a long time, it is better to give some agreeably-flavoured tonic with it, for this prevents the palate and stomach from being palled by repetition, which is very apt to occur when the oil is long taken alone, however well borne and even relished at first. To the great majority of patients it is more agreeable to disguise the taste of the oil; and this may be done by giving it in another liquid, which may also act as an agreeable tonic to the stomach. Some physicians and chemists have endeavoured to render the oil more palatable by the addition of an essential oil or other flavouring

A A

matter; and in this way the taste may be nearly completely disguised. But the great objection to these 'palatable oils' is, that the essential oil, while it covers the taste at the time, considerably increases the tendency to unpleasant eructation afterwards. This effect is still more marked in the 'etherised cod-liver oil,' which is advocated on the ground of its stimulating the pancreatic secretion, and thus assisting the formation of an emulsion in the duodenum; but its pungent disagreeable taste, and the frequent eructations it gives rise to, have in our experience prevented private patients from continuing its use for any length of time. The best way is to take the oil floating on a well-flavoured tonic, such as the compound infusion of orange-peel, with the addition of a little diluted mineral acid, and either sweetened with syrup, or rendered more bitter by the addition of a little tincture of hop, calumba, quassia, or cascarilla, according to the fancy of the palate or the requirements of the stomach. The bulk of the whole dose should be small, so that it may be swallowed at a single draught; therefore the quantity of the vehicle should not exceed a tablespoonful, or half an ounce, with a teaspoonful of oil, which is to be gradually increased to a tablespoonful. The dose of oil should rarely exceed a tablespoonful twice or three times a day: when a larger amount is taken at a time, it generally either deranges the stomach or liver, or some of it passes unabsorbed by the bowels. The mineral acid may be varied according to circumstances. The nitric generally suits best in inflammatory cases, and those attended with much lithic deposit in the urine; but its tendency to injure the teeth is an objection to its long continuance. The sulphuric is more eligible where there is a liability to hæmoptysis, profuse sweats, or diarrhœa. The nitro-muriatic acid suits patients best who are subject to liver disturbance.

But in most cases, and for long continuance, I have found reason to prefer the diluted phosphoric acid, which may be termed the most physiological of the acids, tending to derange the chemistry of the body less than the others. The chief advantage of exhibiting the oil in such a tonic as that now recommended, is that, in addition to disguising the taste of the oil, the tone of the stomach is also kept up, so that it bears the oil in full doses and for a long period : and in this respect it is superior to orange or ginger wine, aromatic waters, lemon juice, coffee, milk, and other vehicles that are occasionally used. In cases of peculiar weakness of stomach, with tendency to vomiting, I have often given a $\frac{1}{33}$ or $\frac{1}{74}$ of a grain of strychnia in a solution with each dose with such success, that I have been led to regard strychnia as a specific against the retching of phthisis. Infants and young children generally take the oil without difficulty ; and it is easy to disguise it in a very palatable and attractive form, in an emulsion with mucilage or the yolk of an egg, and a flavoured syrup.

(3). *Time of Exhibition, Diet, &c.*—General experience has proved that the oil agrees best when taken during or shortly after a meal. Formerly, I recommended it to be taken from one to two hours after; but I have lately found that it rises less, and leaves the appetite more free for the next meal, if swallowed immediately after the meal. When taken on an empty stomach, it often causes eructations, with a rancid, unpleasant taste of the oil for hours. In most instances, after the two or three first meals is the best time, as the stomach is, with the body, nore fatigued towards the close of the day; but I have known several persons to take it well at bedtime : these are generally good sleepers, whose sound repose hides any symptoms of disagreement.

With some individuals the oil agrees so well, and so

much improves their digestive powers, that they require little or no restriction in diet; but this is not the case with the majority. The richness of the oil does prove more or less a trial, sooner or later, to most persons, and to diminish this trial as much as possible, it obviously becomes proper to omit or reduce all other rich and greasy articles of diet. All pastry, fat meat, rich stuffing, and the like, should be avoided, and great moderation observed in the use of butter, cream, and very sweet things. Even milk in any quantity is not generally borne well during a course of oil; and many find malt liquor too heavy, increasing the tendency to bilious attacks. A plain nutritious diet of bread, fresh meat, poultry or game, with a fair proportion of vegetables, and a little fruit, and a moderate quantity of liquid at the earlier meals, commonly agrees best, and facilitates the exhibition of the oil in doses sufficient to produce its salutary influence in the system.

Tonic Medicines in Pulmonary Consumption.

ALTHOUGH cod-liver oil is to be looked to as the great antiphthisical remedy, yet various tonic medicines are highly beneficial, both on their own account, as tending to invigorate the functions of the body and to improve the condition of the blood, but also as means of strengthening the stomach and enabling it to bear the long continuance of the oil, and of fulfilling other special indications. And the mutual relation which the oil and tonics bear to each other suggests the expediency of what has been found a most convenient and useful practice, to give the oil in a vehicle containing the tonic. It has been mentioned that the oil ought to be taken immediately after food; it thus is blended with the food during the process of digestion, and so rarely causes the eructations which often follow its use when taken into an empty stomach.

Tonics also, especially when combined with acids, suit the stomach well at this time, although the diffusion through the mass of aliment may somewhat weaken their tonic properties. This is no disadvantage, as the milder tonics generally agree better with consumptive patients, and their strength may be increased where required.

The mineral acids supply the lightest form of tonic, and of these the nitric is that best suited for inflammatory stages of the disease. It appears to be decomposed in the circulation, and does not increase the uric acid in the urine as all the other mineral acids do. But as it sometimes acts on the bowels, it is not eligible when they are loose, and has a decided tendency to corrode the teeth, the phosphoric or sulphuric are better suited for common use. The sulphuric acid has more tonic and astringent power, and may be preferred where there is a tendency to diarrhœa, profuse sweats, or hæmoptysis. In common cases the phosphoric acid is the safest, not that it has any peculiar power connected with its *phosphoric* nature, for it is far too stable in its composition to yield phosphorus or even hypophosphorous acid, but because it is a common constituent in animal structures, and is therefore less disturbing than other acids. It is different with sulphurous acid, which may nevertheless sometimes be used also, and is not disagreeable when combined with a sufficient proportion of syrup or glycerine. It is a very potent chemical agent, having great antiseptic power, and appears to be directly destructive to the low vegetable and animal organisms which infect bodies prone to decay. It has appeared useful in cases of aphthous mouth and fauces, and fœtid or very purulent expectoration, where it may be inhaled in spray as well as swallowed as a medicine.

Hypophosphorous acid has just been noticed, but this is commonly given in union with soda, iron, and quinine.

The hypophosphites of soda and lime were recommended very strongly some years ago by Dr. Churchill, as a most potent remedy in phthisis; in fact, they were so vaunted as to have suffered prejudice from hyperbolical praise; and in various trials in this country were pronounced to be altogether inert. On the other hand, Dr. Thorowgood, Dr. Radcliffe, and others, have found them to possess considerable power as restoratives in weak states of the system; and I have been convinced of their utility as an aid to cod-oil and phosphoric acid in the treatment of phthisis. Like phosphorus, they are inflammable at a low temperature, and any virtue ascribed to phosphorus may be expected from them; and they certainly do not disagree with the stomach and liver, as I have found phosphorus to do in my attempts to exhibit it as a medicine. In two cases of paraplegia where I gave phosphuretted oil in very small doses, in a few days it produced jaundice with tenderness and enlargement of the liver. No such effect has followed the use of the hypophosphite of soda, and its beneficial effects have been shown in this way. Phthisical patients, generally with advanced disease, have long been taking the oil, with phosphoric acid and some tonic, and after improving much in flesh and other respects, come to a standstill, and get no better. Then the addition of the hypophosphite, in the dose of three or four grains to the usual mixture and oil, has produced a very marked improvement in the vigour and appetite of the patient, generally followed by increase of weight and strength. That is the empirical fact, whatever may be its rationale: and it has been proved too often to admit of doubt; and I am therefore very glad to avail myself of the hypophosphite as a supplementary aid in the treatment of phthisis.

In addition to the mineral acids, or independently of them, other more decided tonics are very useful to im-

prove the appetite and digestion, and to increase the
tone of the whole system. It has been already mentioned that the milder tonics or simple bitters, such as
calumba, cascarilla, chiretta, gentian, and salicine are
often preferable to quinine and iron, because they are
borne better and for a longer time without disagreeing;
whereas the stronger tonics frequently increase the cough
and tendency to hæmorrhage, and sometimes interfere
with the regular action of the bowels. But where they
have none of these evil effects, and especially if there is
much weakness, anæmia, or low febrile disturbance,
quinine and iron are doubtless our most effective aids;
and they may conveniently be given in a pill after or
before the dose of oil in its acid mixture, which ensures
the solution of the quinine in the stomach. Their addition to the mixture would render it too nauseous to
some tastes to be a fit vehicle for the oil. Of all the
tonics for strengthening the stomach and preventing
nausea with the oil, strychnia is by far the best; and as
it has no heating property, its addition to the compound
orange infusion supplies the most elegant and effectual
form of *oil-sauce* that I have yet devised. It may save
the need of longer descriptions, to insert in a note some
of the combinations which I have been in the habit of
prescribing as tonics to accompany the oil.[1] I have

℞ Acidi Nitrici dil. ʒss.
Tinct. Calumbæ
Syr. Zingiberis ãã ʒj.
Infusi Aurantii Comp. ad ʒviij.
A tablespoonful to be taken twice
a day with a teaspoonful of pure
cod-liver oil, gradually increasing the
oil to a tablespoonful.

℞ Acidi Phosphorici dil. ʒss.
Tinct. Cascarillæ ʒiss.
Syr. Zingiberis ʒj.
Infusi Aurantii Comp. ad ʒviij
To be given as the former.

℞ Acidi Sulphurici dil. ʒiij.
Tinct. Aurantii ʒiss.
Salicini ɔij.
Syr. Zingiberis ʒj.
Inf. Aurantii Comp. ad ʒviij.
A tablespoonful with each dose of
the oil.

℞ Acidi Phosphorici dil. ʒss.
Liquoris Strychniæ ɔj.
Tinct. Aurantii
Syr. Zingiberis ãã ʒj.
Inf. Aurantii Comp. ad ʒviij.
To be given as the former.

tures is far more agreeable than that of ether and other volatile essences which have been recommended, and they just as effectually promote the pancreatic secretion, without causing eructations, as the latter generally do.

Although I have expressed my thorough belief in the necessity of the constant administration of antiphthisical remedies in the treatment of consumption, yet I am much opposed to the practice of overdrugging in this or in any disease. Therefore it is that I recommend all necessary tonics to be combined with the two inevitable doses of oil, and that no other medicines should be given, unless called for by the urgency of particular symptoms. Thus a great many phthisical patients go on very well for weeks and months together, with their two doses daily, and enjoying all the additional benefit to be gained from generous living, and health-giving air and exercise. And happy is it for them when they are also able to continue in their usual occupations, with proper caution and with a due regard to their invalid state. The antiphthisical treatment requires that there should be no fatigue,

℞ Acidi Sulphurosi ʒvj.
  Tinct. Calumbæ ʒj.
  Glycerini puri ʒiss.
  Infusi Aurantii Comp. ad ʒviij.
A tablespoonful (with a little water if preferred) to be taken with each dose of oil.

℞ Acidi Phosphorici dil. ʒss.
  Sodæ Hypophosphitis ʒj.
  Tinct. Quinæ Comp. ʒiss.
  Glycerini puri ʒj.
  Inf. Aurantii Comp. ad ʒviij.
A tablespoonful with each dose of the oil.

℞ Acidi Phosphorici dil. ʒss.
  Ferri Sulphatis
  Quinæ Sulphatis āā ℈j.
  Spiritus Myristicæ
  Syrupi āā ʒj.
  Aquæ ad ʒviij.
A tablespoonful with each dose of the oil.

℞ Acidi Phosphorici dil. ʒiij.
  Acidi Hydrocyanici dil. ʒj.
  Tinct. Lupuli
  Syr. Zingiberis āā ʒi.
  Inf. Aurantii Comp. ad ʒviij.
To be given with the oil as above, when the stomach is irritable.

no night work, no undue wear and tear, and an accumulation rather than an expenditure of strength from day to day ; but a light congenial employment of body and mind is more invigorating and conducive to health than absolute idleness.

There is a class of agents which may be made useful as antiphthisical remedies in those stages or forms of consumption in which there is a manifest tendency to corruption or even putrefaction in the system. I speak not of gangrene or gangrenous abscess only, in which the ultimate decomposition of animal matter is obvious to our senses, and strongly calls for antiseptic remedies, but to those more numerous cases in which the expectoration is more or less offensive or disagreeable without being putrid. That which commonly occurs in ozœna sometimes also takes place in the bronchial tubes or in phthisical cavities, and calls for the use of correctives used by swallowing, and also by inhalation. In other cases, the perspiration or the fæces have an unusually offensive odour, and give evidence of their containing corrupt or decomposing matter. In all such cases the strengthening or tonic plan may well be supplemented by the addition of certain antiseptics, which have no deleterious influence on the economy. The nitro-hydrochloric or sulphurous acid may be substituted for other acids, and may be given more largely if combined with glycerine, which sheaths the irritating property of the acids. Creasote and carbolic acid, which are pretty much alike in their nature and action, I have also found of great use, and may be used in emulsion with glycerine and mucilage. The latter may also be effectively used by inhalation with water, in vapour or in spray, two or three times a day; the spray will be found most agreeable in the summer, and the vapour in winter. The improvement in the character of the cough and expectoration, will be sufficient inducement to persevere ; and when, from weakness or disinclination, patients get tired of the process of inhalation, it may still be useful to diffuse the vapour through the air of the apartment by means of Siegles' or Maw's vaporisers. The attendants, as well as the patient, may be benefited by this measure. The diffusion of mere watery vapours in the rooms occupied by pulmonary invalids is of great use during the prevalence of an east wind, and, by similar means, an antiseptic agent or oil of wood pine may be added in case of excessive or offensive expectoration.

The only other antiphthisical remedy which it is necessary to mention is arsenic, which has recently been strongly recommended in France. I have tried it only to a limited extent; for, to say the truth, I have been afraid to interfere with the use of the oil and other remedies in which I have more confidence. The only cases in which it has seemed to me to be useful are those of a chronic kind, with some asthmatic complication, especially in conjunction with eczema or psoriasis (as in Case 102). In these both health and flesh seemed to improve under its use. Arsenic possesses tonic properties, allied to those of quinine, and other undetermined influences over respiration and nutrition, which render it well deserving of further experimental investigation.

CHAPTER XXVIII.

PALLIATIVE TREATMENT.

BY DR. C. THEODORE WILLIAMS.

Palliative treatment useful, but subordinate to Antiphthisical—Treatment of the varieties of Cough by sedatives and mild expectorants—Cough mixtures, linctus, lozenges—Time and form of administration—Objections to their use—Pain in the Chest, how caused and how relieved—Plaisters and Liniments—Treatment of Hæmoptysis—Styptics acting on the Blood—Gallic Acid—Tannic Acid—Acetate of Lead, dose and method of elimination—Turpentine—Perchloride of Iron—Styptics acting on the blood-vessels—Digitalis—Ergot of Rye—External treatment by cupping and blisters—Restrictions in diet and use of ice—Treatment of night sweats—Niemeyer's Conclusions—Tonics—Acid sponging—Sulphuric and Gallic Acids—Quinine, and Iron—Success of Oxide of Zinc—Treatment of Diarrhœa and its varieties—Bismuth—Logwood—Sulphate of Copper—Combination of Astringents with Opiates—Opiate Enemata—Tannic Acid—Acetate of Lead—External applications—Constipation—Importance of counteracting it by diet or mild aperients—Treatment of Bed-sores—Preventive and healing measures—Treatment of Laryngeal symptoms—Blistering—Inhalations—Internal applications to the Larynx.

IN the preceding chapters the general treatment of Consumption in its antiphlogistic and antiphthisical aspects has been discussed, and we will now say a few words on the *palliative* treatment of the disease. Measures for improving the general health and strength of the patient and counteracting the consumptive cachexia are of far greater importance than those directed to the mere alleviation of the symptoms; but as these, by the irritation they cause, often induce sleeplessness, feverishness, vomiting, etc., and thus interfere with the general progress of the patient, it is obvious that we must use all means in our power, to allay them, always taking care that our palliative measures do not interfere with the constitutional ones.

Cough is usually the most prominent and troublesome symptom; if loose and slight in amount, it had best be left alone, but when it is hard and frequent, and interferes with the patient's rest at night, it should be allayed by the use of narcotics, the choice of which and its combination with other drugs, must depend on the nature of the cough and the amount of expectoration. When the cough is hard, and the expectoration, though free, only slight in amount, linctuses, containing opium or its salts, codeia or morphia, combined with such simple expectorants as lemon-juice and chloric ether, are most useful. When the cough is very violent, and ends in retching and vomiting, dilute hydrocyanic acid may be added with advantage; and when the expectoration is offensive, glycerine of carbolic acid, or sulphite of soda goes far to correct the foetor, and at the same time assists the expectoration.[1] Sometimes the cough is convulsive, and accompanied by a great deal of wheezy breathing or stridor, it may then be relieved by belladonna, stramonium, or Indian hemp, in doses of a quarter or half grain in a pill at night.

In some kinds of convulsive cough, with difficult expec-

---

[1] A few formulæ are annexed:—

℞ Liq. Morphiæ Acetat. ℨiss.
  Spir. Chloroformi ℨi.
  Succi Limonis ℨss.
  Mucilaginis Acaciæ ad ℥ij.
Dose, a teaspoonful.

℞ Liq. Opii Sedativ.
  Acidi Hydrocyanici dil. āā ℨss.
  Spiritus Chloroformi ℨi.
  Aquæ ad ℥ii.
Dose a teaspoonful.

℞ Liq. Morphiæ Acetat ℨij.
  Glycerini Acidi Carbolici ℨi.
  Oxymellis Scillæ ℨss.
  Mucilaginis Acaciæ ad ℥ij.
Dose, a teaspoonful.

teration, we have found a combination of bromide of ammonium with chloral hydrate very efficient.[1]

Strong expectorants, equally with the old-fashioned emetics, are, as a rule, to be avoided as tending to upset the stomach; but when the expectoration is difficult, or if there be temporary bronchitis and increased bronchial secretion, small doses of squill or ipecacuanha are indicated. When the cough is very hard and troublesome at night, a few drops of laudanum, liquor opii sedativus, or bimeconate of morphia, in an effervescing saline, generally allay the irritation and induce sleep.

Lozenges of morphia, or morphia and ipecacuanha, or opium, are recommended as portable cough sedatives; but it is advisable to restrict the use of these and of the cough mixtures to the night, so as not to upset the stomach, and thus interfere with the antiphthisical treatment pursued during the day. Apart from this objection to their use in the daytime, they are more required at night, their great use being to ensure to the patient a certain amount of refreshing slumber, and thus increase his strength and appetite.

Pain in the chest is another symptom which sometimes requires direct treatment. It is referred to various parts of the chest, but very often to the sub-clavicular spaces. When it is of a dull aching kind and not markedly localized, belladonna or opium plaisters generally give relief. If more poignant, mild counter-irritation with either tincture of iodine, or one of the turpentine liniments, of which the Linimentum Terebinthinæ Aceticum answers best, is advisable. If more severe, and es-

---

[1] R. Ammonii Bromidi
Chloralis Hydratis, ãã ʒiss.
Syr. Papaveris ʒss.
Aquæ Menth. Pip. ad ℥viij.
An eighth part two or three times a day.

pecially if physical examination detects any decided cause
for it in the existence of dry pleurisy, or pleuro-pneumonia,
then let recourse be had to vesication, either by means of
a small blister, which is perhaps the least painful process,
or by means of the liquor epispasticus, which generally
acts very rapidly, or again by either the liquor iodi or
the strong iodine liniment; the last being rather painful
in its action.   A good form of mild vesicant is composed
of three parts of a strong acetum cantharidis to one of
spiritus camphoræ.   This has been largely used in Dr.
C. J. B. Williams's practice with success; the object being
to create slight vesication on a large surface from time to
time, but not to cause a permanent sore.   And this reminds us that we should not omit a mention of setons and
issues, which were formerly in high repute among physicians, and there is little doubt that much good was
obtained from their use, but now that we have at our
command such a variety of means of counter-irritation,
most of which are more agreeable in application, and at
the same time as efficacious in action, it is not wonderful
that the seton, with its attendant discomforts, has fallen
into disuse.

Hœmoptysis when so slight as not to amount to a teaspoonful, hardly requires the use of styptics, but may be
treated by rest, by avoiding excitement and alcoholic
stimulants, and by mild counter-irritation.   Where, however, the quantity expectorated exceeds that amount, or
continues to recur, it should be promptly checked; and
there is the more reason for doing so if a cavity is known
to have formed, or to be forming, in either lung; as
such hæmorrhage is likely to be more profuse, and if
not checked, may end fatally.   A common, and generally a very effectual styptic, is gallic acid, given in
powders either alone or combined with acid tartrate of

potash,[1] and continued every three or four hours while the bleeding lasts. These powders are a convenient and portable form of medicine; and as but little harm follows from their being taken frequently, they can be safely left in the patient's hands; which is more than can be said of some of the more potent styptics.

Tannic acid is a stronger remedy, which we have found more useful in other kinds of hæmorrhage, as epistaxis, hæmatemesis, and hæmorrhœa; but in hæmoptysis it is useful to combine it with gallic acid,[2] if the latter prove insufficient to check the blood flow.

A more powerful styptic is the acetate of lead, but the dose and mode of administration require some care and attention. In order to produce decided effect on the bleeding, it should be given, not in two or three-grain doses, as many practitioners are in the habit of doing, but in doses of five grains at a time, in the form of a mixture with a little excess of acetic acid, every three or four hours, and where the hæmorrhage is very profuse, it may be given every two hours, or indeed every hour. To prevent the constipation, cholic, and the cachexia consequent on the accumulation in the system of so large a quantity of lead, a draught of sulphate of magnesia and sulphuric acid, should be administered every morning. With these precautions large doses of lead have been given for several

[1] ℞ Acidi gallici
Pulv. Sacchari āā gr. x.
Potassæ Tartratis Acidæ ℈i.
Pulv. Cinnamonis gr. i.
The powder to be taken every three or four hours.
[2] ℞ Glycerini Acidi Gallici ʒss.
Acidi Tannici ℈i.
Tinct. Digitalis ʒiss.
Syrupi Papaveris ʒss.
Aquæ ad ℥viii.
An eighth part to be taken every four hours.

days, with the effect of checking very profuse hæmoptysis, and without any bad results.

Oil of turpentine in doses of ten minims and upwards is by no means a pleasant remedy, but may be resorted to occasionally, and the taste be covered by an aromatic infusion, as peppermint or cloves. The tincture of perchloride of iron is recommended in states of extreme weakness.

The above styptics, as also alum and sulphuric acid, check the hæmorrhage by causing coagulation of the blood; we will now notice some which probably owe their astringent power to their contracting the blood-vessels. Digitalis, in doses of half a drachm and upwards, exercises a marked effect, but its use is more adapted to hæmoptysis from cardiac disease, than to this form of hæmorrhage. In cases of consumption, however, where the heart's action is violent, or where the complication of cardiac disease exists, digitalis succeeds best; and in smaller doses it may be well combined with other styptics, as with gallic and tannic acids. Our experience of ergot of rye has been most satisfactory: we have often tried it when other styptics have utterly failed, and with prompt and decided effects; the dose should be at least a drachm of the fluid extract, and a few repetitions of it will soon test its effects, after which, if success has followed, the quantity had better be reduced, and soon discontinued.

Another way of treating profuse hæmoptysis is by dry-cupping the chest, generally in the interscapular and scapular regions; and this method has the advantage of immediate and decisive action, though the effects are not always lasting. A slower process of derivation, but one that answers well, when the hæmorrhage is somewhat reduced by strong styptics, is the application of a blister; and we have by this means spared the patient several doses of astringent medicine, which, for his stomach's sake, must be considered highly desirable.

But we must not forget to enforce the common sense measures for arresting hæmorrhage, which will sometimes prove efficacious without the administration of medicines, and always greatly assist their action.   The patient should be kept in bed, with his body and mind free from all excitement ; his room should be cool, as also his beverages, which may be iced ; and, except in cases of great exhaustion, must be quite free from all alcoholic stimulant.   His diet should be restricted to nutrient liquids, such as cold beef-tea, chicken broth, milk, etc., and he can suck ice freely, but we cannot sanction the application of ice to the chest—a practice which has been known to induce pneumonia and consolidation of the lung of a phthino-plastic kind.

The bowels should be kept freely open, and tonic medicines, for the time, discontinued.

Night sweats should be attended to, as they greatly exhaust the patient, and often interrupt his needful slumbers; but the course of antiphthisical treatment already described sometimes has the effect of removing them without any special remedies being required.   Where it does not do so, there is no lack of agents, of which one or other is pretty sure to answer the purpose; and we cannot understand how Niemeyer[1] could have come to the conclusion, that ' there are no means of relief for this distressing symptom ; ' but we conclude from his mentioning only a few medicines, and these with doubts as to their efficacy, that he had not tried others of proved value.

Where the perspirations are only slight, sponging the chest with toilet vinegar, or dilute sulphuric acid, at night is sufficient ; where more profuse, a night draught of half a drachm of dilute nitro-hydrochloric, or sulphuric, acid

---

[1] *Text-Book of Practical Medicine.*

B B

in glycerine and water, will often answer the purpose. Gallic acid in ten-grain doses once or twice a day, is an excellent remedy, and sometimes the addition of the tincture of per-chloride of iron, or sulphate of quinine, to the daily tonic will have the desired effect; but these two last drugs are apt to increase the cough, and must, therefore, be given with caution. The medicine we have found to act almost as a specific on night sweats is the oxide of zinc, in doses of two or three grains, in the form of a pill at night. This we have given ourselves, and seen other physicians give, to thousands of patients, and the good results have generally been so prompt and lasting, that in few cases has it been necessary to continue its use for any lengthened period.

Diarrhœa is a symptom which, more than any other, demands special treatment, as its continuance for any length of time produces rapid emaciation and prostration, and often places an otherwise improving patient beyond the pale of recovery. The diarrhœa met with in phthisis arises from more than one cause, and must be treated ac-cordingly. If a foul tongue, a bad taste in the mouth, a tenderness in the right hypochrondrium with nausea, and an unhealthy state of the fæces, show that bilious derange-ment exists, a dose of blue pill or grey powder, combined with some mild aperient like rhubarb, is required before any steps are taken to check the diarrhœa. When the purging is slight and accompanied by a decidedly acid state of the in-testinal canal, a combination of limewater,[1] or bicarbonate of soda with a mild astringent, as hæmatoxylum and carbon-ate or citrate of bismuth, is often sufficient, but where the redness of tongue and the persistence of the diarrhœa indicate ulceration to be going on, opium must be given, five to ten minims of laudanum, or of Battley's solution

---

[1] ℞ Aquæ Calcis ʒij.
Decocti Hæmatoxyli ʒiv.
Dose: two tablespoonfuls every four hours.

being added to each dose of the mixture.[1] Stronger and
more effectual remedies than these, are the sulphate of
copper in quarter or half-grain doses, combined with opium
or extract of poppy, but as the administration of the copper
is sometimes followed by griping, it must be given with
great caution, especially in cases where pain or tenderness
in the abdomen is complained of.

When the stomach is irritable, and it is undesirable to
give much medicine by the mouth, opiate enemata may
be used; and these as a rule comfort the patient greatly,
by checking the diarrhœa and subduing the accompanying
pain. They are generally composed of starch or gruel,
containing twenty or thirty minims of laudanum;
and in very obstinate cases, two or three grains of
tannic acid or three or four of acetate of lead may be
added.

It is hardly necessary to remark, that all substances likely
to irritate the intestinal canal must be carefully eliminated
from the diet, and the patient restricted to arrowroot with
milk or brandy in it, and such other wholesome nourishment as he can retain. Warm applications to the abdomen, as poultices containing opium, turpentine stupes, and
hot fomentations, aid in reducing the diarrhœa by diminishing the internal congestion, and lessen the pain occasionally accompanying ulceration; but this process, we
know, may proceed without pain, and indeed, as Dr.
Powell[2] has shown, without diarrhœa.

Though diarrhœa is common in the later stages of consumption, the opposite state, i.e. *constipation*, often

[1] ℞ Liquoris Bismuthi et Ammoniæ Citratis ʒi.
    Liquoris Opii Sedativi fʒii–iv.
    Spir. Myristicæ ʒss.
    Decocti Hæmatoxyli ad ℥viij.
   Dose : An eighth part every four hours.
[2] *Pathological Transactions*, vol. xix. p. 79.

prevails in the earlier ones, and should be counteracted, for two reasons; firstly, because it is impossible for the oil to agree if the biliary and intestinal secretions are not properly discharged, but allowed to accumulate in the intestines, causing flatus, loss of appetite, etc.; and secondly, because phthisical patients are more liable to hæmoptysis when the bowels are costive than when they act regularly.

The simplest method of correcting this state is by introducing into the diet a fair amount of fresh or cooked fruit: or by substituting the use of brown bread for white, the bran in the former acting as a simple irritant to the mucous membrane of the intestines.

Where dietetic means fail, recourse must be had to aperient medicine, the continuous action of a mild purgative being preferred to the prompt but less lasting results of a stronger one. The confectio sulphuris, or an electuary[1] composed of sulphate of potash and confection of senna, taken in a teaspoonful dose every night, is often sufficient; but what we have found most successful is a pill[2] of Barbadoes aloes, containing 1½ or 2 grains of the extract, combined in the more obstinate cases with ½ grain of extract of nux vomica, and taken at bedtime.

Dyspnœa may be relieved, if coming on suddenly, by spirits of ether and sal volatile, or by the inhalation of oxygen; if of a more chronic kind, by a combination of chlorate of potash and nitric acid.

---

[1] ℞ Potassæ Sulphatis
Syrupi Zingiberis āā ʒss.
Confectionis Sennæ ʒi.
Dose: A teaspoonful every night.

[2] ℞ Extracti Aloes Barbadensis gr. iss.
——— Nucis Vomica gr. ¼
Potassæ Tartratis Acidæ gr. i.
Mastichi gr. iss.
Spiritus rectificati q. s.
To be taken every night.

The acid tartrate of potash is added for the purpose of dividing the pill substance, and the mastich and spirit to make the pills keep for a long time.

Bed-sores should be prevented by carefully watching the state of the skin of the back and sacrum, and by placing the patient on a water-bed, of which the half or three-quarter length sizes are generally preferable to the full-length ones. When the skin, though red, is still unbroken, a wash of brandy-and-water, one part in four, has a fortifying effect, but if it is broken, collodion flexile may be applied with a view to form a protecting film, and thus afford the skin an opportunity of healing. This is, however, of little use if means be not taken to remove pressure from the part, which should be left free for dressings. A circular air-cushion will do the former, but at the Brompton Hospital it has been found that these soon get out of order, and cushions of down of similar shape have been substituted. Another method employed is to apply a piece of thick felt plaister or of the material known as 'rhinoceros hide,' perforated with a hole the size of the wound, and then to treat it with water dressing.

Some of the worst symptoms of the disease are those which indicate the different stages of ulceration of the larynx, pricking pain in the region, difficulty of swallowing owing to the swollen or ulcerated epiglottis, hoarseness, gradually amounting to aphonia and from time to time, convulsive dyspnœa. Here, some relief may be afforded by blistering the larynx externally and by inhalations of conium, carbolic acid, or iodine, internally; and we have known great comfort being given by the use of the sulphurous acid in the form of spray, either alone or diluted with an equal amount of water.

Where the epiglottis is much swollen, temporary relief is afforded by scarifying it; and Dr. Marcet[1] has had good

---

[1] *Clinical Notes on Diseases of the Larynx*, x. p. 95. Dr. Marcet's formula is :—

> ℞ Iodi. gr. xx.
> Potassii Iodidi gr. v.
> Olei Olivæ ʒi.

results from applying a solution of iodine in olive oil, to the interior of the larynx with a brush.

Dr. Powell finds a linctus of morphia, chlorate of potash, glycerine, and syrup soothes the swollen epiglottis and renders swallowing more easy; and we have seen some good done by a combination of chlorate of potash, tannic acid, and glycerine applied to the upper part of the larynx with a brush; but we must confess that hitherto no great progress has been made in the treatment of this very distressing group of symptoms of consumptive disease, and we trust that the efforts of practitioners will some day be more successful than they are at present.

CHAPTER XXIX.

DIETETIC AND HYGIENIC MEASURES.

By Dr. C. Theodore Williams.

*Effects of good diet on Consumptive patients—Object of Diet—Importance
of Meat—Exemption of Butchers from Consumption—Raw Meat: when
useful—Blood drinking—Vegetables and Fruits—Objections to Pastry,
Salads, Pickles—Cautions as to the use of fatty and oily food—Bread and
farinaceous articles—Liquid Nourishment—Stimulants—Mode of administration and uses—Varieties and Rules for their selection—Brandy and
Rum best combined with Food—Cooling Drinks—Clothing—Best material
for underclothing—Warm Wraps—Exercise: its Benefits—Active Exercise:
its Object and Varieties—Rowing—Swinging—Gymnastics—Walking—
Passive Exercise: its Varieties—Carriage—Sailing—Their effects—Riding
—Its great Advantages—Habitation—Soil and Site—Locality and Shelter
—Temperature—Ventilation and Drainage.*

THE dietetics of consumption form a very important item
in the antiphthisical treatment, and the careful regula-
tion of the food and drink, according to the capabilities of
each patient, requires the greatest attention. At the
same time it is evident that, though a sketch may be
made of the system to be pursued, fixed rules cannot be
laid down as to the variety or amount of food to be taken
in all cases.

We know that on good diet alone, without any medicinal
aid, consumptive patients have increased in strength and
weight, and of this Dr. Risdon Bennett has published
some striking examples.[1] We have occasionally seen
similar instances among the in-patients of the Brompton

[1] *Medical Times and Gazette*, 1869.

Hospital, and they demonstrate what effect good and plentiful fare may have on those unused to it; but great improvement, on generous diet alone, has not in our experience often occurred. Indeed, the ingestion and apparent assimilation of large quantities of food without increase, and with even decrease, of weight, has often struck us as a remarkable proof of the consuming nature of the disease.

The great object to be kept in view. as Dr. Pollock briefly expresses it, is ' to supply the largest amount of the most nutritious food which can be digested' But this is not always an easy task in a complaint where the appetite is likely to fail and the stomach is prone to derangement.

Whenever it is possible, fresh meat plainly cooked and unalloyed with rich sauces, gravy, or stuffing, should be taken two, or even three times a day, and the diet varied occasionally by the introduction of poultry, fish and game, but a decided preponderance of butcher's meat, not overloaded with fat, should be retained.

A striking proof of the importance of this point is furnished by the rarity of consumption among butchers; and although the airy and open shops in which they live, and the amount of out-door exercise which they take, may contribute to their good health, their exemption from phthisis must be principally ascribed to the quantity of meat they consume, for, in addition to the cooked article taken at meals, they are in the habit of nibbling bits of raw meat while serving their customers,—a practice which explains the comparative frequency of entozoic disease in this trade. We may mention, by the way, that the use of raw meat in consumption has been much advocated in France and Germany; and we have seen some good derived from its use, when the patients were hysterical girls who would not eat; but it is in the wasting diseases of childhood, that uncooked meat is most useful. When mixed up with sugar, in the French method, it forms a palatable sweetmeat, much liked by children, though the absence of cooking renders them liable to worms from this source. Another practice, carried on in the South of France, and which we cannot regard as otherwise than disgusting, is to drink lamb's blood;[1] and when at Hyères we, ourselves, witnessed with a shudder, elegantly dressed French ladies repair daily to the slaughter-house and quaff the reeking draught, but with what result we never learnt.

Fresh vegetables, plainly dressed, and a small amount of ripe fruits, as, for instance, oranges, grapes,[2] apples, and pears, are to be included in the dietary; but rich pastry, savoury dishes, salads, containing much vinegar, pickles of every kind, and the like, are to be carefully avoided, both as tending to upset digestion, and as interfering with the prolonged use of cod-liver oil. With regard to butter, cream, suet, and various other oily or greasy matters, we must bear in mind that the stomach and liver are already somewhat tried by the regular administration of cod-liver oil, one of the most easily assimilated members of this group, but still occasionally giving rise to symptoms of biliousness and gastric disturbance, and it is therefore highly important not to tax these organs further by the introduction of large quantities of fatty or oily material. Great moderation should be observed in the use of these articles, and, as has been mentioned in a former chapter, the quantity of milk should be limited. At the same time it must be remembered that there are individuals who can assimilate almost

[1] Some years ago Dr. Marcet invented some biscuits, composed of the clot of sheep's or bullock's blood and chocolate, which seems to be a less objectionable mode of trying this form of nourishment, if it is to be tried at all.

[2] The ' grape cure,' which is carried on by the lake of Geneva, and at Meran in the Tyrol, is supposed to diminish the excess of fibrin in the blood of consumptive patients.

any quantity of fatty matter, and to these the above re-commendations do not apply; indeed, such can and do sometimes take cream, in addition to the oil, with benefit. Moreover, where much exercise is taken more fat can be tolerated. Bread, eggs, and farinaceous food naturally complete our dietary; but we cannot recommend cheese, as it is somewhat trying to the digestion, and may take the place of more nutritious material.

In cases of very advanced phthisis, when the intestinal canal cannot tolerate, or assimilate solid food, it will be necessary to have recourse to liquid nourishment, in the form of soups, beef-tea, or chicken, mutton, or veal broth, the various meat essences, and panadas, alternating the same with jelly, arrow-root, tous-les-mois, oswego, tapioca, sago, Iceland moss, and other articles of invalid diet, and these last, should be nicely flavoured with lemon or orange-peel, with orange flower or vanilla, so as to render them more tempting. Though we cannot go as far as Dr. Flint in the importance to be attached to the use of stimulants in consumption, yet we highly commend them when taken *with food*, and not alone, at odd times between meals, as is done by many persons—a custom more sociable than wholesome, and specially injurious to the stomach, for the gastric juice is thus stimulated to secretion, and having no food to digest, acts on the walls of the viscus, giving rise to flatulence and loss of appetite. When the meal time comes, the food is not thoroughly relished, and, on account of the waste of the gastric juice, imperfectly digested.

The two principal uses of stimulants in consumption are, firstly, to increase appetite and promote digestion; secondly, to stimulate the heart's action, and thus obviate the tendency to death by syncope.

For the last purpose it is only required in the very advanced stages of the disease; but in the first lies its principal utility, the only drawback being that stimulants are apt to increase the cough and local irritation, but they are less liable to do so if mixed with water. As regards the choice of different kinds, much must depend on the state of the organs of digestion and circulation. If the patient be not of a bilious habit and the cough be not troublesome, malt liquor—in the form of bitter ale, table beer, or even stout—is a capital appetiser ; but in case of liver disturbance, sherry mixed with water, or hock, or chablis, answers the purpose better. If the cough is at all troublesome, the amount of stimulant should be diminished, and sometimes its use discontinued altogether, but the least irritating to the chest appears to be good wholesome claret ; Burgundy and port are rather too fiery for this purpose. Champagne is only to be employed in cases of extreme weakness, and then but for a limited period. Brandy, gin, rum, and whisky, are most useful in the last stages of the disease ; but they are best tolerated when combined with nourishment, in the form of brandy and arrow-root, egg-flip, rum and milk, and other numerous combinations which the physician and nurse have to employ to ensure a proper amount of food and stimulant being taken by the patient. The custom of taking a cup of rum and milk in the morning, before dressing, is very beneficial to weak subjects. The thirst often complained of in the feverish stages of the disease may be met by iced toast-and-water, barley-water, tamarind-drink, seltzer-water, soda-water and milk, and other cooling fluids.

Let us now notice a few hygienic measures, without which the treatment of consumption would be incomplete.

Clothing.—We need not observe that consumptive patients, who are more susceptible than others to the process called ' catching cold,' and in whom it often sets up intercurrent pneumonia and bronchitis, should clothe warmly, though not to such an extent as to produce perspiration or diseased fat.

The most important point to be attended to is the under-clothing, which for at least eight months of the year should be of flannel, lambs' wool, or some other woollen material, and should not only cover the chest completely, but also encase the whole body and lower extremities. The double-breasted lambs' wool jersey answers the purpose well, and should be worn with drawers of the same material, or of flannel, and with woollen socks or stockings. In the summer months a thinner clothing of merino may be substituted, but the change must be carried out with great caution. Over-clothing is also of consequence, more especially when the patient is driving out in a carriage; and in this particular he can hardly be too careful, for with a weak circulation, and but little means of exciting it, he must prevent the chilling effect of radiation from his body by wrapping up warmly in furs and rugs, and if this should be insufficient, by supplying extra heat by a hot flask to his feet.

Exercise.—It may be safely stated, that, in all cases of phthisis, exercise in some form or other is beneficial, and the good derived where the patients are able to avail themselves of it, is very evident, as seen by the increase of appetite, by the quickened circulation, and the sounder sleep which so often follow when exercise is taken by the patient. Whether it should be of the active or passive kind, and what varieties of each are admissible, depends on the stage and type of the disease, and also on the strength of the patient. In the early stages, where the symptoms are not active, where there has been no recent blood-spitting, and where the cough is not hard or frequent, those varieties of active exercise are of most advantage which most effectually expand the upper portions of the chest, thereby bringing into play the upper lobes

lungs, so generally the seat of phthinoplastic
and 'by causing the blood to circulate freely
the pulmonary tissue, they prevent local con-
and fresh deposits, and aid materially in the
of old ones.

What are the varieties of exercise which best accom-
this end? Those in which the upper extremities
raised, and the muscles connecting them with the
brought into activity. When the arm is raised,
numerous muscles which arise from the ribs and are
inserted into the bones of the upper extremity, e.g. the
pectoralis major and minor, the sub-clavius, the serratus
magnus, &c., in contracting, raise the upper ribs, and
increase the size of the chest cavity. This neces-
sitates the inspiration of a larger amount of air. Dr.
Sylvester has called attention to this important principle,
and on it has founded his excellent system of restoring
respiration in cases of drowning, narcotism, etc. He has
also recommended a modification of it in the incipient
stages of phthisis. The forms of exercise which carry out
this principle are : rowing, particularly the pull and back-
ward movement; the use of the alpenstock in mountain
ascents; swinging by the arms from a horizontal bar, or
from a trapeze; climbing ladders or trees. Dumb-bells,
as commonly used, are calculated to develop the arms
more than the chest; and rather tend to depress the latter
by their weight. Various special gymnastic exercises, of
which there is a great choice now-a-days, may more or
less answer the purpose; but there is one form which is
particularly applicable to the object above mentioned,
viz. the *gymnast* invented by Mr. Hodges. To make
this instrument answer the purpose of a chest elevator or
suspender, it should be fixed, not, as it is sometimes done,
at the height of the operator, but considerably above his
head, in or near the ceiling, with the handles reaching

down about to his shoulders, then, by holding the handles, and walking a few paces forwards and backwards, the arms are brought into a species of action, which, while it exercises the whole body, especially tends to expand and elevate the upper part of the chest.

Walking exercise, as a rule, does not work the upper extremities or raise the upper ribs, but acts generally on the system by drawing the blood to the extremities and quickening the circulation through the lungs. In mountain ascents and in fast walking the quickening of the circulation brings the whole lungs into play, and in this way the upper lobes come into full use. If the alpenstock be used in mountain climbing, the beneficial local effects of raising the upper ribs may be combined with the general advantages of walking. Walking exercise can be taken in all stages of phthisis, provided there be no active symptoms present. Even where cavities are formed, if there be no recent inflammation, a limited amount, and performed on level ground, is beneficial, but great care must be taken not to overtax the patient's strength.

Passive exercise may be used by the weak and delicate, even in advanced stages of phthisis, or when it is of the inflammatory type. Open carriage exercise, sailing, or being rowed in a boat, or carried in a hammock, are instances in all of which little muscular exercise is involved, and they may be considered as means of supplying a constant change of air, with the least fatigue, while their effect in improving the circulation and appetite, and in promoting sleep, is often very apparent. But even these make some demand on muscular and nervous power, and must not be carried to the extent of producing exhaustion in weak subjects.

Riding exercise, from the time of Sydenham, has been generally acknowledged to be peculiarly beneficial to consumptive patients who are strong enough to bear it;

and it is difficult to find a form of exercise which so admirably answers the purpose of giving plenty of fresh air and thoroughly warming both body and extremities with so small an amount of fatigue.

Habitation.—The residence of the consumptive patient should be situated on a dry soil of sand or gravel, free from admixture with clay or other material likely to collect or retain moisture. It should stand on slightly elevated and sloping ground, so as to ensure thorough surface drainage. Vegetation should be present in order to keep up the supply of oxygen, and it should not be rank, succulent, or in excess; but short, herbaceous, heathery, and flower-bespangled, like the grass fields of a dry and open country, or the downy herbage of a hill-side or elevated common. Shrubs, such as broom, furze, thorn, and thin copse-wood are welcome, and a few trees scattered or arranged with a view to shelter; but dense woods and large deciduous trees, the chief ornament of park scenery, do not add to the healthiness of the air, but greatly increase its humidity. There is no objection to the neighbourhood of pines, especially on the north side of the dwelling, their dry shade and fragrant odour being very pleasant, and forming the great attraction of certain localities, as Bournemouth and Arcachon; indeed, the turpentine inhalations from this source are held in great repute in many parts of the Continent, and form one of the numerous ' cures ' so congenial to the German mind.

The vicinity of marshy or swampy ground is of course to be avoided, as likely to cause malaria, and even that of low lands and valleys with a clay soil or sub-soil, for moisture is generally excessive in such districts.

Peat bogs, on account of some antiseptic property, do not engender malaria, but are not exempt from the imputation of dampness; and anyone who has witnessed the swarms of midges on a Scotch morass can testify to their capacity of breeding one kind of plague at least. The close proximity of the house to lakes or ponds of fresh water, or of slowly running streams, little below the level of the ground, is not desirable, as the amount of moisture in the air is thereby increased; but this does not apply to the margin of the sea, for there is certainly something corrective, if not antiphthisical, in salt water and the vapour arising from it, which renders sea damp less injurious than land damp.

The house should be protected from northerly and easterly winds, and well open to the south and west. The walls should be thick and the windows large, so as to allow, if necessary, of thorough ventilation; the rooms should be lofty and airy, and the temperature kept as near 60° F. as circumstances will admit of; whilst means are taken to maintain this degree of warmth, others should not be omitted to ensure a frequent and abundant supply of fresh air, either through the top of the window, or through ventilators opening outside, and also for the removal of the impure air. We need hardly add, that the drainage arrangements should be efficient and complete.

CHAPTER XXX.

CLIMATE.

By Dr. C. Theodore Williams.

Immunity of Localities from Consumption not assignable to any one condition of life—Objections to High Altitude Theory—Kirghis—Icelanders and Faroise—Objections to " Koumiss" theory—Twofold causation of Consumption—Influences originating Inflammatory Attacks—Septic Influences—Nature of disease dependent on its causation—Knowledge of Countries where each class prevails : a guide to climatic treatment—Objects of change of climate—Division of Climates into Marine and Inland—Marine—Their stimulating and equable qualities—Caution as to Seaport Towns—Cool and moist British Coast Stations—Dry Climates of Mediterranean Basin—Warm and moist Madeira group—Inland Climates : their great diversity—Division into three groups—Calm and soft—Dry and warm—Climates of elevated regions—Marine Climates suitable for Consumption arising from Inflammation—Choice dependent on degree of irritability of system—Inland localities best fitted for most irritable variety—Climate of elevated regions indicated for Consumption of Septic origin—Restrictions—Residence at high altitudes important as a preventive measure—Ordinary Chronic Consumption best treated by warm stimulating climate in winter, and cool bracing climate in summer—Importance of Exercise—Inland Climate of North America—Sea Voyages—Advantages and disadvantages—Cautions—Certain cases of Consumption unfit for change of climate—Practice of sending Patients in advanced Consumption Abroad condemned.

Climate.—We cannot attempt, in the few remaining pages of this book, to discuss the important subject of Climate, in all its relations to Consumption, but must refer our readers to what we have published elsewhere on the subject.[1] What we aim at doing, now, is to point out the existence of certain indications which should form the

[1] The Climate of the South of France as suited to Invalids, with Notices of Mediterranean and other Winter Stations, and an Appendix on Alpine Summer Quarters, and the Mountain Cure, 2nd edition.

C C

ground for the physician's decision, as to the climate most likely to be of benefit. And here we must premise, that taking a fair survey of our present knowledge of the geography of phthisis, we cannot subscribe to any theory which assigns immunity from the disease to any one condition of life, and to that only, as, for instance, elevation above the sea, or dryness of soil, or to the use of certain kinds of food, as koumiss, blaand, etc. To the supporters of the high altitude theory, the existence of the Kirghis, who are quite free from consumption, living on vast steppes, 100 feet below the level of the sea, is, as Dr. Charlton[1] well shows, an insuperable objection, which is borne out by the inhabitants of Iceland and the Faroe Isles, who live at but slight elevations above the sea, and, as regards their dwellings, under very unhygienic conditions, but are equally free from this disease. To those who consider that the use of koumiss[2] or fermented mare's milk among the Kirghis, and that of blaand or the sour whey from cow's milk among the Icelanders and Feroëse, is the cause of their immunity from consumption, may be opposed the example of the dwellers on the high table lands of the Andes and of the Alps who do not commonly use such beverages.

We may here remark, that in the somewhat revolting diet of the Icelanders and Feroëse, which embraces fish and flesh in an almost putrid condition, there is one article which seems more likely than blaand to explain their salubrity, viz. cod-liver oil, for this, under the name of 'muggy,' is consumed by all classes and largely.

A more probable view, and one more likely to explain the various phenomena presented by the distribution of

[1] *Northumberland and Durham Medical Society's Proceedings.*
[2] We may mention that this drink has lately been tried at the Brompton Hospital on consumptive patients, but that the experiment was not sufficiently successful to warrant its continuance.

phthisis throughout the world, is given in page 106, viz. that its causation is at least two-fold, and possibly more complex. Firstly. The influences which excite and keep up inflammatory affections of the lungs, the products of which are apt to be of a lowly organised kind, tending to contraction or to caseation. Such influences are the pre-valence of cold and damp weather, and frequent changes of temperature. Secondly. Septic influences, which blight and corrupt portions of the bioplasm of the blood, or of the lymphatics, and thus sow the seeds of decay. As, for instance, the combination of warmth and humidity, foul air, bad or insufficient nourishment, weakening diseases, and other general causes. As has been stated, the co-operation of these two classes of causes often takes place and renders the effect more certain, as when a person deteriorated by foul air is exposed to chill, or when the subject of an inflammatory attack is confined in an impure atmosphere and deprived of the healthy influ-ence of fresh air, of light, and of good food.

This two-fold causation of phthisis is rendered more probable by the marked difference in the kind of disease which each class of causes gives rise to. Consumption arising from the first class of influences is generally a limited disease of one or both lungs running a chronic course, and is that which prevails most largely in cold and temperate countries. Consumption arising from the second class is a disease with more marked constitutional symptoms, is generally tubercular, and runs a more or less rapid course. This type, as Dr. Guilbert has well pointed out, is the prevalent one of hot countries; but instances may be found in abundance, in temperate climates, which are traced to some of the above-mentioned septic causes, foul and hot air, bad nourishment, and the like.

It is evident that in our selection of a climate for a patient we should consider the probable mode of causation of the disease, whether it was inflammatory or septic, and frame our decision to some extent on the conclusion arrived at.

Our great object in consumptive disease is to give the patient as pure an atmosphere as possible, of such thermometrical, hygrometrical, and other qualities that it can be breathed freely and safely by him. It should, therefore, be free from extremes, humid or dry, and neither too still nor too windy, and its influence on his frame should be furthered by frequent exercise of various kinds carried out in cheerful sunshine, uninterrupted by rainy, misty, or windy weather.

Let us glance at the principal varieties of climate at our disposal, and examine what forms of the disease each is most likely to benefit. For convenience, let us divide them into Marine and Inland climates.

Marine.—By this term we mean the climates of localities situated on or close to the sea, and deriving their principal qualities from that element. The beneficial influence of sea-side air on scrofula is well established, and Laennec and others entertained a firm belief that it had some curative as well as preventive power over phthisis. All the most favoured winter resorts for consumptive patients in this country are on the sea-coast, and most of those in other parts of Europe are so likewise. It is very desirable to make careful statistical comparisons as to the prevalence and mortality of phthisis and the various forms of scrofula in sea-coast places, compared with those inland. Enquiries that have already been made on these points have obtained discordant results; and further information is required before any conclusions can be drawn. One point deserves mention, as it bears on the present subject. Several of the towns called sea-port towns are not on the open sea, and, although they communicate with the sea, the greater number of the inhabitants are living inland,

exposed to inland damp and marsh, and to the insalu-
brious circumstances of a crowded population, on which
the vicinity of the sea, or of an arm of the sea, can have
no influence whatever. Such are Portsmouth, Plymouth,
Liverpool, Bristol, and others ; and these we do not
designate marine towns, for even those nearest to the sea,
as the three first, have much flat marshy ground behind
them, on which the sea exercises little or no influence,
salt water reaching them only at high tides. Marine
climates vary according to their latitude, meteorology,
soil, and shelter from cold winds, but are all, more or
less, stimulating. They are also more equable than inland climates, and less liable to great or sudden changes
of temperature. Though their stimulating character
depends on the quantity of saline matter contained in
the atmosphere, it is modified by the temperature and the
amount of moisture present. As examples of these, where
a large amount of humidity is combined with a moderate
degree of temperature, we may cite the British and Irish
warm coast stations—Torquay, Penzance, Dawlish, Ventnor, Bournemouth, Hastings, Worthing, Tenby, Cove of
Cork, and others. Another class of the marine climates
are those where a higher mean temperature is combined
with a far smaller degree of moisture, the stimulating
influence being thus considerably increased. Such are
the Mediterranean winter resorts — Malaga, Hyères,
Cannes, Nice, Cimiez, Mentone, San Remo, Ajaccio,
Palermo, Malta, and Algiers. A contrast to these is the
group of Madeira, the Azores, the West Indies, and other
islands, where a high mean temperature is combined with
a large amount of moisture, and thus the stimulating influence is considerably reduced, and indeed nearly neutra-
lized by it.

Inland.—These depend for their principal features on
their latitude, elevation above the sea level, proximity to

mountain ranges, soil, and shelter from wind, and vary
greatly according to the differences they display in each
of these qualities.   They have not, like the marine class,
any one common feature, as that of a stimulating character, for they may be bracing, or relaxing, according to
circumstances. Three groups may be formed out of them:
(1). Mild climates remarkable for their stillness of atmosphere, such as Pau, Amélie les Bains, Bagnères de Bigorre,
and Pisa.   (2.) Warm and dry climates, as Upper Egypt
and Syria, parts of South Africa and Australia.   (3.) Climates of elevated regions, varying according to the elevation of the locality and its latitude. Such are the climates
of the table lands of the Andes, of the high plateaus of
Mexico in America, of the Alps in Europe, and of the
Himalayas in Asia, varying in altitude from 3,000 to
10,000 feet, and remarkable for their dryness, purity of
atmosphere, and, at the same time, for their low temperature.

   When consumption is of inflammatory origin, it is our
object to remove the patients from the action of those
influences which have produced, and may again produce,
inflammatory attacks, to place him in a well-sheltered
locality, and at the same time to apply a certain amount
of stimulus to the system, and enable it to develope tissue
of a more healthy standard.   For this purpose marine
climates are invaluable; and our choice between the
British, Mediterranean, and Madeira groups, for a winter
residence, must depend, apart from other considerations,
chiefly on the degree of irritability which the vascular
system and the pulmonary and intestinal mucous membranes show. When this is slight, or when it is absent altogether, the dry climates of the Mediterranean basin are of
great benefit, both for the purpose of preventing fresh inflammatory attacks, and of stimulating and invigorating
the constitution, and thus correcting phthinoplastic ten-

dencies. The climate of the various winter stations in
the sub-Alpine Riviera can be recommended for members
of consumptive families : for patients who have shown evidence of lymphatic phthinosis : for cases of chronic sorofu-
lous pneumonia, and for the common forms of chronic
phthisis ; all which classes of disease derive great benefit
from a winter passed in this region; and even some
patients in whom the irritability is rather more marked
may do well in this region if they confine themselves to
the softer and less stimulating climate of Hyères, Cimiez,
and Cannet.

Cases, however, in which the irritability of the vascular
system is more prominent than the wasting tendency, as
described in Chapters VIII. and XII., often do not thrive
well in such bracing and exciting places, and for these the
moister and cooler British coast stations answer better ;
but even they are sometimes too stimulating, and their
large number of windy and rainy days are a great obstacle
to invalids taking proper exercise. Here it is that the
soft marine climate of Tangiers or of Madeira supplies
what is wanted, though the relaxing character of the
latter is an objection, but it is to be met by the patient
keeping up as much as possible on the hills of that
island.

A cooler substitute is to be found in the calm inland
climates of Pau, Amélie les Bains, and Pisa, and a dryer
one on the banks of the Upper Nile and the inland climates of Southern Africa and Australia.

For consumption originating in septic influences, a
climate of great purity and dryness would seem to
be indicated, and this is to be best found at considerable
heights above the sea level. The remarkable results observed by Archibald Smith, Guilbert, and Hermann Weber,
of residence in elevated regions on cases of phthisis contracted in hot enervating valleys, in the impure atmosphere

of large cities, and in unhealthy employments, arising, in fact, from causes more or less septic in kind, incline us to recommend the trial of mountain climates in this form of consumption, where it is possible to remove the patient so far, and where inflammatory complications are absent. These open and more bracing climates prove most beneficial in the more scrofulous and phthisical varieties, where degeneration and wasting of the bioplasm are marked from the beginning.

Unfortunately, many subjects of the constitutional forms of phthisis are too rapid in their downward course to admit of their being removed from this country at least, to the lofty regions of the Alps or Andes ; but, if it were possible to foresee, either from a knowledge of the family history, or from examination of the individual's frame, that he is more likely than other people to be attacked by this variety of the disease, it would be highly desirable to fix his residence in some elevated mountain district, as a precautionary and preventive measure, and it need hardly be remarked that such persons should be brought under the influence of the antiphthisical measures of pure air, and cod-liver oil and tonics early, more especially at the dangerous age of the cessation of growth.

We must bear in mind that in this country the great mass of consumptive cases either originate in, or are complicated with, inflammatory attacks ; and it is with the view of affording the patient immunity from these, and of enabling him to take abundant exercise that we recommend, in most cases of chronic consumption, a dry warm climate during the winter, with as much stimulating element in it as he can well bear, and when summer approaches and the sheltered winter station becomes hot and oppressive, we advise a change to the cooler and more bracing climate of the Alpine health resorts, such as Bormio, Comballaz, Rigi Kaltbad, Monte Generoso, and other high stations, where he can remain till the approaching winter renders his return to the warm station desirable.

The great purity and somewhat exciting quality of the air in all these places has a vivifying influence on the bioplasm, and on all the vital functions, and generally produces a change soon in the colour and spirits of the patients, and in time on their strength and flesh also. But in order to ensure the good effects of the air, exercise must be regularly taken, and as patients are seldom strong enough to walk for the requisite time in the open air, riding or driving should be much resorted to.

We may here remark, that even patients, who are deemed fit cases to pass the winter in high level resorts, will be wise to commence their sojourn in the elevated district in summer, and thus become gradually inured to the vigorous climate, and reap all the good which can accrue from it.

It is the custom in America to send consumptive patients for the winter to dry inland localities, of no great elevation, as St. Paul's in Minnesota, and certain parts of Canada; and we have seen patients who have wintered there, but up to this date the evidence collected by us has not been altogether favourable to these climates, of which we imagine the dryness to be the best feature.

One of the most approved methods of giving a phthisical invalid change of air is by a long sea-voyage, as, for instance, to Australia and back; and facts are tolerably numerous to testify to its beneficial effect, not only in the very early stages of the disease, but even where limited cavities have formed. This mode, however, of change of climate, is liable to some drawbacks, which are: want of opportunities for exercise, very variable weather and temperature, sometimes bad accommodation and food, and often *ennui* and home sickness. If the patient can go in comfort, pleasure, and hope, and start in the month of

October, provided that his disease is not very extensive, he may reap considerable benefit.

Before we close this short notice of climate in relation to consumption, we ought to mention what patients ought not, in our opinion, to be sent abroad. These are, cases of acute phthisis, both tuberculosis and scrofulous; pneumonia, if the latter be in an acute stage, though if its progress, as happens sometimes, be rendered more chronic, the patient may possibly be excepted from our rule.

While patients with lungs in various stages of the disease may benefit greatly by going abroad, provided the amount of lesion be not very extensive, we must add our warning to that of other medical writers against the cruelty and madness of allowing those, whose extreme state precludes all hope of recovery and who are obviously near their end, to exchange the comforts of a home in their native land for the miseries of foreign exile, for it is far better for them to sink into their graves surrounded by all that art can suggest and affection supply, to assuage their sufferings, than to close life by a death-bed in a strange land, and often among strange people, to whom many of the luxuries which smooth the dying pillow are unknown. Some patients, who have been greatly reduced by inflammatory attacks, or by hæmoptysis, have the appearance of being in extreme phthisis, but an examination of their lungs, will show that they are not really so. These are the patients who are said to have been placed on board ship, in a dying state, and to have recovered, and it would not be well to place an absolute veto on such treatment in their cases.

In conclusion, we would state that too much must not be expected from climate alone, in the treatment of so formidable a disease as pulmonary consumption; but that when its influence is joined to that of medicine and hygiene, much may be done towards mitigating, arresting, and even curing, the dread malady.

INDEX.

LONDON: PRINTED BY
SPOTTISWOODE AND CO., NEW-STREET SQUARE
AND PARLIAMENT STREET

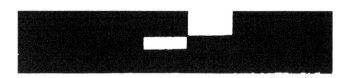

LINDSAY & BLAKISTON'S

Medical, Dental, and Scientific

PUBLICATIONS.

☞ Sent by mail, free of postage, upon receipt of the retail price.

AITKEN'S Science and Practice of Medicine. Second American from the Fifth London Edition. Containing a colored Map showing the Geographical Distribution of Disease over the Globe, a Lithographic Plate, and numerous Illustrations. Two vols., octavo. Price, in Cloth, $12 00; Leather, $14 00

The American Editor, Dr. MEREDITH CLYMER, has added to this edition new matter equal to 500 pages of the English edition, including many new articles on subjects with special reference to the wants of the *American Practitioner.*

ALTHAUS' Medical Electricity, Theoretical and Practical. A new enlarged Edition. Illustrated. 5.00

ACTON on the Functions and Disorders of the Reproductive Organs. From the Fifth London Edition. 3.00

ANSTIE on Stimulants and Narcotics. With Special Researches on the Action of Alcohol, Ether, and Chloroform on the Vital Organism. 3.00

BYFORD'S Practice of Medicine and Surgery. Applied to the Diseases and Accidents Incident to Women. Second Edition, with additions and Illustrations. Price, in Cloth, 5 00 Leather, 6 00

BYFORD on the Chronic Inflammation and Displacement of the Unimpregnated Uterus. A new Enlarged, and thoroughly revised Edition. 3 00

BIDDLE'S Materia Medica. For the Use of Students. Fourth Revised and Enlarged Edition. With Illustrations. 4 00

BEALE on the Microscope in its Application to Practical Medicine. Third Edition. Revised and enlarged, with 500 Illustrations. 7.00

BEALE'S How to Work with the Microscope. Fourth Edition. 400 Illustrations. 7.50

BEALE on Kidney Diseases, Urinary Deposits, and Calculous Disorders. Third Edition, very much enlarged. Containing upwards of 400 Illustrations copied from Nature.   10.00

do.   **Protoplasm or Life Matter, Mind.** A New Edition, enlarged. With Colored Plates.

do.   **Disease Germs.** Their Supposed Nature, with Colored Plates.   1.75

do.   do.   do.   Their Real Nature, 24 Plates, many of them colored.   4.00

do.   **on Vital Theories and Religious Thoughts.** 6 Plates.   2.75

do.   **Archives of Medicine.** Part 17, vol. 4.   1.50 Previous volumes supplied to order.

do.   **Mystery of Life.** Two Colored Plates.   1.50

BEASLEY'S Book of 3000 Prescriptions. A new Revised and Enlarged Edition.   4.00

do.   **Druggists' General Receipt Book.** Sixth American Edition, Revised and Improved.   8.50

do.   **Pocket Formulary.** 8th London Edition.   3.00

BARTH & ROGER'S Auscultation and Percussion. From the Sixth French Edition.   1.25

BOUCHARDAT'S Annual Abstract of Therapeutics, Materia Medica, &c., for 1867.   1.50

BULL on the Maternal Management of Children in Health and Disease. ▼   1.25

BIRCH on Constipated Bowels. The various Causes and Different Means of Cure. Third Edition.   1.00

BRAITHWAITE'S Epitome of the Retrospect of Practical Medicine and Surgery. 2 vols.   10.00

do.   **Retrospect.** Half-yearly, $2.50 per annum, in advance; or $1.50 for single parts.

BRITISH and Foreign Medico-Chirurgical Review. London Edition.   Price per annum, 10.00

CHAMBERS' LECTURES, Chiefly Clinical, illustrative of a Restorative System of Medicine. From the Fourth London Edition.   5.00

CHEW'S Course of Lectures on the Proper Method of Studying Medicine.   1.00

CAZEAUX'S Great Work on Obstetrics. A Theoretical and Practical Treatise on Midwifery. Including the Diseases of Pregnancy, Parturition, &c., &c. From the Seventh French Edition. With 175 Illustrations. Royal Octavo.
Price, in Cloth, 6.50; Leather, 7.50

CANNIFF'S Manual of the Principles of Surgery.
4.50

CLEAVELAND'S Pronouncing Medical Lexicon. A new improved Edition. 1.25

CARSON'S History of the Medical Department of the University of Pennsylvania, from its foundation in 1765, with Illustrative Sketches of Deceased Professors, &c. 2.00

COHEN on Inhalation. Its Therapeutics and Practice. With Cases and Illustrations, 2.50

DILLENBERGER'S Handy Book of the Treatment of Women's and Children's Diseases. With Prescriptions. 1.75

DUCHENNE on Localized Electrization. With Notes and Additions by the Translator, and numerous Illustrations.

DIXON'S Guide to the Practical Study of Diseases of the Eye. With Test Types and Illustrations. A New Edition, thoroughly revised. 3.50

DURKEE on Gonorrhœa and Syphilis. The Fifth Edition, revised and enlarged. With Portraits and Colored Illustrations. Octavo. 5.00

FULLER on Rheumatism, Rheumatic Gout, and Sciatica. A New Edition preparing.

do. on Diseases of the Heart and Great Vessels. Second Edition.

GANT'S Science and Practice of Surgery. Illustrated. One vol., octavo.

GARDNER on Sterility. Its Causes and Curative Treatment, Octavo. 3.00

GOFF'S Combined Day-Book, Ledger, and Daily Register of Patients. Quarto. Half Russia. 12.00

GRAVES' Clinical Lectures on the Practice of Medicine. A New Edition. Edited by J. MOORE NELIGAN, M.D. 6.00

GROSS' American Medical Biography of the Nineteenth Century. 3.50

GARRATT'S Guide for Using Medical Batteries. With Illustrations. 2.00

GREENHOW on Chronic Bronchitis. 2.00

HEWITT'S Diagnosis and Treatment of Diseases of Women. Second Edition. With Illustrations.
Price, in Cloth, 5.00; Leather, 6.00

HOLMES' Surgical Diseases of Children. Second Edition. With Illustrations. 9.00

PEREIRA'S Physician's Prescription Book. Fifteenth Edition.
Price, in Cloth, 1.25 ; in Leather, with Tucks and Pocket, 1.50

Physician's Visiting List. Published annually.
For 25 Patients weekly. Tucks, Pockets, and Pencil, . . 1 00
　50　"　　"　　"　　"　　"　. . 1 25
　75　"　　"　　"　　"　　"　. . 1 50
　100　"　　"　　"　　"　　"　. 2 00
　50　"　　"　2 vols. { Jan. to June, } " . . 2 50
　　　　　　　　　　{ July to Dec.. }
　100　"　　"　2 vols. { Jan. to June, } " . 3 00
　　　　　　　　　　{ July to Dec., }

INTERLEAVED EDITION.

For 25 Patients weekly, Interl'd, Tucks, Pockets, &c., . . 1 50
　50　"　　"　　"　　"　　"　. . 1 75
　30　"　　"　2 vols. { Jan. to June, } " . 3 00
　　　　　　　　　　{ July to Dec., }

PRINCE'S Orthopedic Surgery. With Illustrations. 3.00

PRINCE'S Plastic Surgery. With Illustrations. 1.50

RINDFLEISCH'S Pathological Histology, translated from the German. 208 Illustrations. 1 volume, octavo.

RADCLIFF'S Lectures on Epilepsy, Pain, Paralysis, &c. With Illustrations. 2.00

ROBERTSON'S Manual on Extracting Teeth. With Illustrations. Second Revised Edition. 1.50

RANKING'S Half-Yearly Abstract of the Medical Sciences. Per annum, in advance, $2 50. Back numbers or volumes furnished.

RENOUARD'S History of Medicine, from its Origin to the Nineteenth Century. 4.00

REPORTS on the Progress of Medicine, Surgery, and the Allied Sciences. Octavo. 2.00

RUPPANER'S Principles and Practice of Laryngoscopy, &c. With Engravings. 2.00

RYAN'S Philosophy of Marriage. In its Social, Moral, and Physical Relations, &c. 1.00

REESE'S Analysis of Physiology. Second Edition. Enlarged. 1.50

REESE'S American Medical Formulary.. 1.50

REESE'S Syllabus of Medical Chemistry. 1.00

STILLE'S Epidemic Meningitis; or, Cerebrospinal Meningitis. Octavo. 2.00

STILLE'S Elements of General Pathology. Second Edition. (In preparation.)

SCIENTIFIC BOOKS.

BEETON'S Book of Household Management, with 72 Colored and 600 other Illustrations. Demi-Octavo, Half Roan.
3.25

COOLEY'S Toilet and Cosmetic Arts in Ancient and Modern Times.
3.00

OTT on the Manufacture of Soaps and Candles. With Illustrations.
2.50

PIESSE'S Whole Art of Perfumery, A new Revised and Enlarged Edition. With Illustrations.
3.00

OVERMAN'S Practical Mineralogy, Assaying, and Mining. 12mo.
1.25

PIGGOTT on Copper Mining, Copper Ores, &c.   1.50

MORFIT'S Chemical and Pharmaceutical Manipulations. Second Edition. 500 Illustrations.
6.00

BRANSTON'S Handbook of Practical Receipts. 1.50

CAMPBELL'S Manual of Scientific and Practical Agriculture. 12mo. With Illustrations.
1.50

DARLINGTON'S Flora Cestrica. Third Edition.   2.25

MILLER on Alcohol, Its place and Power, and LIZARS on the Use and Abuse of Tobacco. The two in one volume.
1.00

Descriptive Catalogues of our publications, together with a CLASSIFIED list of all other important Medical publications, American and English, furnished free, by mail or otherwise, upon application.

Foreign Medical Books and Periodicals imported promptly to order, and at the lowest rates.

LINDSAY & BLAKISTON,

Medical Publishers and Booksellers,

25 S. SIXTH ST. (2d Floor),

PHILADELPHIA.

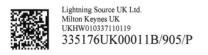
Lightning Source UK Ltd.
Milton Keynes UK
UKHW010337110119
335176UK00011B/905/P